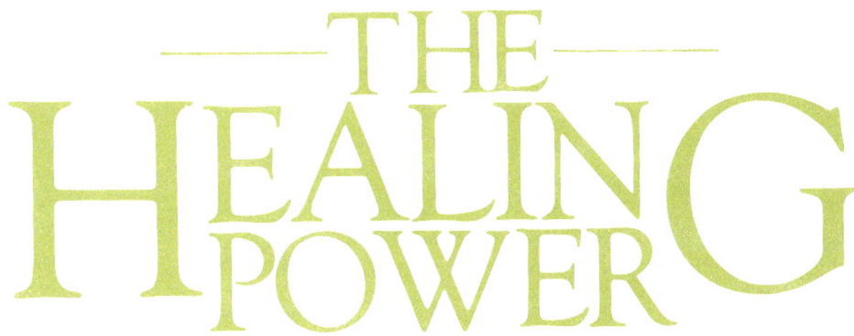
THE
HEALING
POWER

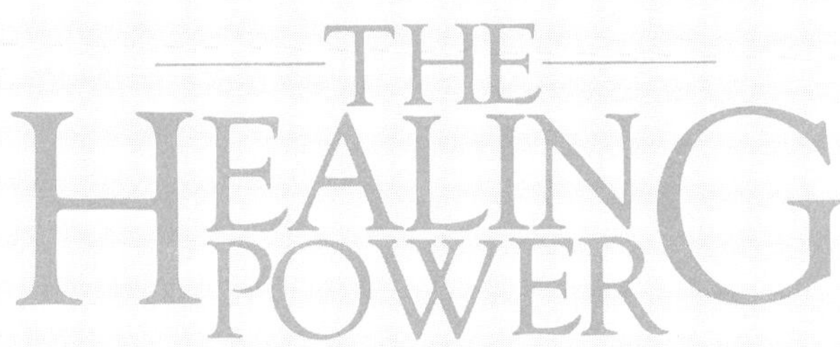

THE HEALING POWER

a handbook of
alternative medicine
and natural health

NEVILL DRURY
with contributions by John Newton & Merren Parker

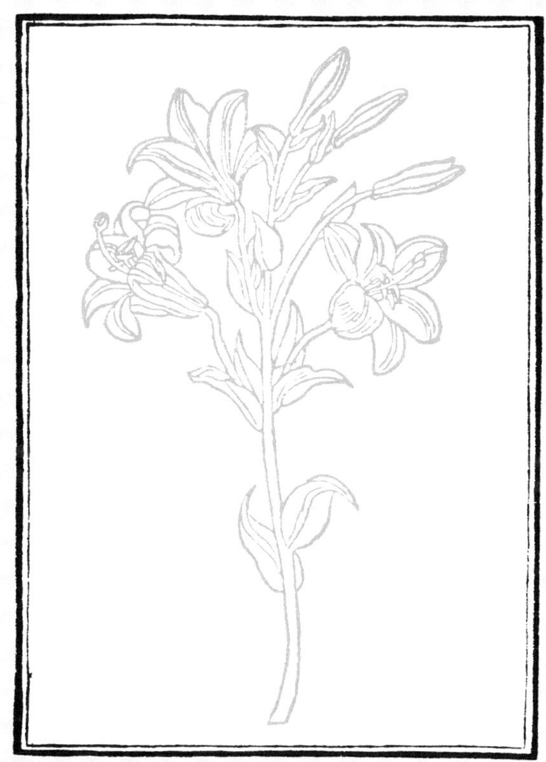

Frederick Muller Limited
London

Related books by the same author:
THE SEARCH FOR ABRAXAS (with Stephen Skinner)
THE PATH OF THE CHAMELEON
FRONTIERS OF CONSCIOUSNESS (ed.)
DON JUAN, MESCALITO AND MODERN MAGIC
THE OCCULT SOURCEBOOK (with Gregory Tillett)
INNER VISIONS
OTHER TEMPLES, OTHER GODS (with Gregory Tillett)
THE SHAMAN AND THE MAGICIAN

Picture Credits:
(These are given with page number followed in sequence by illustrations in descending order from left to right)

Collection N. Drury: 10, 12, 14, 17, 19, 30, 46, 47, 48, 50, 57a, 67, 75, 95, 97, 106, 117, 142, 169, 211; News Limited, Sydney: 15, 28a, 201; John Newton (including photographs kindly lent by interviewees): 18, 33, 37, 52, 54, 74, 78, 91, 109, 146, 163, 204, 209; Alan Fisher: 19, 57b, 58, 81, 108; Dover Publications, New York: 20, 68, 182, 198, 199a, 210a,b; Mode Magazine, Sydney: 22, 23; Austin Levy: 28b; John Flynn and Martin Cohen: 29; Mind Force Australia: 38, 39a,b, 42, 112; John Fairfax Ltd., Sydney: 60; Vitamin Supplies Ltd., Sydney: 62; Xandria Williams: 64; Merren Parker (including photographs kindly lent by interviewees): 65, 73, 85, 122, 205; Gerald Rosenove: 66, 140a,b; Dr David Phillips: 70; Alexander Street Herbal Centre, Sydney: 84, 99; Dorothy Hall and Thomas Nelson, Melbourne: 100, 101: Graydon Rixon: 103a,b, 124, 125, 161, 202; American Journal of Acupuncture: 104, 105a,b; Ann O'Donovan Ltd., Melbourne: 115; Francesca Naish: 116; Russell Atkinson: 121, 214a,b; Fred Weston: 129; Harper & Row, Publishers, 132, 187, 188a; Malcom and Zoe Hagon: 134; Time Magazine: 166; Amos Hollis: 174; Peter Eedy: 179; The Woodstock Aquarian, New York: 188b; Vital Magazine, Sydney: 191; Ann Skea: 194, 197; Daniel Weber: 196; Gregory Tillett: 199b, 200; Search Centres Ltd and New Awareness Centre, Sydney: 207, 208; Julie Chenery: 212; Simply Living Magazine: 149, 152; Otto Rogge: front cover illustration
Any inadvertent error or omission in the picture credits will be corrected in future editions of this book

THE HEALING POWER
First published in Great Britain 1981
by Frederick Muller Limited, London, NW2 6LE

British Library Cataloguing in Publication Data
Drury, Nevill, b. 1947
The healing power
1. Therapeutic systems
1. Title II. Newton, John
615.53 R733
ISBN 0 584 97078 1
ISBN 0 584 97106 0 pbk
Designed by Judy Hungerford
Printed in Hong Kong
I. Therapeutic systems
I. Title II. Newton, John

CONTENTS

FOREWORD

This volume is a handbook of alternative medicine and natural health that has been compiled as a working resource. There is no doubt that in many Western countries there has been increasing dissatisfaction with orthodox forms of medical treatment despite extraordinary scientific advances in many areas of medical research and health-care. Unfortunately, in an area of complex technology, the individual aspects of health-care often seem to be diminishing. Hospital complexes are often monolithic and uninviting, a vast variety of synthetic drugs pours routinely onto the market from the giant pharmaceutical companies to increase our dependencies and create 'needs', and sophisticated but impersonal equipment is used to monitor body processes. In short, orthodox medicine has moved steadily towards becoming a science and away from being an art. Holistic health practitioners are more concerned with individual treatment for the individual person, and in this sense seek to rediscover the art of medicine.

The new movement echoes E.F. Schumacher's sentiment that 'small is beautiful' and holds that traditional accumulated medical knowledge has served mankind for centuries and in many ways is preferable to complex modern treatments that may have long-term effects that no-one can anticipate. On the whole, the increasing interest in alternative medicine and natural health represents an admitted retreat to the past. Man himself, say the holistic practitioners, has not changed substantially – only his environment has. So the time-honoured intrinsic healing processes of mind and body remain valid, and it is up to us to see past the complexity that orthodox medical treatment presents to an essentially holistic view that man can heal himself through natural processes, drawing on natural resources.

It is true that some of the alternative therapies included in this book are modern, chiropractic, osteopathy and polarity balancing among them. But manipulative treatments have been documented since the times of the ancient Chinese, Greek and Egyptian cultures, and energy flow is a recurring theme in the Oriental healing arts. Many of the new therapies are simply presenting old knowledge in new, systematic formats. Psionic medicine and Kirlian diagnosis, meanwhile, draw on technological expertise to monitor intrinsic and natural energy patterns in the human body.

This book presents some of the healing modalities that offer an alternative to orthodox medicine. Familiar Western techniques of medicine – sometimes called 'allopathic' – posit an external source of disease that similarly requires treatment of an external nature (medicines, pills, ointments) to combat the disease entity in the organism. Practitioners of natural medicine, on the other hand, take the view that most forms of disease derive from imbalances in the human organism and that if these imbalances can be rectified, disease is automatically eliminated. Health is natural, disease unnatural. The holistic practitioner aims simply to restore the natural state and many naturopaths reject the very idea of specific disease categories : 'there are no diseases . . . only sick people'. There is also the very real criticism that many synthetic drugs suppress symptoms and could force disease deeper into the body — from one organ to another — affecting the delicate mind/body balance. A cure of one particular symptom is no guarantee that imbalance may not surface elsewhere in the body. Accordingly natural health practitioners often emphasise that they are treating the whole person, not just the most obvious ailment or disease aspect.

The Healing Power does not seek to endorse the alternative therapies presented here so much as to present them for consideration. Many of the therapies are appropriate in conjunction with orthodox medicine and offer new insights for health treatment.

It seemed a good idea to place some emphasis on the healing practitioners themselves since their attitudes and backgrounds are of considerable interest. While there have been several excellent overviews of alternative medicine published in recent years, the healers themselves have been neglected in most of them.

We have also included a resource directory so that you — the reader — can make contact with practitioners of a healing morality that may be especially suited to you. Our sincere hope is that you will find this book a useful one.

Nevill Drury
M.A. (Hons.) Dip.Ed.

Sydney, 1981

ACUPUNCTURE

According to an ancient Chinese legend, acupuncture owes its origin to a particular man who developed a severe headache while lifing some heavy rocks. The pain from the headache was so disorienting that he lost his concentration and dropped one of the rocks onto his foot. Immediately his foot began to throb with pain and bleed but paradoxically his headache stopped. It is said that the practice developed whereby the rock was replaced by a small sharp stone which could be pressed into the skin to produce the same curative effect, and eventually the rock was in turn replaced by a variety of needles. Early acupuncture needles were made of stone, bone, bamboo, copper, iron and silver and are now constructed from stainless steel. It is an interesting fact that the location known as 'Liver 3' near the big toe is used even today to relieve headache and migraine . . . so perhaps there is some foundation to the legend!

An early account of acupuncture treatments is given in the historical *Shi Ji* by Szuma Chien who lived during the Han Dynasty, and also in the *Biographies of Pien Chueh and Tsang Kung* dating back almost 2000 years ago.

Pien Chueh, who was also known as Chin Yueh-jen, was born in Mochou in what is now Hopei Province. He was allegedly skilled in acupuncture, massage and herbal remedies. On one occasion he is said to have been in the State of Kuo (now Honan and Shensi provinces) with two of his apprentices when he heard that the Prince had lapsed into unconsciousness. Funeral preparations were already underway as Pien Chueh hurried with his colleagues to the palace. Pien Chueh examined the Prince and noted that he was still breathing weakly. Diagnosing a coma state, Pien Chueh instructed one of his apprentices, Tzu Yang, to administer acupuncture. The Prince began to revive. Meanwhile the other apprentice applied herbal fomentations to both armpits. Soon the Prince was able to sit up in bed. Pien Chueh recommended that he take a course of herbal medicine for twenty days and he subsequently recovered.

The earliest acupuncture needles that we know about specifically were made of stone and were called *bian shi* (stone piercer); *chan shi* (stone borer) and *zhen shi* (stone needle). A famous doctor named Yu Fu is supposed to have treated his patients with these and there are also various instances of their use cited in the ancient Chinese *Canon of Medicine*. With the development of metal-working in China, acupuncture needles were made of iron and silver and there were nine of them:

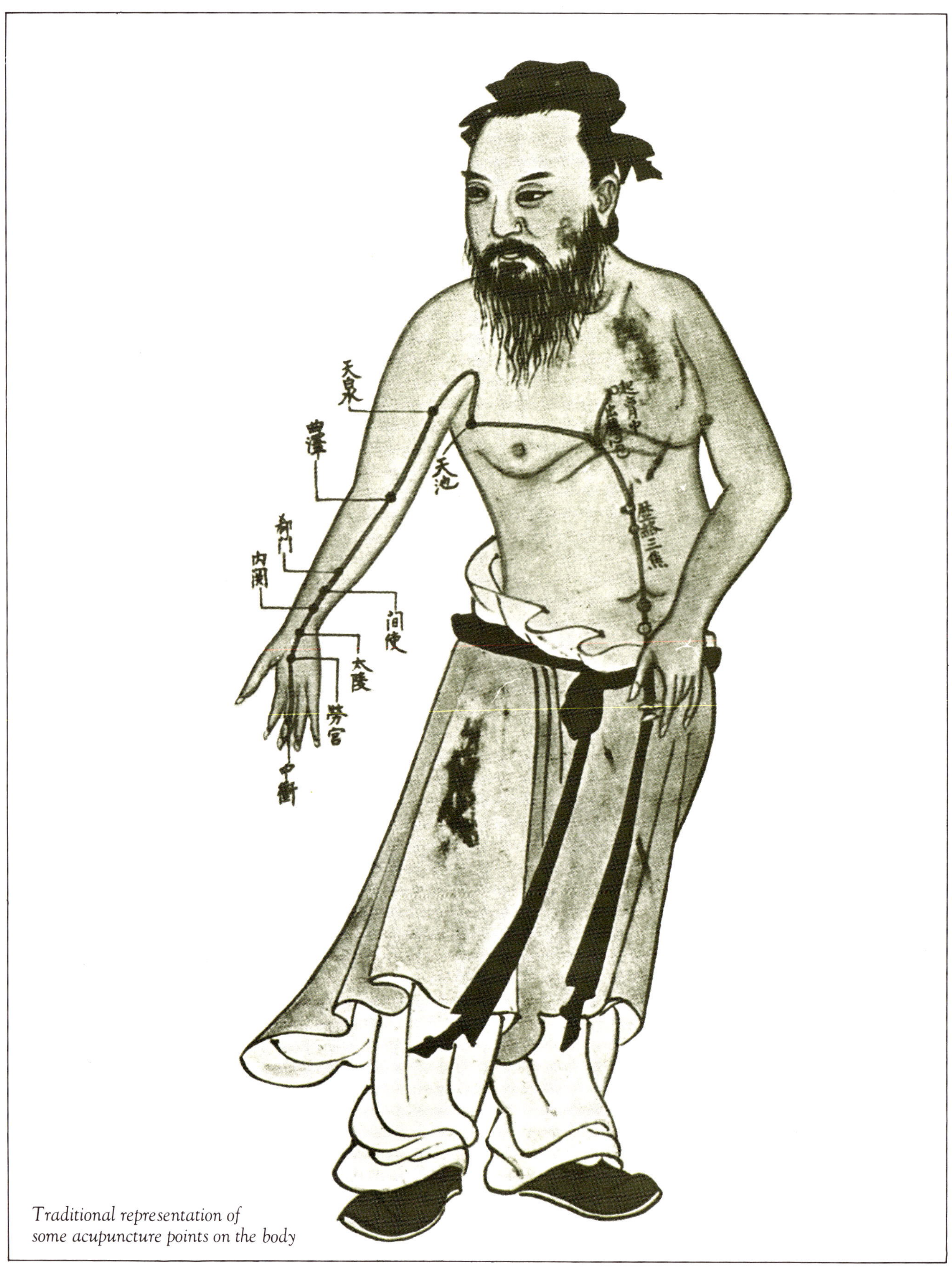

Traditional representation of some acupuncture points on the body

- the Arrowhead needle, for superficial pricking
- the Round needle, for massaging
- the Blunt needle, for pressing
- the Sharp Three-Edged needle, for pricking veins
- the Sword-like needle, for releasing pus
- the Sharp and Round needle, for rapid pricking
- the Filiform needle, for general use
- the Long needle, for puncturing thick muscle
- the Large needle for treating arthritis

Several of these needles are no longer used and the Filiform has been refined from its early shape; the Three-Edged needle however, remains in a similar form. A set of ancient metal acupuncture needles was discovered in 1968 in the tomb of Liu Sheng dating from the Second Century B.C. and shows that in some cases the implements of acupuncture have remained unchanged through the centuries.

Appropriate acupuncture points on the body for inserting the needles were only gradually discovered and later the concept of lines of force connecting these points was established. Ancient texts refer to the *kong xue* (converging spot) and *shu xue* (transmitting spot) and also to systems of channels and collaterals. The acupuncturist Huangh Mi completed a work in A.D. 265 listing needle points on the head, face, thorax, abdomen and back, and by the time of the Tang Dynasty (618–907) the state of knowledge was considerably more advanced. The Imperial Medical College had one professor of acupuncture, one assistant professor and ten instructors. Acupuncture charts dating from this period were also coloured and isolated points on the body from front, back and side views. The physician Sun Szu-Miao (581–682) detailed the twelve channels in five colours, with the eight interweaving ones depicted in green.

At the very heart of acupuncture practice are the philosophical and mystical concepts of *Yin* and *Yang*, and *Ch'i*. Often depicted by the symbol of a circle divided by an S-shaped line, the *Yin-Yang* is representative of the flux of polarities ever-present in all things. The light side of the circle, *Yang*, is active, positive and masculine, while the dark side or *Yin* is passive, negative and feminine . . . a distinction aimed at expressing the vital mystery of continuity and transformation rather than a statement of pure chauvinism! *Ch'i* energy is the very essence of the life-force and flows through channels in the body which the acupuncturist terms 'meridians'. These are not normally identified with either the central nervous system or the blood circulation vessels per se although, as will be seen later, there is an acknowledged degree of overlap.

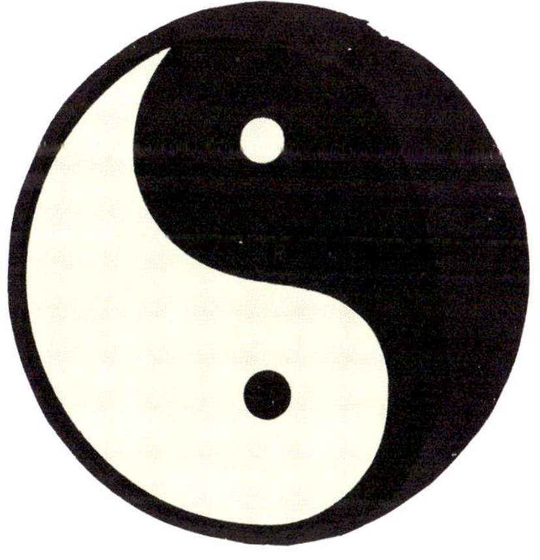

Yin and Yang: opposite polarities within the circle of being

The amount of *Ch'i* in the body varies from time to time and the ratios of *Yin* and *Yang* are also in flux. If an imbalance occurs and causes sickness, it is the task of the acupuncturist to use his needles to restore the appropriate, harmonising balance.

Traditionally each part of the body is thought to have both *Yin* and *Yang* qualities, however a division is made into the five elements and these are associated with the five so called Ts'ang organs: Liver (wood); Heart (fire); Spleen (earth); Lungs (metal) and Kidneys (water). There are also two metaphysical organs which are referred to in acupuncture practice as the 'Triple Warmer' and the 'Gate of Life'.

The first of these is sometimes called 'Three Burning Spaces' and is thought of as a regulator of both the organs and the flow of vital fluids. It is a Yin organ. The Gate of Life, on the other hand, is a Yang organ and underlies the sexual impulse. Most abstractly, it is linked to notions of 'happiness and joy'.

When we consider the main meridians of the *Ch'i* energy we find that in traditional Chinese thought the great divisions of the body each have Yin and Yang aspects and each encompasses two major meridians:

Body section	*Meridian*	*Organ*
Sunlight Yang	Arm Sunlight Yang	Large Intestine
	Leg Sunlight Yang	Stomach
Greater Yin	Arm Greater Yin	Lungs
	Leg Greater Yin	Spleen
Lesser Yang	Arm Lesser Yang	Triple Warme
	Leg Lesser Yang	Gall Bladder
Absolute Yin	Arm Absolute Yin	Gate of Life
	Leg Absolute Yin	Liver
Greater Yang	Arm Yang	Small Intestine
	Leg Greater Yang	Bladder
Lesser Yin	Arm Lesser Yin	Heart
	Leg Lesser Yin	Kidneys

It is interesting to note that in early Chinese medicine the brain was not very highly regarded and so does not feature in the above classification!

The twelve meridians listed above are the main, but by no means the only, points of treatment. There are also numerous branch meridians and also the fifteen 'Luo' channels connecting the main meridians to each other. Generally it is estimated that acupuncturists use 59 meridians and around 1000 acupuncture points in their work. The early texts usually refer to only 365 points, however.

When an acupuncturist begins his diagnosis he feels the 'pulse' associated with each meridian and will subsequently use his needles to rectify any imbalance discovered.

With interest in acupuncture developing in the west, controversy stills surrounds the long term effectiveness of treatment and the debate continues about what is actually occurring.

Dr Felix Mann, who popularised interest in Chinese medicine in Britain in the 1960s, believes that acupuncture channels are 'visceral, cutaneous and nervous reflexes' which may be sensitive 'trigger' points on the skin. Meanwhile Canadian Professor Ronald Melzack has recently concluded that there is a 71% correlation between trigger points and traditional acupuncture points used to relieve pain. If a point is stimulated for a time by needles or electrodes, the pain in the affected organ subsides. Melzack found that 58 acupuncture points lie on cerebrospinal nerves and 69 in the outer walls of major blood vessels. The correlations between acupuncture meridians and nerve tracks has also been confirmed by Chinese-born, Australian acupuncturist Dr Pui Sinn, who notes, for example, that:

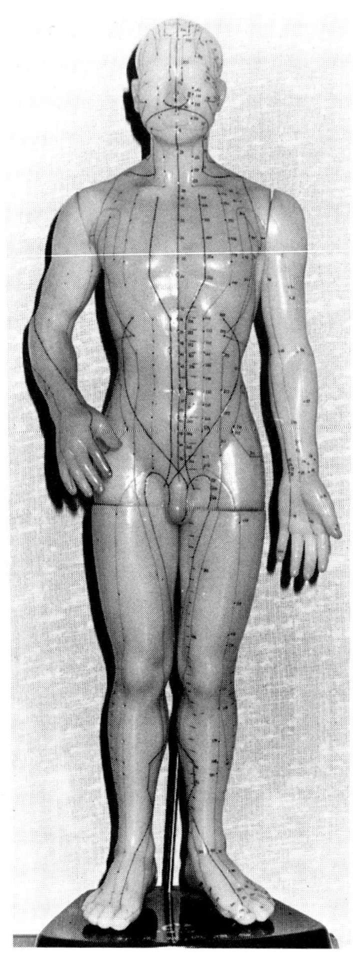

Acupuncturist's model showing major meridians and points

- The heart meridian lies along the internal cutaneous nerve and ulnar nerve.
- The bladder meridian lies along the sciatic nerve.

- The circulation/sex (Gate of Life) meridian lies along the median nerve, and in general, 'a great number of acupuncture points are located right over the trunks of cutaneous nerves or border adjacent cutaneous nerves'.

British doctor Julian Kenyon, who is also an acupuncturist, believes that acupuncture activates 'electrical pathways' which weave through the neuroglia, the connective tissue of the nervous system, and produce effects that way. Certainly we require some sort of explanation like this to explain why a needle inserted near the big toe can relieve migraine!

Acupuncture certainly is not a universal cure-all; it is of little use, for example, where body tissue has begun to disintegrate as with cases of cancer. Where it does seem to be most effective is in relieving pain, and research is continuing into its potential for inducing anaesthesia for surgery.

Gradually acupuncture is gaining more acceptance from orthodox doctors and the benefits of ancient Chinese medicine are being acknowledged as a useful adjunct to the more familiar techniques of diagnosis.

DR DAVID TAI

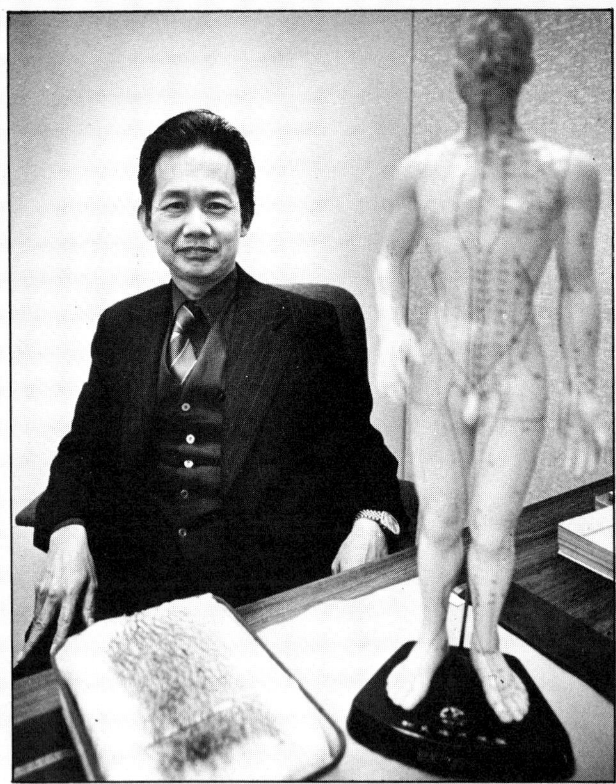

Dr David Tai runs his acupuncture practice from an impeccably modern suite in a new office block close to the Chinese Haymarket community in Sydney. But if the environment is thoroughly contemporary, the medicine itself derives from an ancient Chinese context. Interestingly, Chinese-born Dr Tai is a convert from western medicine to the Taoism and acupuncture of his forefathers, rather than the other way around, and that in itself makes his story an unusual one.

Born in 1933, David Tai moved with his parents to Sumatra at an early age and spent most of his youth there. Despite the fact that he had a traditional Chinese mystical heritage — his grandfather was a Taoist who meditated in seclusion regularly and his mother's father was a herbalist — young David had no inclination at that stage to follow in their footsteps. Instead he came steadily under the influence of a local German doctor who encouraged him towards more orthodox medical pursuits. So it was that when David Tai decided to return to mainland China to further his studies his inclination was to western medicine rather than the traditional Chinese systems of thought. Following a matriculation year in Shanghai he went on to the University of Peking where he graduated with such distinction that he was invited to join the teaching staff. For three years he held an academic position and visited country regions occasionally as a locum. He was developing a keen interest in surgery but became puzzled when certain operations he observed had unexpectedly limited success. Then an event took place which changed his total attitude towards western and traditional Chinese medicine.

David Tai had had an accident and injured his lower back; western style medical injections failed to relieve the pain. Meanwhile a colleague who specialised in acupuncture offered to help. Dr Tai recalls that this doctor obviously wanted to make a good impression on behalf of the traditional healing arts and inserted needles in particularly strong energy zones. One of these locations was the centre of the upper lip and there were others in the hands and back. Dr Tai felt an immediate effect, a very strong energy impulse like a healing current followed by instant relief. The effect was akin to a religious conversion. Feeling was believing! He consequently decided that he had neglected a large body of traditional knowledge and slowly began — at the age of 31 — to study those topics like acupuncture, herbalism and moxibustion which his western-style training had ignored.

He was fortunate that his position as a doctor allowed him to extend his research and now, as he visited different hospitals and institutions, he observed how moxibustion was used for 'toning' the body and how acupuncture needles were inserted to alleviate pain. It was also a time, during the last years of the Maoist regime, when considerable encouragement was being given by the government to the investigation of acupuncture and anaesthesia. Dr Tai says that he has observed major surgery being performed with total dependence on acupuncture for the anaesthetisation of pain and he feels that it is enormously beneficial for the patient to be able to communicate with the doctor during the operation. Nevertheless, despite the coverage in the press, such instances of surgery with acupuncture alone are comparatively rare and quite often western-style drugs are used in conjunction with traditional healing techniques. It is often necessary, for example, to use sedatives to reduce tension in the patient. Some people also react nervously to the idea of acupuncture needles entering the skin. Dr Tai believes it is very important for patients to get used to the sensation of the needle penetration for it is, as he says, 'part of the acupuncture effect'. Do the needles ever cause pain? 'No', says Dr Tai — at least, not if the correct technique is applied by the doctor. The 'acupuncture effect' is not in itself a painful sensation and the needles rarely cause a feeling of discomfort unless the practitioner has incorrectly sterilised them with alcohol.

Dr Tai has been living in Sydney since 1976 and says it took him almost two years to adapt his acupuncture techniques to suit westerners. In fact, he believes that the individual nature of acupuncture treatment has been underplayed by many of his colleagues. When in China Dr Tai found that many differences in body structure could be found even in such regional locations as Canton, Southern Mongolia and Shanghai, and the early Chinese texts on acupuncture accurately reflected these variants. He finds that in Australia he has had to experiment with his acupuncture techniques and adapt them to the western metabolism and physique.

Like a true healer, Dr Tai also emphasises that it is vital for any acupuncturist to gauge the energy flow of the patient, and that the healing process can be a very draining experience for the practitioner. On one occasion during his medical career he nearly died himself from energy loss suffered during a healing session. Consequently he also tries to take care of his own mind and body processes. Every day he spends at least 30 minutes meditating, finally following the traditions of his maternal grandfather whose contemplative approach he ignored when he was young.

Dr Tai is an engaging, humble man who hopes to broaden the appeal of acupuncture for the Australian public. He intends some time in the future to establish an acupuncture college in the country and also work in new areas of research. One of his projects, for example, is to develop the use of acupuncture to assist paraplegics, in some cases helping patients to walk again.

With acupuncture gaining increasing recognition in the west, we are indeed fortunate to have a man like Dr Tai giving such study added impetus in this country.

DR PUI SINN

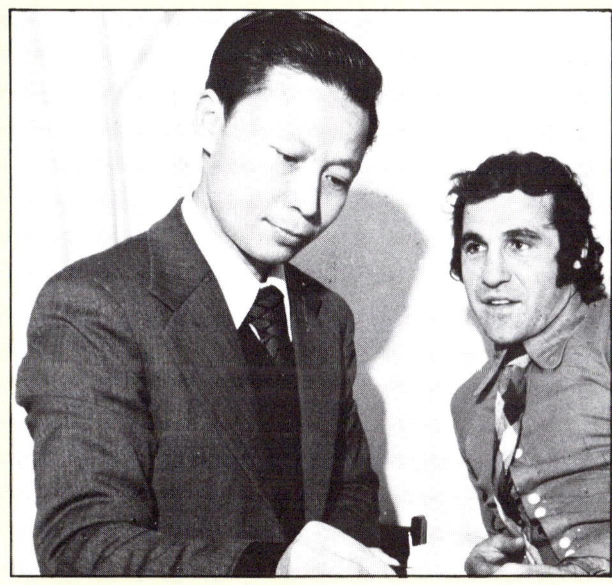

Dr Pui Sinn has lived in Australia for 11 years and was one of the first qualified Chinese doctors to practise acupuncture in this country. In his role as the Director of the Acupuncture Institute in Sydney, he treats patients with his shiny stainless steel needles at four clinics located in the metropolitan area. He has a relaxing manner, inserting the needles as mildly as possible and smiling and joking while he does so. Perhaps this is to overcome the inhibitions many westerners would have if they consciously pondered the act of being pierced by a fine steel needle. According to Dr Sinn, for acupuncture to work effectively it is preferable for the patient to be thoroughly relaxed; however it is often used with people who are tense since one of its noted effects is to relieve muscle tension.

In recent times Dr Sinn has helped treat a number of conditions through acupuncture. These include migraine, spasm, arthritis, lumbago, neuralgia, asthma, hypertension, gout, sciatica and various muscular complaints. His methods have also been effective treating cases of overweight and drug withdrawal symptoms.

For example, it is estimated that around five percent of Sydney's overweight population has tried acupuncture and many have found the methods highly successful. Recently Dr Sinn treated a young Sydney hairdresser who went to him weighing 11½ stone (73 kg). On her first visit Dr Sinn inserted needles above her stomach, in her legs and in her ear. He also inserted an 'ear staple' and advised her to wiggle it three times a day to activate the appropriate nerve. Within four weeks the young lady was pleased to report that she had lost 1½ stone (10 kg) and she felt confident of reducing her weight further.

The instances involving drug withdrawal symptoms are also impressive. On several occasions doctors have referred patients who are suffering withdrawal from heroin and other hard drugs. Dr Sinn believes that the acupuncture needles cause a chemical change in the body and transmit messages to the brain which result in inhibiting the pain responses. Acupuncture is also often able to relieve the sickness associated with the withdrawal: 'By placing several needles at the right points,' Dr Sinn commented, 'we can kill the withdrawal pains by stimulating nerves which cancel out the pain.'

Dr Sinn was born in Canton and studied both traditional Chinese and western medicine at Sian Medical University in Sian Shensi Province. His training also encompassed herbal medicine but since arriving in Australia he has neglected this aspect of his work because many traditional Chinese herbal ingredients are not readily available here.

Several doctors, from Royal Prince Henry Hospital and elsewhere, have come to seek his advice, particularly on acupuncture techniques of inducing anaesthesia for application in surgery. He has also earned several friends amongst sportsmen. When Rugby League footballer Denis Pittard severely injured his knee it seemed that he would miss several vital games. Dr Sinn's acupuncture treatment completely healed Pittard's knee and he was playing football again within a week.

Dr Sinn admits that acupuncture remains something of a mystery to him. Even though he has a thorough knowledge of the 1020 meridian points and the anticipated effects of his needles in various combinations he is still baffled why it works. He feels that western medicine is beginning to accept it more readily nevertheless, particularly because of its use in major surgery. Hopefully in future years eastern and western medicine will be practised more uniformly alongside each other. Dr Sinn is certainly helping to bring this process about.

ALEXANDER TECHNIQUE

The essence of the Alexander Technique is posture: learning how to stand and move so that an appropriate relationship exists between the neck, head and back. Although this may seem extremely basic, a surprising number of ailments derive from poor posture, and it was such an ailment that led to the discovery of some of the techniques in the first instance.

F. Matthias Alexander (1869–1955) was born in Wynyard, Tasmania and as a young man showed considerable talents as an actor and recitalist. He had arduous day-time jobs to endure, however, including tin mining which affected his health and general well-being. Alexander was puzzled by the fact that during his amateur recitals he would sometimes totally lose his voice, and he sought orthodox medical opinions which were not very helpful. He was advised to use throat sprays but these were very unreliable. Then he resorted to studying his own posture in a mirror and he noticed that the position of his head was affecting his entire pattern of body movement. He seemed to be letting his head sag, depressing his larynx. He found that by consciously lifting his head vertically that he was able to improve his vocal disorder.

Gradually Alexander adopted the view that the body should move with maximum balance and co-ordination so that only minimal effort was made for any given activity. In his belief that good posture aided natural breathing patterns and blood circulation, and eased pressure on the vertebrae, Alexander stressed that there was one basic movement – the Primary Control – from which proper body movement flowed. His formula was 'let the neck be free to let the head be forward and up, and the back widen and lengthen'. Relaxation was essential to allow each part of the body to loosen up and contribute to the specific activity.

Alexander was a temperamental man and a poor teacher; he had to be coaxed to pass his methods on to trainers and students. He wrote four books, *Man's Supreme Inheritance* (1910), *The Use of the Self* (1918), *Constructive Conscious Control* (1933), and *The Universal Constant in Living* (1942), but these works lacked the practical perspective provided by his students and followers since.

A noted contemporary practitioner of the Alexander Technique, Sarah Barker, has devised seven basic actions which flow from the 'basic movement' of raising the head upward. These are:

1. *Leaning forward and backward while sitting:* Here the essentially vertical direction of the head and body is maintained in the sitting position. One does not crouch over, for example, during the act of eating from a dish.

2. *Moving the arms:* The arms are extended horizontal to the ground in front of the chest, then raised above the head and lowered to rest on the thighs. Emphasis is placed on 'lengthening' the arms while the shoulders move upward and outward.

3. *Walking with ease:* The head moves 'upward and away from the body'. One walks with an easy rhythm, the head and shoulders erect.

4. *Moving the legs:* The right leg is raised until the thigh is parallel to the floor. It can be lifted and lowered several times. However, while this is occurring, the head should be eased vertically away from the body, allowing it to 'follow'. The lifting should not be exaggerated, for there is a tendency to compensate by leaning on a hip. The line of the hips should be parallel to the floor.

5. *Heel and toe:* The toes are placed on the floor while the heel is raised and lowered. Subsequently the action is reversed so that the heel is fixed, and the toes are raised and returned to the ground. The lengthening process is held in the imagination so that one visualises tension easing out, and the movement become freer and more relaxed.

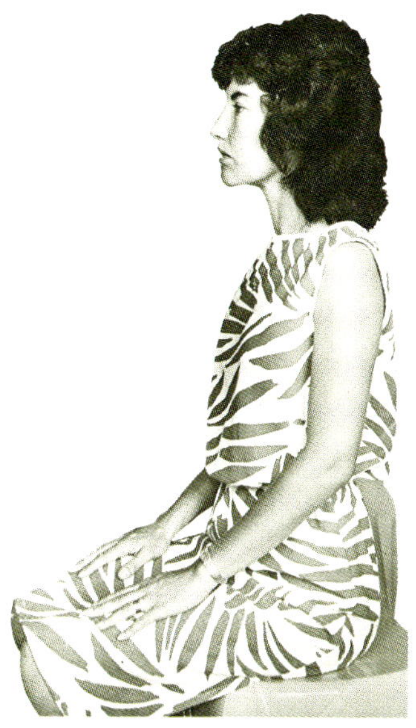

Alexander Technique . . . an appropriate relationship between neck, head and back

6. *Knee bending:* The feet are a shoulder's width apart. Both knees are bent while the body remains perpendicular to the ground. The hips and ankles should not be bent.

7. *Standing up and sitting down:* One develops the ability to use the minimum amount of effort in rising from the seated position to the standing one. As one leans forward with a straight back, the weight shifts to the feet allowing easy transfer. If one 'pushes' in rising from a chair, however, there is an adverse tightening effect on the body.

Among the alternative health therapies, the Alexander Technique is one that has received widespread acclaim from both the medical profession and the public. Professor Frank P. Jones of Tufts Institute for Psychological Research researched the Alexander posture methods over a 25 year period and subsequently endorsed them, and Professor Nikolaas Tinbergen of Oxford University praised them during his acceptance address for the 1973 Nobel Prize for medicine. Famous novelist Aldous Huxley commended the Alexander methods in his works *Eyeless in Gaza* and *Ends and Means*, and there has since been a resurgence of popular interest in the approach.

It is natural that this should occur. With new perspectives opening up in the fields of holistic medicine and mind/body relationships it is appropriate that the Alexander Technique, which stresses the direct relationship between body movement and mental balance, should receive greater recognition. Dr Wilfred Barlow, a doctor as well as an advocate of Alexander's posture methods, believes the latter are especially suitable for situations involving rheumatic, spinal and breathing disorders, although in terms of preventing possible bodily ailments their scope is, of course, even broader.

Practitioners of the Alexander Technique are now found in a large number of Western countries.

FRANCES ROBINSON

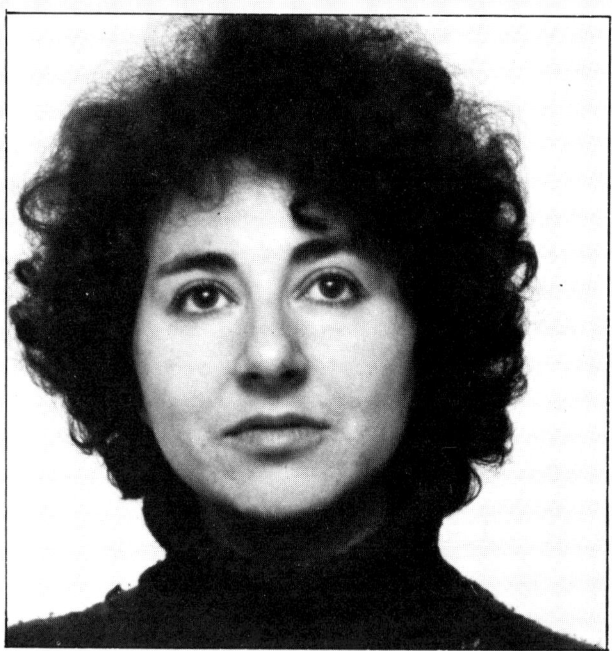

Frances Robinson came to the Alexander Technique at a period when she was re-thinking the whole course of her life. The work she had been doing, first as a secretary, than an assistant producer at the BBC, did not satisfy her and she gave it up. Then followed a period of self-exploration, an opportunity to do many of the things she had no time for previously. Among these new activities, she joined a self-defence class for judo exercises and instruction in the martial arts. When she attempted the various movements and exercises involved, she found it extremely difficult to carry them out. 'I didn't seem to have the right control over myself, I couldn't release my body physically because I was too tense mentally.' She was, in fact, in a similar predicament to that of many of the pupils who come to her today.

In retrospect she realises that much of her tension arose from dissatisfaction with the work she had been doing. Giving it up, she says, was in keeping with the Alexander philosophy which teaches 'stop doing the things that are wrong for you'. It was through the leader of the judo class, an Alexander teacher, that she became interested in the method and decided to take lessons. She trained with Peter Scott, a foremost Alexander teacher, who had himself trained with F. Matthias Alexander. She recalls that after many lessons on one occasion she was on holiday at Scotland staying in a very old cottage. Her heel caught on one of the woodwormy stairs and she fell down the twisted flight of stairs. 'However, an amazing thing happened — just at the moment of falling I was able to remind myself to leave my neck free (an important feature of the Alexander Technique). This didn't of course, prevent me from falling, but it did enable me to consciously relax into the fall. When I picked myself up at the bottom of the stairs, I directed myself again to leave my neck free. I suffered no shock, no broken bones, not even a bruise from the fall.'

After completing her training she set up practice first in London and later in Bournemouth. She sees her work as 'teaching the technique of change'. She explains that in order to change you have to stop doing the 'old things'. Posture will only become right when you begin to send yourself different mental messages. The trouble is, she points out, that the things people do in their everyday activities *feel* right but that doesn't mean that they are right. Because of these habitual patterns of thinking and posture, which have become second nature, people often don't even want to change. Many of those who come to see her with conditions such as asthma, stuttering or depression are rarely aware that it is what they are doing to themselves that is at the root of their problems. That awareness, as it develops, starts the process of self-healing. She tells of a pupil who had been an asthmatic for years and came for a lesson while he was having an asthmatic attack: He was rigid with tension, his torso was puffed up and he was pumping away with his upper arms to try and get more air into his lungs. I reminded him to leave his neck free, and I also worked with my hands to renew the previous experience I had given him of the improved head, neck and back co-ordination. Within a minute or so he was able to give his own direction to free his neck. Immediately the panic and tension began to subside and his breathing became normal. He had brought his attack under control and from then on his asthmatic attacks diminished in intensity and frequency.

Most people, she finds, dis-coordinate themselves, or in Alexander terms 'mis-use themselves'. They stiffen their necks (again and again she emphasises the importance of 'leaving the neck free') and that causes the head to go back and down.

Frances Robinson, through the Alexander Technique, offers them an alternative. Even though most of their lives they have learned to send messages from their brain that produce over-tension and bodily dis-coordination, with help they can be taught to send the right messages that will restore the balance. Many of those who turn to the method are actors or musicians. After they have been playing for years, she says, often their backs, or their shoulders, or hands seize up. Some of them suffer from concert nerves or lack of confidence. They realise that they must do something about it if they are to continue their careers and they come to her for help. Many of them, after treatment, speak of feeling less tired or that the tone of their playing has improved. Singers frequently find that they have more breath than they thought was possible. Frances Robinson finds deep satisfaction in her work. 'Results aren't achieved overnight. It's a gradual but exciting process working with a pupil.

The novelist Edna O'Brien has said of the Alexander Technique, 'It has given me the possibility of harmony'. In her work Frances Robinson tries to bring harmony to her pupils in the place of discord.

AROMATHERAPY

The term 'aromatherapy' was coined half a century ago by the French chemist René Maurice Gattefossé but the actual art and practice it refers to dates back to the times of the ancient Egyptians. Basically, aromatherapy is concerned with the use of essential oils that derive from flowers, plants, trees and resins and which can be used to treat the skin, to cause stimulation or relaxation, to prevent infection or maintain bodily resistance to disease. The oils can be taken through the mouth, inhaled or massaged into the pores of the skin and include a variety of chemical categories such as esters, aldehydes, ketones and terpenes. However it is important to note that we are dealing here with the *essence* of a plant rather than the whole plant itself and that this aromatic oil may be contained in different parts of the plant even at different times of the day. Since the essences circulate in the plants they may be found, for example, in the flowers during the evening and in the leaves by day.

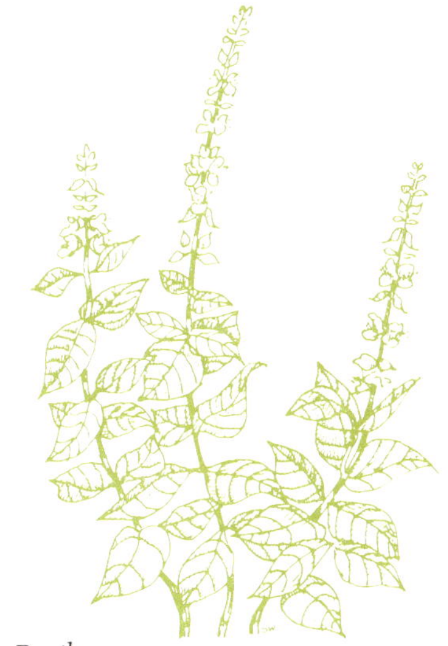

Basil

In modern society the emotional impact of various essences has been acknowledged and applied by the makers of cosmetics and perfumes, and the oils also find their way into tonics and inhalants. However if we consider that it takes a tonne of rose petals to make 1 kg of rose essence we can see that the oils used in aromatherapy are both highly prized and very expensive.

Although aromatherapy is sometimes compared to herbalism it is in fact closer to the Bach Flower Remedies since it is the ethereal nature of the highly volatile essences that causes the mental and emotional effects in the human organism. On the other hand herbalists very rarely use essences and there is often a different healing effect between a herb and its essence.

The ancient Egyptians were particularly knowledgeable in the medicinal uses of essences and when Tutenkhamen's tomb was opened it was found to contain among other things a number of pots which had been used to hold myrrh and frankincense. The use of essential oils for skin care and health has also been linked with the cultures of ancient China, the Middle East, Tibet and India as well as Greece and Rome. In modern times a few notable pioneers have advanced our knowledge of aromatherapy considerably.

Rene Gattefossé actually discovered the beneficial effects of plant essences by accident. He was working in his laboratory and burned his hand while engaged in an experiment. A dish of lavender oil was nearby and he used it to soothe his hand and was amazed at the speed with which his burn

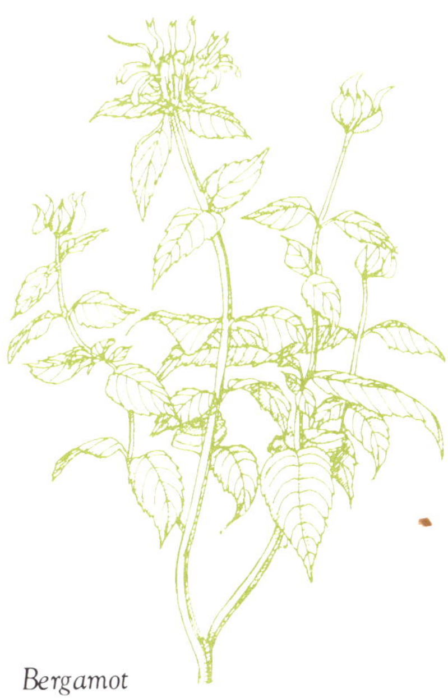

Bergamot

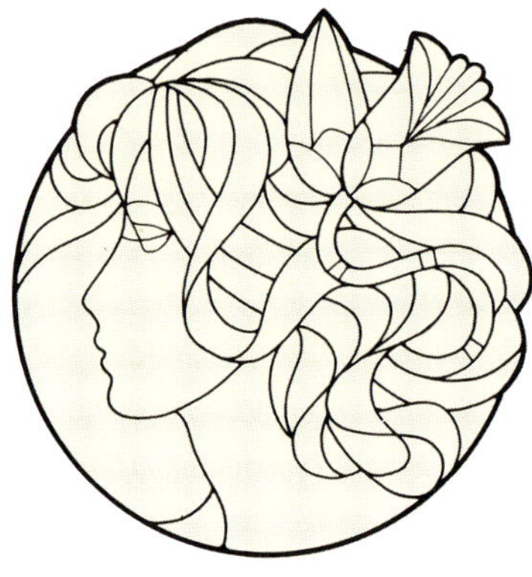

healed. Gattefossé later noted that such essences could be used as cosmetic agents and also to treat skin conditions like dermatitis. They also seemed to possess anti-bacterial qualities and could therefore be potentially useful against infections.

A colleague of Gattefossé, M. Goddissart, established an aromatherapy clinic in Los Angeles and developed a treatment for skin cancers using lavender oil. In 1938 he also reported that he was obtaining excellent results in using essences to treat gangrene, osteomalacia, wounds and facial ulcers, all of which were healing in rapid time. Dr Jean Valnet, who authored the influential book *Aromatherapy,* also used similar techniques to Goddissart during the Second World War to heal wounds and scars. More recently the French biochemist Madame Marguerite Maury developed the techniques of applying plant essences and focused on the process of 'rejuvenation'. She found that aromatherapy stimulated the reproduction of skin cells and restored the elasticity of muscle tissue, enabling the skin to remain healthy and comparatively unwrinkled. Mme Maury also believed that the abundant free electrons of aromatic essences were able to influence physiological functions and that it was by this method rather than by some chemical process that the oils actually worked. In 1962 she was awarded the Prix International d'Esthetique and in 1967 the C.I.D.E.S.C.O. Prize for her work into aromatherapy preparations.

During a healing session a sample of the patient's blood is analysed to determine the essential oil required. Occasionally radiesthesia (dowsing with a pendulum) is also used for the same purpose. An individual treatment is then prepared and these oils and creams may be used by the patient at home. Often the therapist provides a massage, concentrating on the back and spine and perhaps employing acupressure methods. Other parts of the body such as the arms, hands, neck and feet may also be massaged and the patient's individual oil is used. There are over two hundred essential oils and numerous possible combinations to suit the patient's individual requirements. The table shows a listing of familiar ailments and proposed aromatherapy treatments.

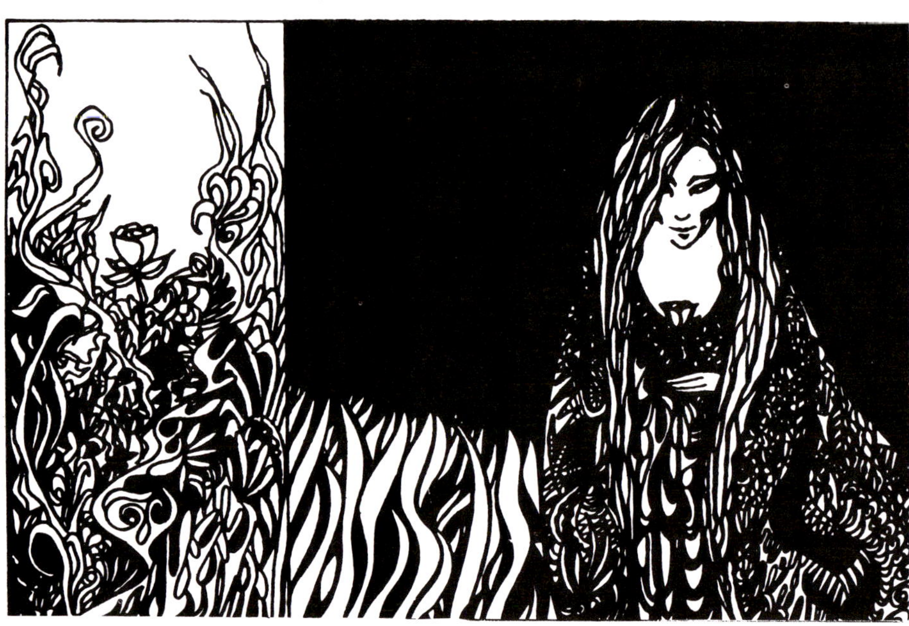

The evening essence of a flower . . .

ESSENTIAL OILS FOR THERAPEUTIC USES (INTERNAL OR EXTERNAL) IN AROMATHERAPY

ACNE		Cajeput, juniper, lavender
ACIDITY	of the stomach	Lemon Mint
ARTHRITIS		Garlic, juniper, lemon, marjoram, onion
ASTHMA		Aniseed, cajeput, eucalyptus, garlic, hyssop, lavender, lemon, marjoram, mint, niaouli, onion, oregano, pine, rosemary, sage, savory, thyme
BITES		Lavender, sage
BOILS		Chamomile, lemon, onion, thyme
BREATHING	Difficult	Hyssop
BRONCHITIS	Chronic	Cajeput, eucalyptus, garlic, hyssop, lavender, lemon, mint, niaouli, onion, oregano, pine, rosemary, sage, sandalwood, savory, thyme, turpentine
BURNS		Chamomile, eucalyptus, geranium, lavender, niaouli, rosemary, sage.
COMPLEXION	Care of	Lemon
CONSTIPATION		Rosemary, turpentine
COUGHS		Aniseed, eucalyptus, hyssop
CRAMPS	Gastric and intestinal in children	Chamomile
DIARRHOEA		Chamomile, cinnamon, clove, garlic, geranium, ginger, juniper, lavender, lemon, mint, nutmeg, bitter orange, rosemary, sage, sandalwood, savory, thymol
DIURETIC		Cypress, juniper, onion, rosemary, sage, turpentine
EARACHE		Cajeput, garlic
FLU		Chamomile, cypress, eucalyptus, fennel, garlic (preventative), hyssop, lavender, lemon, mint, niaouli, nutmeg, onion, pine, rosemary, sage, thyme
GUMS	To maintain and fortify	Fennel, lemon, sage
HAYFEVER		Cypress, hyssop
HEADACHES		Lavender, lemon, menthol, mint
HEART	Nervous and cardiac problems	Rosemary
HEPATITIS		Lemon, mint, rosemary, sage, thyme
HICCUPS		Tarragon
HIGH BLOOD PRESSURE		Garlic, lavender, lemon, marjoram, ylang-ylang
INDIGESTION		Aniseed, basil, bergamot, chamomile, cinnamon, clove, coriander, fennel, garlic, ginger, hyssop, juniper, lavender, lemon, mint, nutmeg, onion, sage, savory, tarragon, thyme, verbena
INSOMNIA		Basil, chamomile, lavender, marjoram, bitter orange, thyme
LARYNGITIS		Niaouli, onion
MIGRAINES		Basil, chamomile, eucalyptus, lavender, lemon, marjoram, mint, onion, rosemary, turpentine
PERIODS	Difficult	Carraway, juniper, lavender-cotton, sassafras
RHEUMATISM	Chronic	Cajeput, chamomile, cypress, eucalyptus, garlic, hyssop, juniper, lavender, lemon, niaouli, onion, oregano, pine, rosemary, sassafras, tarragon, thyme, turpentine
RHEUMATISM	Muscular	Oregano, rosemary, thyme
SCIATICA		Turpentine
SKIN	Dermatitis	Cajeput, chamomile, hyssop, juniper, geranium, sage, sassafras, thyme
SINUSITIS		Eucalyptus, lavender, lemon, mint, naiouli, pine, thyme
ULCERS	of the stomach and intestine	Chamomile, lemon
VARICOSE VEINS		Cypress, garlic, lemon
WARTS		Garlic, lemon, onion, thuja
WRINKLES		Lemon

ANNE SEYMOUR APPS

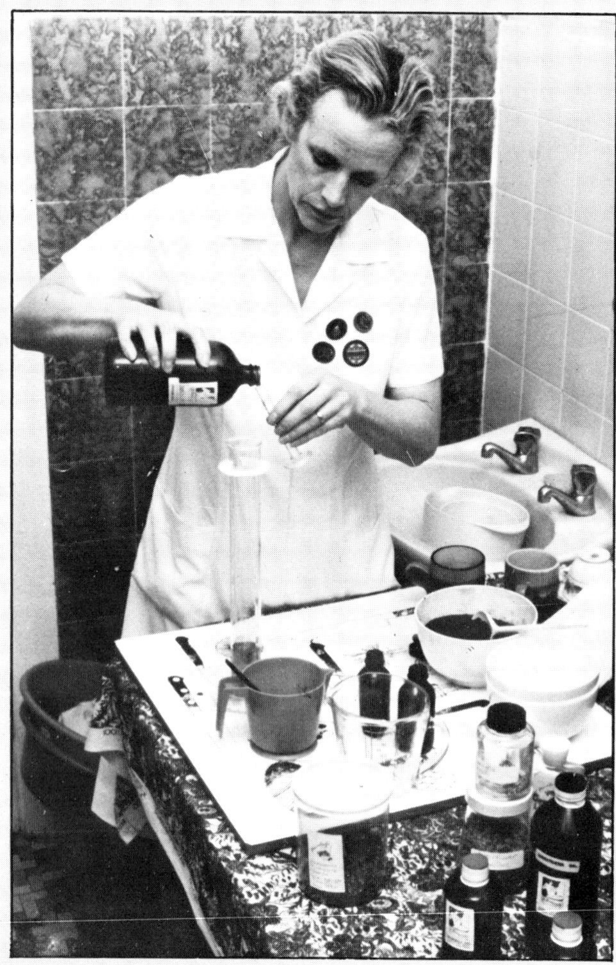

Anne Seymour Apps preparing a treatment

An attractive woman in her forties, Anne Seymour Apps arrived in Canberra in 1979 after working in London with Madame Micheline Arcier, one of the world's leading authorities on aromatherapy. Anne believes that the Essential Oils which are used in this practice not only help the skin, face and body, but render the whole organism less vulnerable to illness and disease. We live in an age of stress and an excess can bring about a multitude of physical disorders, perhaps up to 85% of them being of a psychosomatic origin. Aromatherapy like acupuncture, acupressure and some varieties of yoga, makes use of the energy field surrounding and permeating living organisms, and reduces tension, allowing the healthy flow of energy through the body. Aromatherapy is undoubtedly linked to the philosophy of 'looking well, feeling well' and it is no surprise that Anne regards her approach as a bridge between the medical profession and beauty therapy. Her qualifications in this area are impeccable. She is a Fellow of the Society of Health and Beauty Therapists (London), a Member of the British Association of Beauty Therapists and a Member of the Association of Advanced Beauty Therapists, holds a City & Guilds Further Education Teaching Certificate and Beauty Therapists Certificate as well as being Madame Arcier's Deputy in Australia.

From her Aromatherapy, Herbal and Natural Skin Care Centre in Manuka, a Canberra suburb, Anne provides a series of aromatherapy treatments for clients which last up to two hours each. She has tended to specialise in using aromatic oils for tension, insomnia, stress, migraine, skin allergies, massage, varicose veins, and for preventing stretch marks caused by pregnancy. Anne points out that although aromatherapy as such is comparatively recent, the knowledge of the beneficial properties of aromatic plants and oils can be traced back to the ancient Egyptians who knew that many healing oils could be used to invigorate or soothe the mind and body. In our city atmosphere especially, our skin has to cope with considerable external stress – the effects of dirt-laden air, extremes of temperature and humidity, and the effects of air conditioning and central heating – and these factors can upset the skin's normal metabolism causing excessive dryness or oiliness. Anne has found that on the whole her clients are women probably because they are often more concerned with their skin and facial qualities than men, but she is quick to point out that the techniques of aromatherapy apply equally well to men . . . and many men need such help because they are similarly prone to the stresses of city living, especially if they hold executive positions.

Over the years Anne has helped many clients through her techniques, and several of these had explored other avenues of medical help before coming to her. One was a lady whose social life and appearance were important to her but who was becoming increasingly emotionally drained by the idea of menopause. She became overweight and depressed and her morale began to deteriorate. After explaining the characteristics of menopause Anne treated her with a variety of herbal teas for fluid retention (Uva Ursi, Cherry stalks and Dandelion); for her blood circulation (Sage and Rosemary) and for relaxation (Balm and Lime blossom). She then prescribed tissue salts to supplement these and also Zinc and the vitamins E, B and C. The client came for one aromatherapy session a week and was also encouraged to engage in relaxing cultural pursuits like literature, music and yoga. Some aromatic essences for blood circulation were also given for internal use at home and others were for rubbing into the skin both in the morning and at night. Anne felt that the best body oil in this case was a blend of Sage, Lavender and Geranium, to help firm up the body tissues as the client's body weight and fluid retention were reduced. The lady concerned, who was nearing 50 at the time of treatment, is now much improved and her physical and mental well-being is self-evident to all who see her.

Another client had been depressed from an early age and her speech and general manner were being affected. She had seen several psychiatrists who had treated her

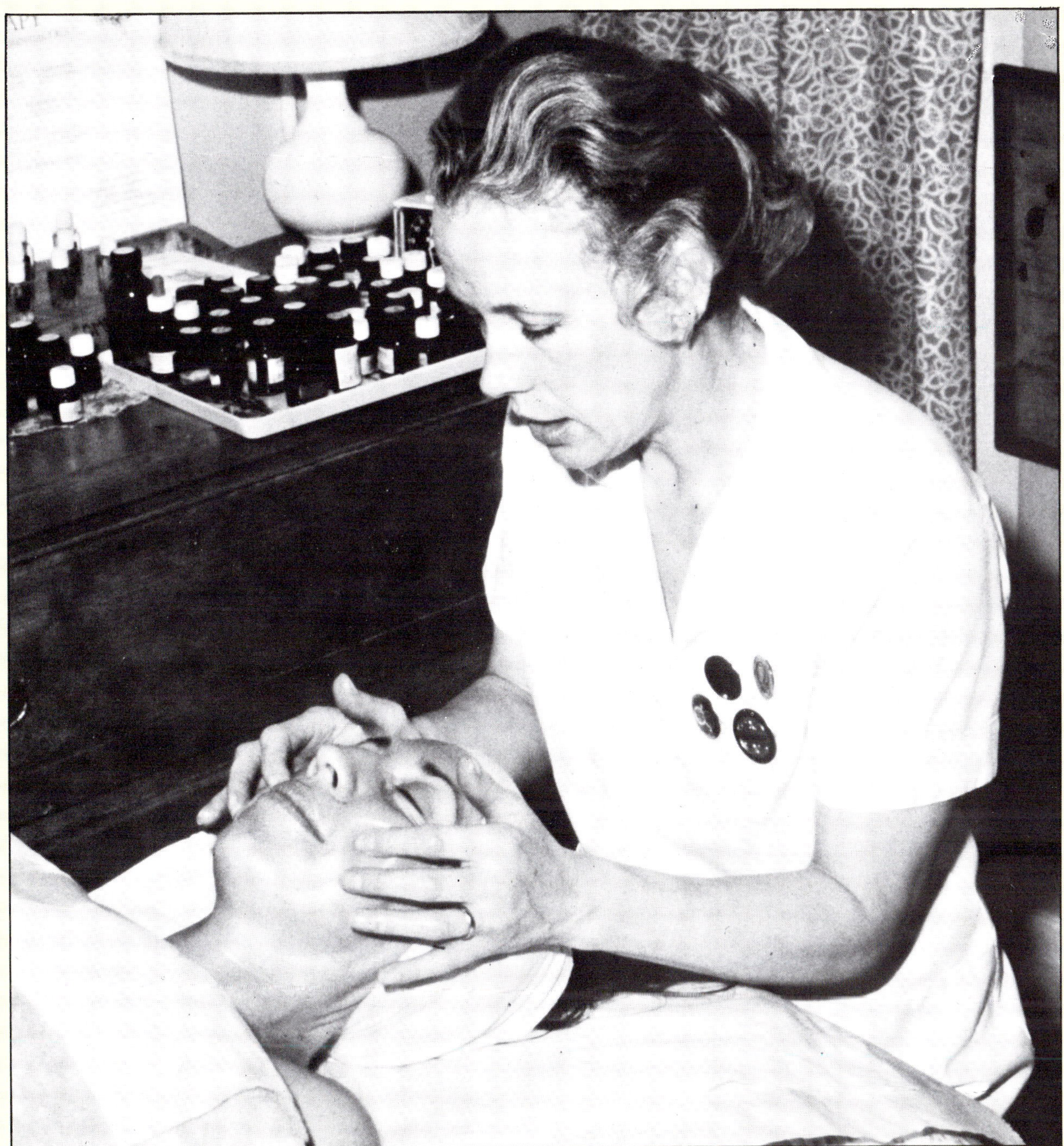

Soothing the skin . . .

without success. Anne recommended vitamins B, C, A and D, and Zinc and strong essences like Juniper and Lavender to lift her up. She also had herbal teas to fortify her (Hawthorn, Rosemary) and Lime-flowers to calm her. The aromatherapy helped her to relax and gradually she began to develop new routines and regain confidence in herself.

Anne continues to have personal clients but she is also an educator and lecturer. Aside from numerous talks and demonstrations in clubs and associations and on radio and television she trains students in aromatherapy both from a theoretical viewpoint and also in terms of practical applications. She prefers her students to have had a background in nursing, beauty therapy or physiotherapy and offers the Micheline Arcier Aromatherapy Diploma for a course extending 60 hours in duration and culminating in written, practical and oral examinations.

Already Anne Seymour Apps has become Australia's most notable aromatherapist and recently gave a workshop at the Third Australian Mind, Body and Healing Festival. We will be hearing a lot more about her work in the future.

ASTROLOGICAL DIAGNOSIS

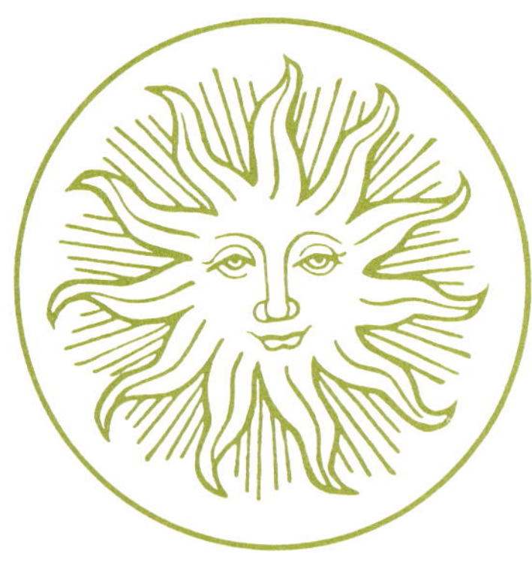

Astrology is among the most ancient of sciences and has traditionally been linked with divination. Although in modern times astrology has come to be seen as a symbolic guide to human potentialities and biorhythms quite aside from its popular image as a fortune-teller's art, in early societies it was closely linked with portents of the future.

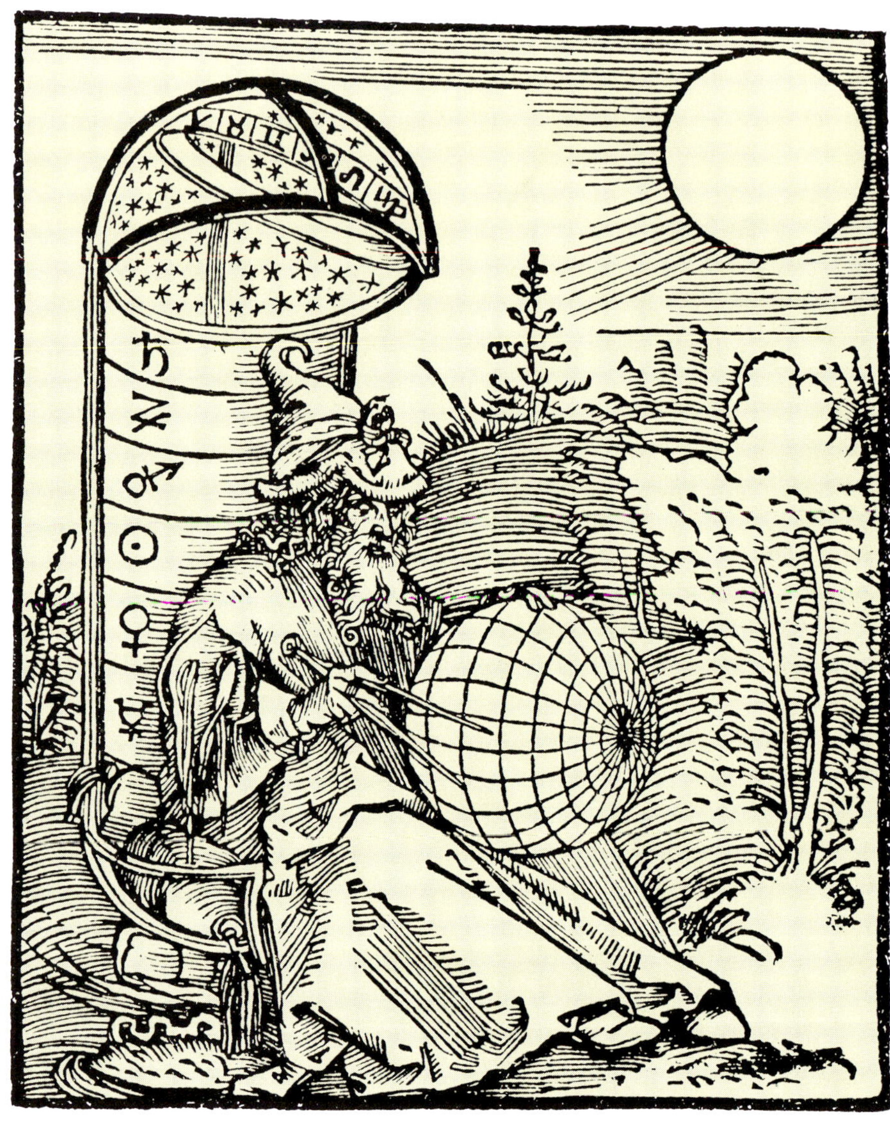

A traditional astrologer: woodcut by Albrecht Dürer

Among the Babylonians and Assyrians special priests were assigned to study signs and omens, and the deities Shamash the sun-god and Adad the storm-god were also gods of divination. Although among these people the liver was regarded as the chief organ of life and the livers of sacrificial animals were examined accordingly, the signs of the heavens were most important and the movements of the sun, moon and planets were among the most noteworthy ways of determining divine will and providence. The individual horoscope did not develop until later when astrology and astronomy held equal status in ancient Greece and Rome. Astrology was declared to be an exact science in predicting both public and personal affairs and even supplanted the famous Sibylline oracles. Tiberius believed that astrology helped him foretell the destiny of his consul Galba, and when Claudius was dying from the effects of poison Agrippina took care to announce his demise at a time the astrologers would find favourable to Nero.

After the Roman period the Arabs revived astrology and in 827 the *Megale Syntaxis* of Ptolemy was translated as the *Almagest* by Al Hazen Ben Yusseph. The conquest of Spain by the Moors carried astrology into Europe where it was sanctioned by Alonzo of Castile, also noted for his scientific researches. It also flourished as an art in England from an early time where it was pursued by such figures as the venerable Bede and the scholar Alcuin, and later by Roger Bacon and the noted astronomer and astrologer Dr John Dee, who was invited to calculate the most favourable date for the coronation of Queen Elizabeth I.

Traditional astrology aligns the twelve signs of the Zodiac with certain human characteristics and with diseases which affect different parts of the body. In brief these can be listed as follows:

Aries (dry/hot) *Disposition:* warm, hasty, passionate.
Diseases: those of the head and face, small-pox, epilepsy, apoplexy, headache, ringworm, paralysis, measles, convulsions.

Taurus (cold/dry) *Disposition:* melancholy, slow to be angered but violent when aroused.
Diseases: those of the neck and throat, scrofula, tonsilitis and tumours.

Gemini (hot/moist) *Disposition:* sound in judgment, lively, playful, skilful in business.
Diseases: those of the arms and shoulders, aneurisms, frenzy and insanity.

Cancer (cold/moist) *Disposition:* phlegmatic, weak in constitution.
Diseases: those of the breast and stomach, cancers, consumption, asthma and dropsy.

Leo (hot/dry) *Disposition:* fierce, sometimes cruel, but also capable of being open, generous and courteous.
Diseases: those of the heart, the back and the vertebrae of the neck, fevers, plague, jaundice and pleurisy.

Virgo (cold/dry) *Disposition:* amiable, benevolent, witty, and studious but not persevering.
Diseases: those of the viscera or internal organs eg. the intestines.

Libra (hot/moist) *Disposition:* courteous and just, balanced, peaceful.
Diseases: those of the kidneys.

Scorpio (cold/moist) *Disposition:* emotional, with strong desires and aspirations.

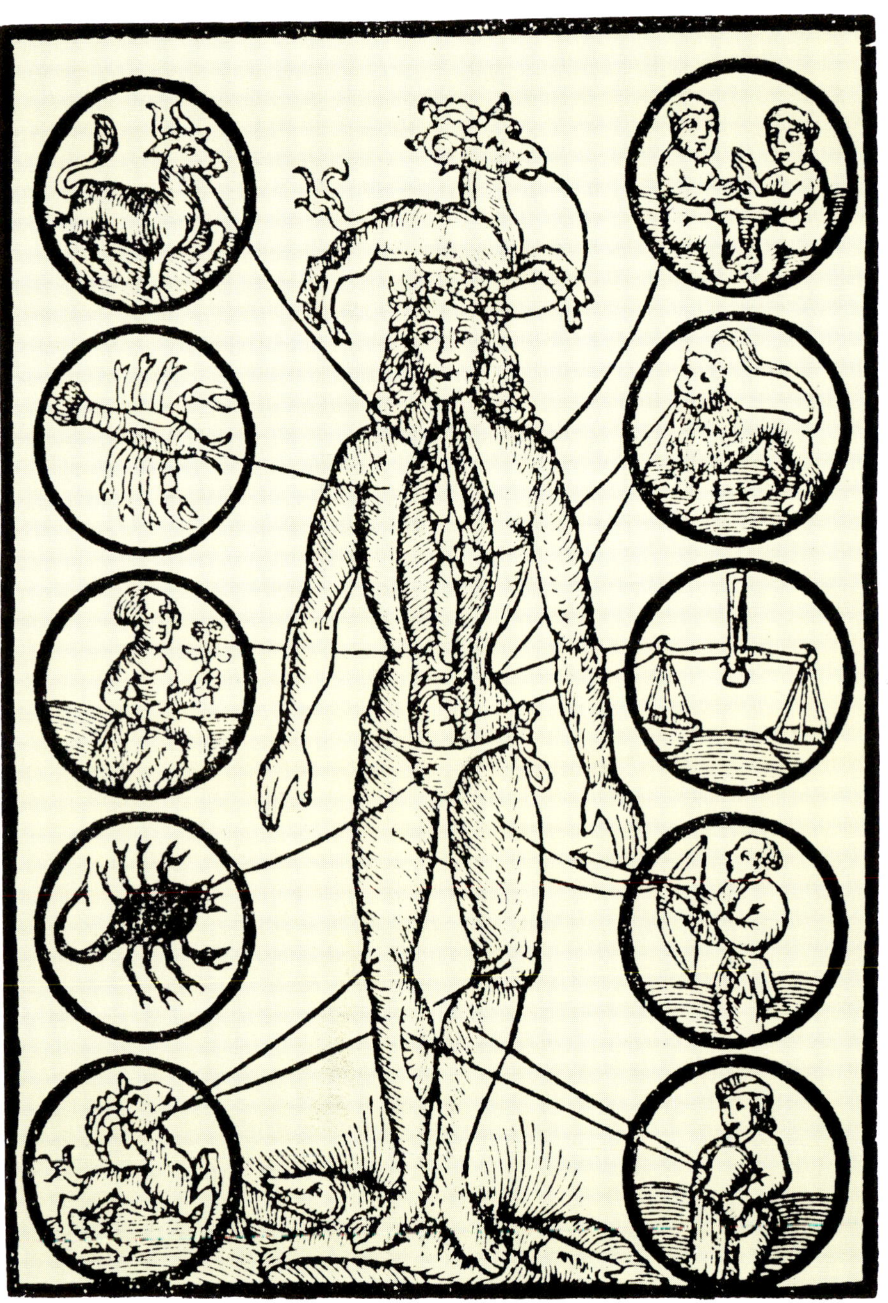

Astrological links between signs of the Zodiac and organs in the body, from a 17th century almanac

Diseases : those of the sexual organs.

Sagittarius (hot/dry) *Disposition:* strong and sporting but often hasty and careless.
Diseases: those of the hips and muscles, gout and rheumatism.

Capricorn (cold/dry) *Disposition:* cheerful, talented and upright.
Diseases: those of the knees, all cutaneous diseases (eg. leprosy) and melancholy ailments like hysteria.

Aquarius (hot/moist) *Disposition:* fair, open and honest.
Diseases: those of the legs and ankles, lameness, swellings and cramps.

Pisces (cold/moist) *Disposition:* weak and vacillating, well-meaning but devoid of energy.
Diseases: those of the feet.

An interesting example of the use of traditional astrology in treating medical ailments was related by Rudyard Kipling in an address to the Royal Society of Medicine. It concerns an English herbalist and astrologer called Nicholas Culpeper:

Nearly three hundred years ago Nicholas Culpeper, an astrologer physician, was in practice in Spitalfields, and it happened that a friend's maid-servant fell sick, which the local practitioner diagnosed as plague. Culpeper was called in as a second opinion. When he arrived the family were packing up their beds, preparatory to going away and leaving the girl to die. He took charge. There was no silly nonsense about taking the pulse or looking for the characteristic plague tongue. He only asked what hour the young woman had taken to her bed. He then erected a horoscope and enquired of the face of the heavens how the malady might prove. The face of the heavens indicated that it was not plague, but just smallpox, which our ancestors treated as lightly as we do. And smallpox it turned out to be. So the family came back with their bedding and lived happily ever after, the girl recovered, and Culpeper said what he thought of his misguided fellow practitioner. Among other things he called him a man of forlorn fortunes with sore eyes . . .

While traditional astrology is obviously simplistic in its categories, some contemporary astrologers believe that analysis can show the kind of diseases that a person may be susceptible to. In a recent article, astrologer John Addey describes how Charles Harvey, President of the British Astrological Association, traced the occurrence of haemophilia in descendants of Queen Victoria for whom birthdates were available. He found that afflicted descendants showed planetary or mid-point positions either exactly in conjunction with Queen Victoria's Saturn or Mars/Saturn mid-point, or at exact 45° intervals round the Zodiacal circle. This is significant because of the importance in the horoscope of mid-points between pairs of planets. Saturn and Mars/Saturn mid-points symbolise the hereditary haemophiliac deficiency ('blood disease').

Dr Michel Gauquelin in his book *Cosmic Influences on Human Behaviour* has written of his experiments to use the date and time of birth of 25,000 parents and children to show that where planetary positions were present in the charts of one of the parents there was a statistically significant tendency for the same position to arise in the charts of the children. Where a position was represented in the charts of *both* parents the tendency for it to show in the child's horoscope was *twice* as strong. So in this sense astrology is able to show genetic tendencies in children.

Former President of the Australian Astrological Research Society, John Flynn, has recently noted that although astrology has in times past been seen as a means of predicting causality, in fact it symbolises life-cycle patterns and basic potentialities. In this way it is valuable as a tool for self-analysis.

For example, astrological systems have been devised for predicting monthly fertility in women. The Czechoslovakian gynaecologist Dr Eugene Jonas noted that every woman's cycle is predicated on the angle of her sun and moon at birth. This natal angle repeats approximately thirteen times a year. Jonas discovered that the fertility cycle identified by the angle is a 96-hour period and that as a life-cycle rhythm for predicting possible conceptions it

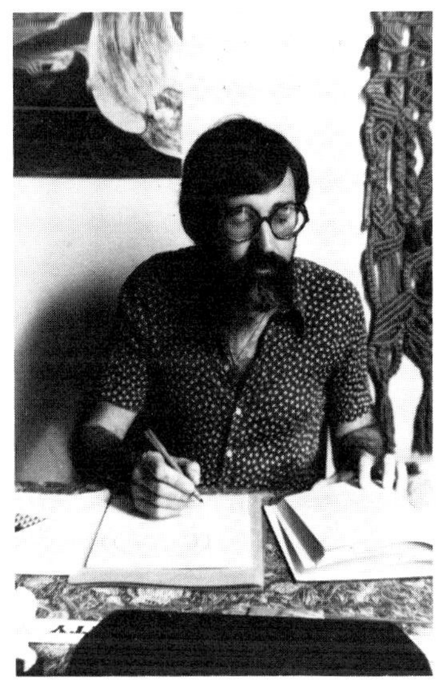

Australian astrologer John Flynn

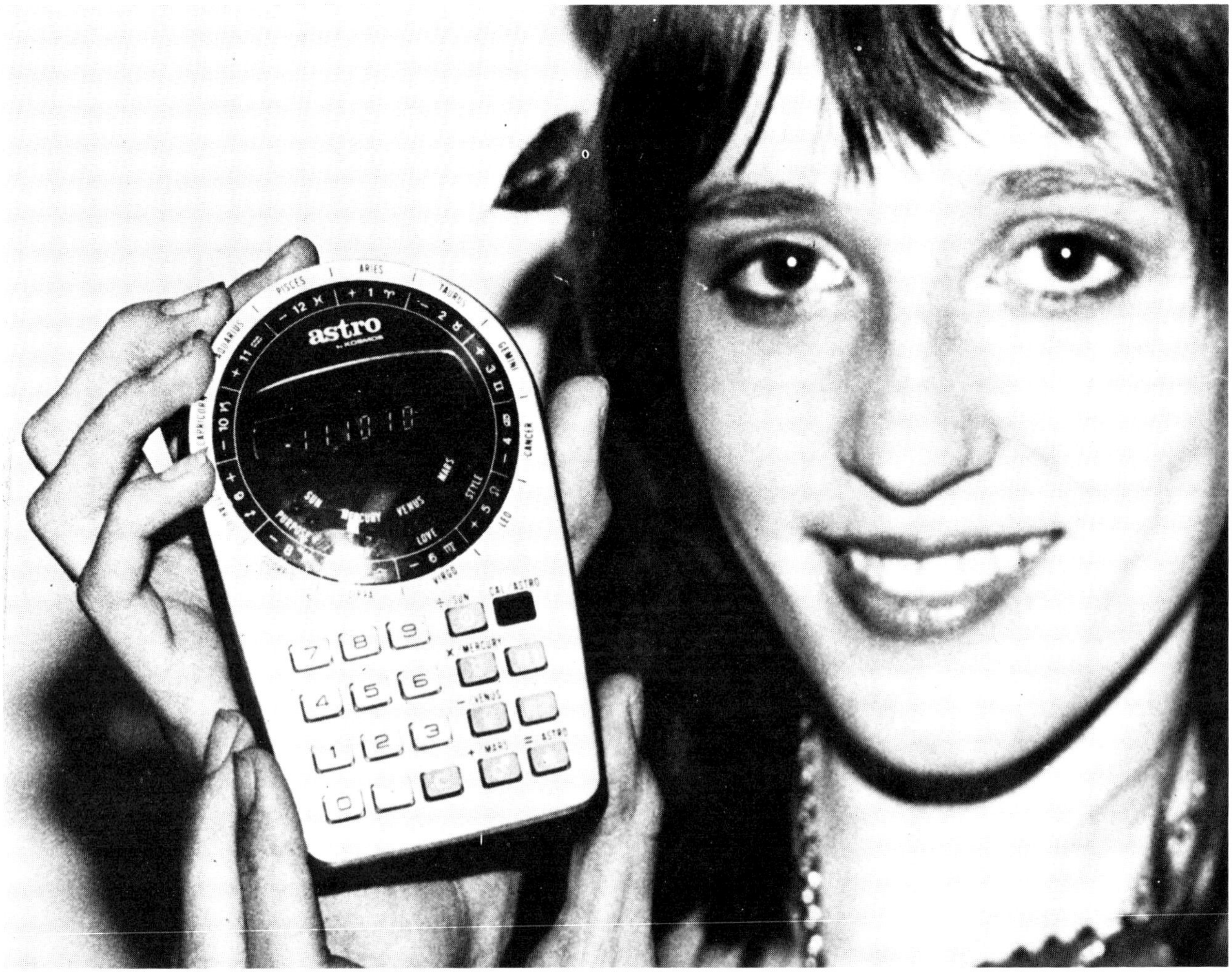

'Astro': a pocket-sized astrological computer

is 85% reliable. When combined with the rhythm method this reliability rate rises to 98%.

These days if anyone wants a chart for analysis of astrological clues to one's disposition and susceptibility to disease (planetary pairs and mid-points) it is quite an easy matter, since astrological charts can now be produced by mini-computer.

American astrologer Jeff Jawer recently demonstrated a pocket-sized astrological computer called *Astro* that is able to provide details of astrological compatability and personality analysis. Meanwhile in Australia computer astrologer Austin Levy has established a service called Astrosearch which employs an impressive range of hardware, including a mainframe PDP-II Digital computer and a Commodore microcomputer with an on-line disc storage and printer. The end result is a computerised horoscope which is produced so promptly that it allows the astrologer more time to spend on diagnostic analysis.

Astrology may draw on ancient concepts but it has thoroughly adapted itself to the requirements of the twentieth century.

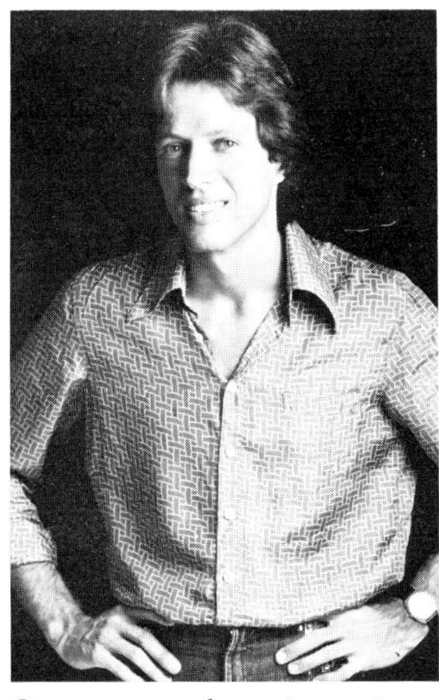

Computer astrologer Austin Levy

AURA ANALYSIS

The aura is regarded traditionally by mystics and psychics as an energy field surrounding the human body. It is often described as an oval cloud of light radiating different colours which change with the mood and emotional balance of the person concerned.

The aura has been noted through history, particularly as a sign of spirituality, and Christ, Moses and St John of the Cross were all said to radiate a bright light or halo. The famous alchemist Paracelsus seemed to be aware of the aura as a guide to inner well-being and noted : 'The vital force is not enclosed in man but radiates round him like a luminous sphere . . . In these semi-natural rays the imagination of man may produce healthy or morbid effects. It may poison the essence of life and cause diseases or it may purify it after it has been made impure and restore the health'. Paracelsus appears to have anticipated by several centuries the concept of psychosomatic disease and the mind/body relationship central to holistic medicine.

Modern notions of the aura, however, have been largely influenced by theosophical concepts and, in particular, the writings of one man – C.W. Leadbeater. Two books, *Thought Forms* and *Man Visible and Invisible* published in 1901 and 1902 respectively, proposed that matter is solid, liquid, gaseous and *etheric* while *spirit* is all-pervasive. Leadbeater described the three 'bodies' on the etheric plane as 'astral', 'mental' and 'causal'. The first of these levels reflected emotional feelings and was subject to considerable change, the second was a deeper state more permanent in nature and the third equated to some extent with the religious notion of the soul as a vehicle for evolution. Leadbeater believed that these bodies presented themselves as ovoids of light known as the aura. While they were not visible to most people, trained sensitives or natural psychics could perceive the auric colours and analyse the personality traits and emotions indicated by them.

The symbolic meaning of the colours is as follows:

rose – pure affection; *brilliant red* – anger and force; *dirty red* – passion and sensuality; *lemon yellow* – high intellectuality; *orange* – selfish intellect, pride and ambition; *brown* – avarice; *green* – variable from deceit and jealousy through to sympathy for others; *blue* – religious sensitivity and devotion; *purple* – psychic awareness, spirituality and mystical consciousness.

The aura remained essentially elusive until efforts were made in the 1920s by the British scientist Walter J. Kilner to develop a special type of glass called a Kilner screen which would enable non-psychics to perceive the aura.

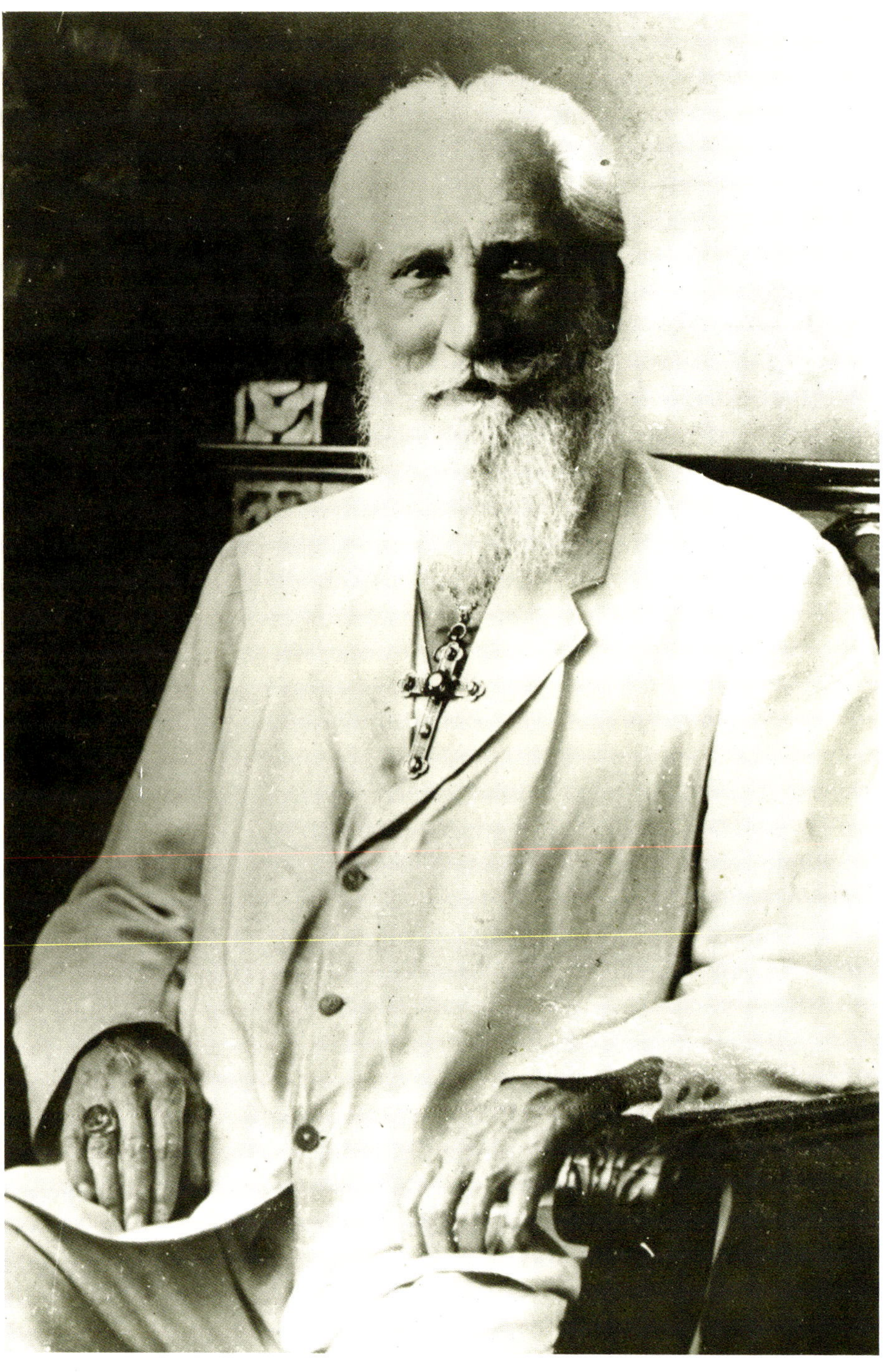

C. W. Leadbeater: pioneer of aura analysis

More recently the development of Kirlian techniques, which allow spectacular photographs to be made of the energy fields surrounding the human organism and other living things, has led to speculation that such energy patterns equate with the earlier notion of the aura. While this is by no means proven there does appear to be some overlap and the vibrant qualities of the Kirlian 'aura' certainly depend upon the presence of life-energy in the organism being photographed. This lends support to C.W. Leadbeater's concept of an 'etheric or vital body' unifying the life energy pouring into, and supporting, the physical body.

BATES METHOD

Dr William H. Bates (1860–1931) was a leading eye physician and ophthalmologist in New York and taught in the New York Postgraduate Medical School. After years of practice, during which he examined more than 30 000 pairs of eyes, he came to regard vision as being at least 50% mental process and believed that when the well-being of his patients improved so too, quite often, did their eyesight. He did not follow the view that defective vision was due to damage to or deterioration of the lens of the eye. Much of Bates' work hinged on the alleviation of stress, for he concluded that the process governing the visual act of accommodation (i.e. responding to close and distant objects) depended not on the lens but on the two oblique extrinsic muscles encircling the whole of the eyeball.

The basic idea of what is now known as the Bates Method is to teach people to make use of their eyes in a relaxed manner. Bates had been finding that some of his patients continued to complain about headaches and eyestrain and many had to continue to have their prescriptions for glasses strengthened. Then on one occasion while he was in his office relaxing after a busy period, Bates took his own glasses off and cupped his head in his hands, covering his eyes. After about quarter of an hour, feeling revived by the peaceful darkness, he removed his hands and became aware that all sensations of colour were intensified in his surroundings.

As a result of his own experience, Bates initially developed *palming*: the patient covered the closed eyes with the palms of the hands, crossing the fingers on the forehead to avoid pressure on the eyeballs. Some practitioners combine this with meditation in which the subject conjures to mind internal, imaginary scenes and shifts focus from objects which are near to those which are distant within the inner vision. This practice of alternating focus to objects near and far also applies, of course, to the external world. It strengthens the muscles and improves the functioning of the eyes. Bates also believed that the defective eye blinks too rarely. The normal healthy eye blinks both gently and frequently so he advocated that his patients should cultivate conscious blinking. This improves the vision by lubricating the eyeball and counteracts the harmful effects of staring.

Bates also believed that sunlight was an ingredient in improving vision but that the sun should play on the outer surface of the closed eyelid. The head could be moved gently from side to side during this process, and this in turn could be followed by palming. *Sunning*, as this was known, was essentially a meditative relaxation process and the act of swinging the head from side to side allowed a free-form, spontaneous feeling to arise.

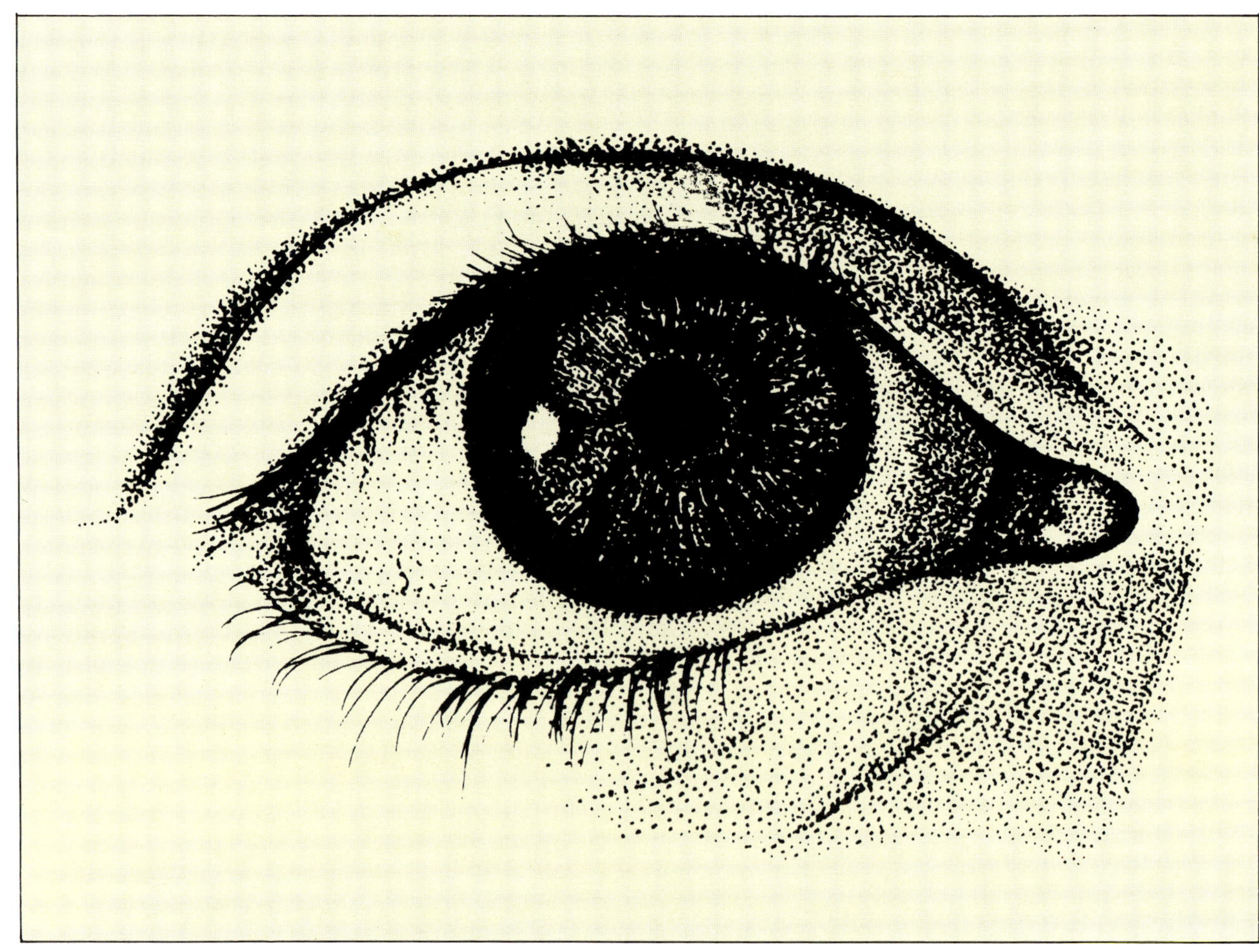

Aldous Huxley, who initially needed powerful glasses to see and write, was one of the Bates Method's most noted successes. In his work *The Art of Seeing* he reaffirmed Bates' view that vision was both mental and physiological. Referring to ophthalmologists in general he noted : 'They have paid attention exclusively to eyes, not at all to the mind, which makes use of the eyes to see with . . . My own case is in no way unique; thousands of other sufferers from defects of vision have benefitted by following the simple rules of that Art of Seeing which we owe to Bates and his followers'.

EVELYN B. SAGE

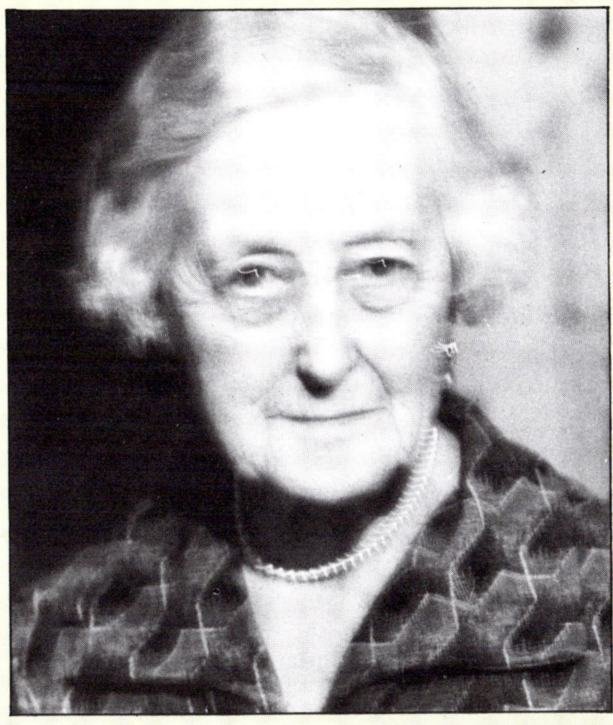

For more than thirty years, from her home in a quiet North London avenue, Evelyn Sage has been teaching her pupils that declining eyesight and the wearing of eyeglasses are not an inevitable accompaniment of advancing years. Spectacles, she tells them, are an 'optic crutch' and the more you depend on them the weaker the eyes become.

At the age of 80, she is a good example of her therapeutic philosophy. She needs no glasses and in a good light has little difficulty in reading the small print of a telephone directory. However, this was not always so. In her forties, when she was an employee of the Bank of England, not only did she wear spectacles but as a result of eyestrain suffered severe headaches. A friend suggested to her that she read a book called *Perfect Sight Without Glasses* by an American ophthalmologist named William H. Bates. She did so and began to practise the methods it recommended. Soon she was able to discard her glasses and the headaches no longer troubled her.

Evelyn Sage became so fascinated with the Bates method that she decided to leave her work at the Bank and train as a Bates practitioner. After completing her training with two English Bates practitioners, she set up a practice in 1950. Her clientele grew and over the years pupils have come to her from all over the world with every type of eye problem. One of her recent pupils was a Dutch concert pianist, the victim of a mugging, whose hands and eyesight were so badly damaged that she had to give up her career. She was advised to visit Evelyn Sage, who arranged for her to see an osteopath to correct a neck lesion which had resulted from the attack, and then began treating her. After six weeks in England and five treatments her sight has so improved that she has been able to resume her concert performances.

Evelyn Sage employs the methods advocated by William H. Bates, a leading eye physician who taught at the New York post graduate medical school and hospital. When he died in 1931 he had revolutionised knowledge and treatment of the eye. Bates disputed the long held belief that all defective vision was due to irreversible damage to or deterioration of the lens of the eye. He wrote: 'Accommodation, which is the process that governs near vision, like reading, and distant vision, like spotting the lightning conductor on top of the church spire, is not a function of the lens, as hitherto believed, but of the four extrinsic muscles which encircle the whole of the eyeball'. This discovery had a profound and practical result. It meant that visual defects need no longer be considered incurable. Eye muscles, like other muscles, could be trained and retrained. The essence of all such training is mental relaxation. Evelyn Sage puts it this way: 'You don't have to *do* anything to see. People try too hard. What they need to do is learn to relax' and that is what she teaches them to do, by using methods that induce relaxation in the eye muscles. These include palming, swinging and blinking. Palming is done by covering the closed eyes with the palms of the hands, fingers crossing on the forehead, to avoid pressure on the eyeballs. This simple procedure is one of the most effective ways of relaxing the eyes and mind and promoting better vision. Swinging not only relaxes the eyes but counteracts the damage done by the strain of staring. It is done by standing with the feet about a foot apart, then turning the body to the right, at the same time lifting the heel of the left foot. Neither the head nor eyes are moved and no attention is paid to the apparent movement of stationary objects. The left heel is then placed on the floor, the body turned to the left, and the heel of the right foot is raised. The movement is continued, alternating, for about five minutes. Blinking the eyes also helps to break the staring habit, and rests and lubricates the eyes.

In addition to these basic methods, Evelyn Sage teaches her pupils to breathe correctly, with expansion of the rib cage. If you don't get enough oxygen, she explains, eyesight is affected. Often she will arrange for a pupil to see an osteopath to correct any neck problem that is causing tension. She also recommends the Alexander Technique, as an aid to good posture, which is a factor in good eyesight. Many eye defects she believes are the result of fear, anger and anxiety, all of them emotions that produce tension. She receives letters from all over the world seeking advice, but she will not treat by correspondence. She insists on seeing pupils personally.

Now in her eighth decade, Evelyn Sage still works a five day week. 'I shall never retire', she says, 'I love my work and love helping people'. There are many who will gratefully testify that she has helped them to regain the precious gift of good eyesight without glasses.

BIOENERGY

The concept of *bioenergy* grows out of the views of Wilhelm Reich (1897-1957) who came to view therapy as a process of allowing the free flow of energy throughout the body. In his book *Character Analysis* Reich dealt with basic character types and discussed the relationship between defences which were revealed in therapy and what he called 'bodily armour'. According to Reich, bioenergy would travel through the body in various circuits but would be trapped wherever muscles – for example, in the neck or pelvis – became tense, tight or hardened. Repressing the emotions rather than expressing them could lead to a tightening of specific groups of muscles in an armouring process and this layering of tensions would accumulate over the years, leading to poor health and physical diseases. Such blockages also destroyed natural feelings and inhibited sexual responses, which Reich felt to be most important. The sexual act represented a fusion of male and female with a pulsing of energy passing through both – a total release in orgasm of inner tensions. Sexuality thus had a major healing function and was perhaps the original natural medicine!

While sexual orgasm represented freedom, specific character traits reflected repression. Conflicts from an earlier period of life left traces in the character in the form of rigidity. Increasingly Reich's psychiatric work dealt with freeing the emotions, such as joy, anger or anxiety, by working with the body, analysing posture, body awareness and muscle tension. Reich concluded that physical and psychological armour were essentially identical. While he was engaged in this work Reich discovered that the loosening of chronically rigid muscles often resulted in such physical sensations as prickling, itching and emotional arousal and he came to regard these sensations as reflecting the movement of bioenergy in the body.

Out of this context grew two therapeutic approaches – the Bioenergetics of Alexander Lowen and the Biodynamic Psychology of Gerda Boyesen.

Lowen was associated with Reich from 1940 and in 1956 established the Institute of Bioenergetic Analysis. Bioenergetics focuses on integrating mind and body processes so that the person is able to experience a heightening of energy flow and with it the discovery of the pleasure found in self-awareness. Physical tensions are alleviated by paying attention to the psychological problems causing them.

Lowen's approach lays emphasis on three areas : *Grounding*; *Breathing* and *Character Structure:*

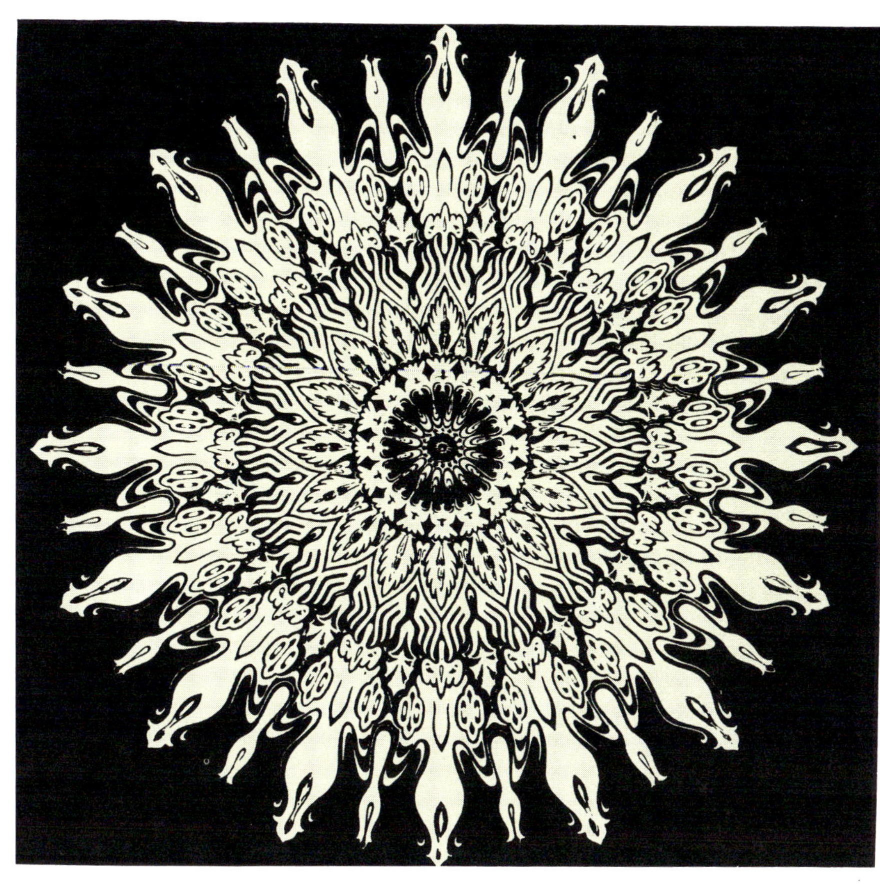

Mandala design: energies of life

Grounding This focuses on the dependency of people on others and tries to bring through the true sense of identity. When a person is grounded, he or she needs to be in a specific stance with the feet on the ground and energy flowing freely in a circuit which reinforces a positive link with the earth.

Breathing Breathing patterns often reveal defensive blockages, some of them deriving from muscular tensions. As regular breathing patterns are developed, the sensory awareness of feeling and being alive is enhanced, and with it the feeling of pleasure. The therapist develops awareness of breathing by placing the patient's body under stress, e.g. by using a bioenergetic breathing stool or by having him kick the legs forcibly while lying prostrate on a mattress.

Character structure Bioenergetics recognises five major character types and most people manifest aspects of all five, not one alone:

Schizoid character: Represented by muscular patterns of holding the body together as a result of the fear of its falling to pieces. Social behaviour is not in harmony with body awareness.

Oral character : The muscular pattern reveals a fear of abandonment or isolation. The person needs to find significance in all his relationships.

Psychopathic character : Here a muscular pattern of holding up against the fear of failure is revealed. A sense of superiority is common and the therapist has to guide the person towards interdependency and away from notions of automatic dominance.

Masochistic character : The muscular pattern derives from tension caused by

blocking feelings of rights and needs. The person has to learn to admit certain needs and put them in certain instances, before the needs of others.
Rigid character: Exemplified by a muscular pattern of holding back against emotions. The therapist endeavours to develop a unity of intellectual and sexual drives and the sense of acceptance in the person concerned.

In summary, Bioenergetics seeks to release defence structures and develop the sense of well-being and pleasure.

The School of Biodynamic Psychology was developed by the Norwegian therapist Gerda Boyesen and similarly pays special attention to the interplay between mind and body processes. This therapeutic approach uses massage and body movement techniques and works on the premise that a neurotic person embodies his neurosis in physiological processes.

Gerda Boyesen has developed Reich's views on 'muscle armouring' into a cyclical framework. She believes that the heightening and dissipation of emotions are accompanied by a range of physiological effects and in a normal person when the wave has passed the organism should return to normal. She is concerned, however, that in many people residual effects remain and has developed the idea of 'psycho-peristalsis' to clear out emotional tensions or blockages. These show up when body fluids fail to circulate efficiently or when tissues are not properly cleansed. As a result bioenergy cannot flow and vitalise the body.

Gerda Boyesen's methods include special massage techniques to eliminate body armouring, stethoscopic analysis of the abdomen to check on peristaltic sounds during massage, and a response by the therapist to the body tissue where these sounds demonstrate energy blockages. The therapist teaches the patient to acknowledge 'stimuli from within' and learn to recognise repressed feelings literally coming to the surface. Finally, the non-neurotic personality is freed from its blockages and learns to express itself.

Gerda Boyesen notes: 'The unique principle expressed in the therapy is the confidence in the individual's vital and creative self — the primary personality. The body itself wants to rid itself of the neurosis. This is an (often unconscious) biological drive which impinges from within. And it is just a matter of penetrating the first layer of resistance to contact this drive'.

GERDA BOYESEN

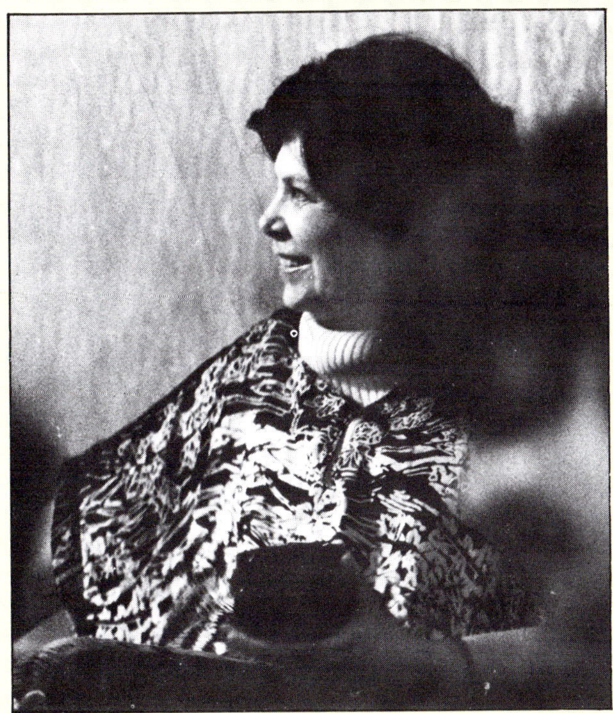

Perhaps the seven mountains that surround the Norwegian town of Bergen, where Gerda Boyesen was born, symbolised the challenges that she would face in her professional life. She has rarely failed to rise to them. A woman of boundless energy and enthusiasm, in her work as a psychologist, physiotherapist and researcher into bioenergy and bioenergetics, she has always been motivated by a deep compassion for the suffering of those emotionally crippled by their upbringing.

To understand that motivation it helps to know how it began. At the age of five with her family she came to Oslo and its show – 'I grew up with skis on my feet'. She attended Oslo University – where she was later to become Chief Psychologist – to study social economy but soon realised her interests lay elsewhere. She says of herself, 'As a child I was a model, the sort that uncles and aunts dote upon, a junior tennis champion, a quick learner, bookish, intelligent and obedient'.

But underneath the image all was not as it seemed. She was inhibited and introverted and shrank from touch, paradoxically so, as much of her future work was to be linked with the healing contact of the human hand. I am immensely grateful, she says, for the neurosis I experienced during those years, for the insight and understanding it has given me into the pain of others.

In her early twenties she read a book by a Norwegian professor of Psychology called *Neurosis and the Neurotic Character*. It contained, she realised, the evidence about herself that she had been waiting for. In the best traditions of the adage 'Physician, Heal Thyself', she presented herself to the author of the book and announced, 'I am neurotic, I want to be treated'. The professor's waiting list was too long but she was eventually accepted for Reichian analysis with Ola Rakness, one of Norway's leading psychologists and the principal co-worker of Wilhelm Reich in Europe. This was not only to have a profound effect on her personal life but also helped to form the basis of much of her future work. Reich's discoveries about cosmic energy, which he called orgone, she describes as the most basic and essential finding in connection with physical and mental well-being. It was to have a deep influence on her own research and practice in bioenergy.

Then began a period of intense activity in which she combined studying for a degree in psychology at Oslo University, and analysis with Rakness, with her role as housewife and mother of three children. These activities complemented each other perfectly. She also took a diploma in physiotherapy at the Oslo Orthopaedic Institute. Then at the Bulow-Hansens Institute she trained in a method of massage which has been described by the therapist Moshe Feldenkrais as being a 'psychoanalysis of the body'. It had the effect of releasing anxiety and other blocked emotions, and it forms the basis of the methods she uses today.

During her years in Norway, among the many positions she held were clinical psychologist at Dikemark mental hospital and psychological consultant at the Vinderen psychiatric clinic, where she later worked as full-time clinical psychologist. In 1969 she came to live and work in England, where she set up in private practice. It was in 1971, when she attended seminars led by visiting American practitioners of bioenergetics that she realised the theory and methods they demonstrated coincided with her own work in Norway. She began to integrate bioenergetics with her experience in psychotherapy and physiotherapy to formulate the techniques of Biodynamic Psychology, that she has introduced in the centres she has established.

In these developments she is helped in her work by her daughters Mona Lisa and Ebba, and her son Paul. Her Biodynamic therapy works to restore the body's natural self-regulating function. It does so with a combination of the specialised massage she employs, breath-release methods and the expression of repressed emotional material.

In 1976 she opened the Boyesen Centre for Biodynamic Psychology in London. Here, bioenergetics and biodynamic psychology is used in individual therapy, group work and as part of various training programmes. She also holds seminars in Germany, Holland and Switzerland, and has set up centres in France, Australia and Los Angeles. She plans to develop self-healing groups where the participants can learn simple massage methods to use on themselves. She speaks with enthusiasm of her future work and looks forward to applying her methods to the most intractable psychiatric conditions. Of all challenges it is the ones that present the biggest problems that she relishes most.

BIOFEEDBACK

Important research has been done both in the United States and Britain on biofeedback training which has been defined simply as 'a procedure that allows us to tune-in to our bodily functions and, eventually, to control them'.

Following on from Professor Neal Miller's work at New York's Rockefeller University it is now apparent that the distinction between the so-called voluntary and involuntary processes in the body is not as clear as previously thought. Man can learn to exert conscious control over 'involuntary' or 'autonomic' functions like heart-rate and blood pressure.

Biofeedback machines monitor changes in the electrical activity at the surface of the skin which in turn reflect increases in muscle tension. These changes are interpreted electronically as light flashes, clicking noises or some other sensory signal, and allow subjects to respond to processes occurring in their own bodies. Some equipment even allows a person to produce his own 'light and sound show' which is aesthetically pleasing as well as informative.

Biofeedback was pioneered in the United States by Dr Joe Kamiya in San Francisco. He monitored a person's alpha brain waves with an electroencephalograph (EEG) device that produced a pleasant sound only at certain levels of alpha. Kamiya discovered that subjects could learn to generate or suppress alpha waves and that when alpha was enhanced it led to feelings of inner well-being. Biofeedback has more recently been used in hospitals to control abnormal heart rhythms, indicate stomach acidity and control migraines.

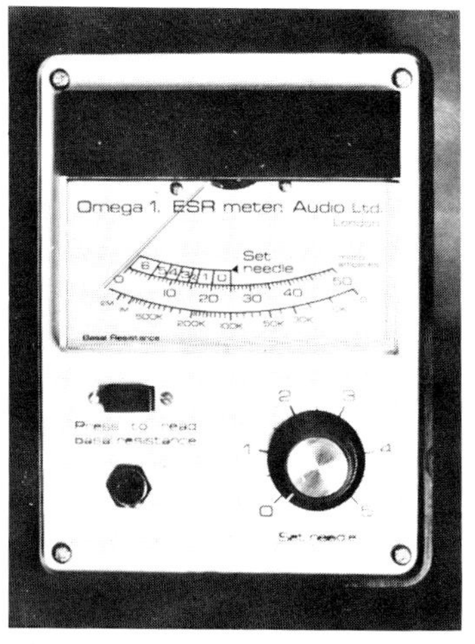

Electrical Skin Response Meter

In England a number of biofeedback devices have been designed and produced by C. Maxwell Cade and Geoffrey Blundell. Cade now conducts courses which combine Yogic meditation techniques of relaxation and biofeedback technology. For example, the Electrical Skin Response Meter is connected to the palm of the hand and measures the electrical skin resistance which in turn indicate degrees of tension. Cade has shown how biofeedback can be used to check personal levels of high blood pressure, muscle tension, blood circulation and cortisone levels. Unused cortisone reduces the body's immunity to disease, while continuously tensed surface muscles may lead to fibrositis. The alpha state appears to unite the modes of the two brain hemispheres, balances the attention between external and internal states of awareness and is accompanied by high electrical skin resistance.

One of the devices which can be used to monitor mental states is the so-called Mind Mirror, a type of EEG machine which shows reactions of

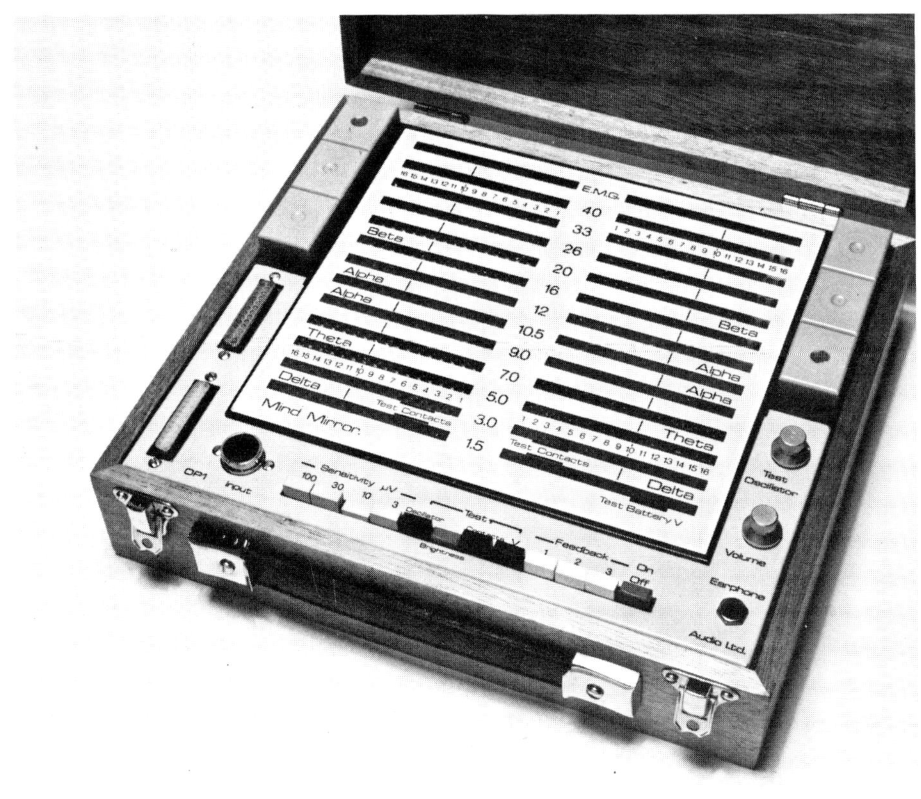

The extraordinary Mind Mirror

mood and thought. Geoffrey Blundell, who developed the device through the auspices of Audio Ltd, notes that research with the Mind Mirror has confirmed links between different levels of consciousness and certain combinations of alpha, beta, theta and delta. Blundell and Cade believe that four distinct states of consciousness can be distinguished :

Tense body/tense mind: Low ESR - beta EEG = *panic states*
Relaxed body/relaxed mind: High ESR - alpha/theta = *meditation*
Aroused body/relaxed mind: = *mediumistic trance*
Relaxed body/aroused mind: High ESR - alpha, beta, theta = *Zen meditation.*

The Mind Mirror measures the rhythms from each side of the brain and allows the blend of the two to be seen as a pattern. What Cade calls the 'awakened mind' is achieved when the meditative levels of consciousness do not remain solely internal but can be externalised into everyday life.

Quite aside from its meditative functions, biofeedback can also be used to remedy a number of different medical and health problems. In their book *Beyond Biofeedback*, Elmer and Alyce Green of the Menninger Foundation report that such techniques have been effective in treating migraines, gastrointestinal disorders, asthma, neuromuscular disorders, epilepsy and cerebral palsy. It has also been used to remedy cases of anxiety, high blood pressure, heart disease and tension headaches:

Anxiety

Biofeedback lets a subject know whether relaxation techniques are proving effective. Dr Paul Grim conducted a session with 96 nursing students who had been initially tested for anxiety levels. They were then asked to lie quietly on a bed while biofeedback equipment that amplified their breathing

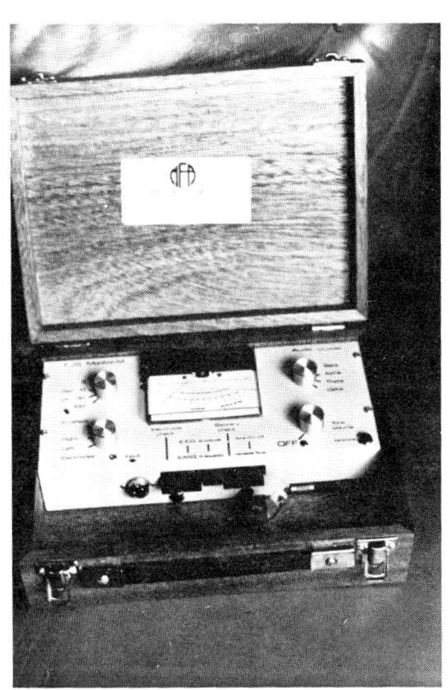

Monitoring EMG . . .

was connected. Grim asked the students to relax and let go of muscle tension while they listened to the magnified sounds of their own breathing.

The effect was that the nurses learnt to breathe more smoothly, and when Dr Grim tested the anxiety levels after biofeedback he found that they had dropped substantially.

High blood pressure

Dr David Shapiro of Harvard Medical School conducted an experiment with a group of young men to try to lower their blood pressure through biofeedback. Each subject was placed in a cubicle with controlled levels of light and sound. A cuff for measuring blood pressure was attached to the arm and a microphone inside the cuff amplified blood pressure activity in the brachial artery.

When the subject was comfortable he was asked to watch a blue light signifying the commencement of a trial period in which he had to maintain a flashing red light and sound tone for as long as possible. The more often the red light flashed the greater the degree of control the subject was exerting over his blood pressure. Every time a subject achieved a score of 20 light flashes he was allowed a five-second flash of a *Playboy* pin-up girl. Shapiro found that under such circumstances the subjects soon became adept at controlling and lowering their blood pressure!

Heart disease

Doctors Bernard T. Engel and Thomas Weiss of the Baltimore City Hospital undertook a study to determine whether eight heart patients could learn to control serious irregularities in heartbeat by mental discipline alone.

Each patient lay comfortably in bed connected to a cardiotachometer which converted the heartbeat into electrical signals which in turn translated into red, yellow and green lights on a panel at the foot of the bed. In mimicking the driving rules of the road, the patient had to slow the heartbeat when the red light was on, increase it when green showed and 'drive at middle speed' when the yellow light came on.

Some of Dr Engel's patients achieved a 20% speeding or slowing of their hearts and irregular heartbeats were eliminated. Patients also found later when they were disconnected from the biofeedback equipment that they could still regulate the heartbeat without artificial aids.

Tension headache

Thomas Budzynski and Johann Stoyva of the University of Colorado undertook a study project that built on the work of two British researchers who had shown that the resting levels of the muscles of the forehead are higher in tension headache patients than normal. Tension headaches are often caused by the contraction of the muscles in the scalp and neck. Budzynski and Stoyva felt that if patients could learn to relax these muscles, the pain could be alleviated.

In a controlled experiment in 1973, 18 patients who had suffered from severe headaches for six to nine years were selected and divided randomly into three groups. Group A received EMG (electromyographic) biofeedback which involved an auditory response in the form of a clicking sound which related to the degree of tension in the forehead (faster click rate = increased tension); Group B received 'pseudo-feedback': tape recordings not of their own responses but those of Group A; and Group C had no training but were asked to keep headache charts.

Groups A and B received 16 sessions of training and also had to practise relaxation twice a day outside the laboratory. Group C members were told their training would commence in two months time.

Overall, the use of drugs (pain-killers etc.) to alleviate pain among the headache sufferers declined dramatically in *all* Group A patients and in two Group B patients during a three month follow-up period. After 18 months it was clear that in the group experiencing genuine biofeedback (A) there was a 75% decline in headache activity.

Clearly biofeedback has enormous potential in its applications for health care in modern society. Gay Luce and Erik Peper put it this way:

Biofeedback promises to return us to a more holistic kind of medicine in which the patient will acquire more responsibility for, and power over, his own health, no longer finding himself treated as a defective organ, but as a person in a context, with a life style and habits that affect his own body. Biofeedback puts the emphasis back on training, rather than the 'miracle pill' or surgery, and indicates that the mind itself can be trained to do most of the things that mind-changing drugs are used for.

PAUL McISAAC AND DAVID GOROVIC

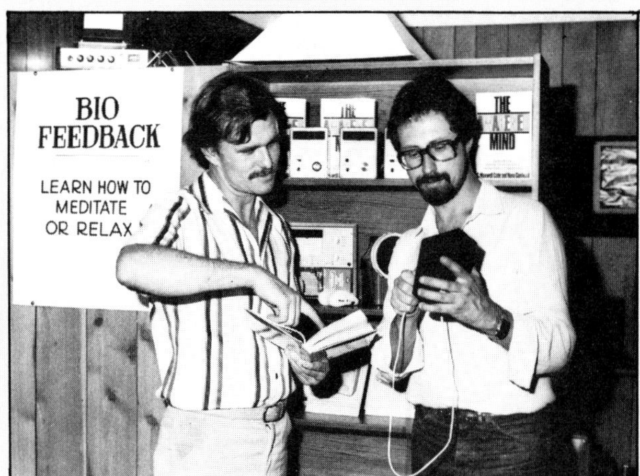

Before founding Mind Force Australia, Paul McIsaac made film documentaries, freelanced for Film Australia and worked in the printing division of Australian Consolidated Press. Although he had earned himself a film grant and had studied graphic arts he felt somehow that this was not his personal direction. In fact, in his own words, at the age of 23 Paul felt 'chronically introverted' and somewhat confused. Earlier, in his teen years he had gone through a passionate and emotional flirtation with eight different types of Christianity ranging from the Seventh Day Adventists to Pentacostalism. Now he felt drawn towards philosophies expressing an inner calm. He became interested in Eastern thought but pursued it privately, absorbing most of his knowledge of meditation from books. While he still felt too introverted to join a meditation group he gradually acquired new personal insights and a more positive direction.

In 1976 a friend showed him a magazine reference to biofeedback equipment developed in England by Geoffrey Blundell. Paul wrote to Blundell requesting background information and with a friend later purchased ESR and temperature meters. The personal biofeedback results were impressive: Paul felt that he had to work on himself initially, and found the meters very informative in terms of supplying data on physiological responses. Shortly afterwards he attended a conference at Cumberland College in Sydney, at which Elmer and Alyce Green, the well known American exponents of biofeedback, discussed new techniques and applications. Meanwhile he had been granted Australian distribution rights to the biofeedback equipment developed by Geoffrey Blundell and Maxwell Cade – initially for a year, but later as an exclusive arrangement. Today Mind Force Australia distributes this equipment to both private purchasers and university departments but Paul's interests extend far beyond that.

Early on his home had become a gathering place to discuss the applications of biofeedback but Paul soon felt he wanted to establish the meditation courses which now currently run on a weekly basis. The classes are restricted to ten members per group and Paul finds there is increasing general interest in combining meditation with biofeedback. Recently he gave a course specially to a group of female yoga teachers who wanted to explore areas of overlap.

Personally, Paul finds biofeedback more specific than many other techniques since direct information is supplied on mind/body states. He finds it 'ten times more effective' than ordinary meditation for example, and holds to the maxim that 'with knowledge man may understand himself'.

Paul McIsaac has recently been joined by Russian-born psychologist and biofeedback therapist David Gorovic. David grew up in the Ural Mountains of Western Siberia, went with his family to Poland and emigrated to Australia with his mother after his father died. In high school he showed an aptitude for science and felt he might become an engineer. His studies at the University of New South Wales were intermittent. He pursued various courses in engineering, computing, commerce, philosophy and psychology, dropping out to work for a computer firm and recommencing at university on three different occasions. His study of philosophy had interested him in questions of the relationship between mind and body and he went on to read such works as Maxwell Maltz's *Psycho-Cybernetics* and John Lilly's *The Human Biocomputer*. Lyall Watson's *Supernature* and *The Romeo Error* were turning points and aroused in him a lasting interest in the life principle. He followed it by studying new findings on ESP – and heard for the first time about biofeedback research. Soon afterwards he also began to practise Tai Chi, attend meditation classes at the university, and learn about macrobiotic diet.

It was while working at a community health centre as part of the practical requirement for his psychology degree that he first observed biofeedback equipment in operation. After taking a course in its applications he realised its relevance in showing human consciousness levels and structuring meditation and relaxation practices.

He has used biofeedback equipment therapeutically ever since and would like to broaden general knowledge about it by including it in health education programmes in schools.

Mind Force Australia has been established to run courses and demonstrate the effectiveness of biofeedback to the public at large. Many people come to Paul and David seeking instant cures, forgetting that biofeedback itself is only a learning process. With the equipment a person learns to respond and develop skills of consciousness regulation. Instead of depending on an external source like a doctor, one learns with biofeedback to become more aware of the control that can be exerted over individual patterns of health. In other words, biofeedback helps people to help themselves . . .

BIORHYTHMS

Basically the concept of biorhythms draws on a theory that everyone is affected, throughout life, by three internal cycles – physical, emotional and intellectual – that determine the amounts of energy available to the human organism.

The *physical* cycle, which affects resistance to disease, strength, co-ordination and other body functions, takes 23 days to complete. The *emotional* cycle which includes such factors as sensitivity, mood, perceptions and mental well-being, passes through 28 days, and the *intellectual* cycle which includes memory, alertness and the logical aspects of intelligence, takes 33 days.

The cycles begin at a common point at birth and from 'zero' rise into a high, positive phase increasing the energies available and then reach a half-way point after which they begin to decline. The second half of each cycle tends to be negative as the energies diminish. Finally each cycle reaches zero-point and begins to build again.

Because the cycles are of different lengths they very rarely coincide. They cross the baseline at exactly the same time only at birth and after 58 years, 67 (or 68) days. People are thus subject to a mixed blend of available energies and this influences their effectiveness in their lifestyle and occupation.

To the extent that biorhythms appear to affect behaviour, knowledge of likely 'up' and 'down' days is a way of anticipating a positive, creative period of activity or warning against a particularly negative phase. Biorhythms therefore offer 'preventative' perspectives since one would not want to make important decisions or put oneself at risk during an acutely negative period. By the same token, the 'highs' of the biorhythm cycle are periods of perceptive and sensitive creativity – a time for performing. Truly 'critical' days make up only 20% of one's life and these are times when we should all be careful and take things easily.

Biorhythms were jointly discovered by two scientists working separately: Dr Hermann Swoboda, professor of psychology at the University of Vienna, and Dr Wilhelm Fliess in Berlin who became president of the German Academy of Sciences. When working with his patients Swoboda noticed that creative ideas seemed to recur in certain rhythmic phases. Later he also kept records of patterns of inflammation and fevers, heart attacks and bouts of asthma. Finally he began to discern physical and emotional cycles of 23 and 28 days respectively – two distinct biorhythms – and documented his work in several books, including *The Periods of Human Life* (1904) and *The Critical*

Days of Man (1909). He was awarded an honorary degree by the University of Vienna and a medal by his home city, in recognition of his work.

Wilhelm Fliess attended the University of Berlin and later became a member of the Berlin Board of Health. Fliess similarly found evidence of the 23 day physical cycle and the 28 day emotional one, and over a sixteen year period wrote four books on the case for recognising biorhythms. Fliess died in 1928 before receiving the public acknowledgment his work deserved.

Later a third biorhythm – the intellectual – was discovered by another pioneer in the field, Alfred Teltscher, an Austrian doctor of engineering. Teltscher tested the intellectual performances of his students to see whether rhythmic cycles presented themselves, and made a very detailed statistical analysis of examination performances at the Innsbruck high school and college. The cycle of 33 days was discovered and later verified.

'Critical' days occur twice in any of the given cycles : for example, in the emotional pattern of 28 days they occur at two-week intervals. With this in mind it is not surprising that research has been done to determine whether such negative points in the cycle can be correlated with an increase in accidents, industrial errors or other man-made disasters. We should remember in considering the following findings that chance would provide a 20% occurrence of accidents on the critical days concerned.

Hans Schwing, who earned his doctorate from the Swiss Federal Institute of Technology in Zurich, undertook a study based on data from insurance companies on 700 people involved in serious accidents. He concentrated on accidents where personal judgment, reflexes and decision-making processes and not mechanical failure were decisive.

When he calculated how many of the events had occurred on critical days he found that out of 700, 401 had occurred on single, doubly or triply-critical days: that is to say, 57% of the people involved in the study. The other 299 accidents occurred on mixed-rhythm days.

Overall, Schwing's survey showed that accidents are five times more likely on critical days than on others, and death was almost eleven times more likely to occur on a critical day than otherwise.

On occasion specific patterns of biorhythms have proved catastrophic. Airline accidents provide very pertinent data because flight recorders allow researchers to analyse whether mishaps have occurred as a result of pilot error or mechanical failure. Dr Robert Woodham of the Guggenheim Aviation Safety Center discovered in a survey of accidents with private planes that almost 80% occurred on one of the pilot's critical days. In one tragic instance involving a commercial airliner, when TWA Flight 514 (1 December 1974) came in to land in Washington D.C., it descended far too quickly and crashed into the Blue Ridge mountains. The pilot *and* his crew had all misjudged the heights of the surrounding mountains by 500 feet. Subsequent analysis of the biorhythms of those involved in flying the airliner showed that the flight controller was undergoing a physically critical day which probably dulled his perceptions, the captain was experiencing negative physical and emotional phases and the co-pilot was negative in all three cycles and was only two days off a double-critical point.

In another area of research, Russell K. Anderson who headed a safety engineering firm found, when examining 300 industrial accidents caused by

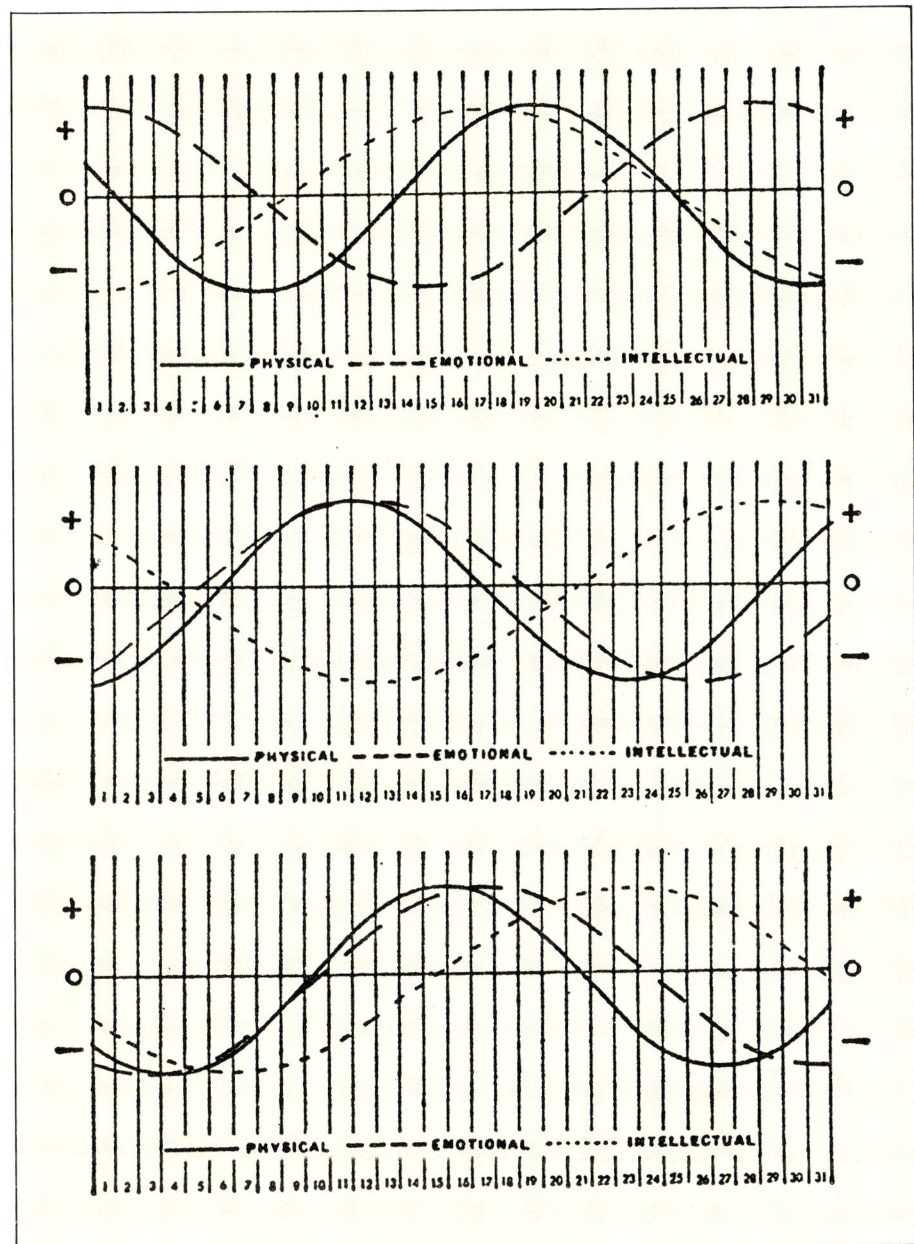

Biorhythm patterns for flight staff involved in the tragic air crash of TWA Flight 514. The critical and negative aspects predominate

human error, that 70% had occurred on critical days within the cycle and the greatest number took place when two rhythms crossed at a base-line or zero point.

Does this mean we should all go through life morbidly aware of the dangers that critical biorhythm phases portend? Well – it would pay to be careful, but of course there are also the high points to remember! Biorhythms are the natural cycles of life, and as with all energy patterns they have both positive and negative aspects that we should all heed.

CHIROPRACTIC

Although the physical manipulation techniques of chiropractors and osteopaths are often thought of as a modern development, comparable practices were employed in several ancient cultures. The Chinese *Kong-Fou*, which dates from around 2700 B.C., refers to manipulation as a healing technique and it was also practised by the ancient Greeks, Romans, Egyptians, Syrians and Aztecs. Hippocrates, the Greek physician who established a school of healing on the island of Cos, and is regarded historically as the 'Father of Medicine' noted:

One or more vertebrae of the spine may or may not go out of place . . . They might give way very little, and if they do, they are likely to produce serious complications and even death, if not properly adjusted . . . many diseases are related to the spine.

The word 'chiropractic' derives from two Greek words, 'cheiro' and 'practikos' and were combined together to suggest the meaning 'done by hands'. The phrase was coined by Daniel David Palmer who is credited with being the founder of modern chiropractic.

Palmer was born in Port Perry near Toronto although he later practised his new medical techniques in Burlington and Davenport, Iowa. He had become a student of Paul Caster, a healer who used techniques of 'animal magnetism' derived from the teachings of Anton Mesmer. Palmer worked with these methods for a full ten years before discovering chiropractic.

On 18 September 1895, a man named Harvey Lillard came to see him in his Davenport office. Lillard was extremely deaf and could not hear the sound of wagons passing in the street. He told Palmer he had become deaf quite suddenly 17 years earlier when stooping in a cramped position at work. When Palmer examined Lillard's back in a routine way he found a prominent vertebra out of position. Lillard confirmed that this particular location had been a source of considerable pain at the time he had lost his hearing. Using a manipulative technique Palmer repositioned the bone and Lillard stated that his hearing immediately improved. Following further treatments Palmer was able to restore Lillard's hearing to its original normal level.

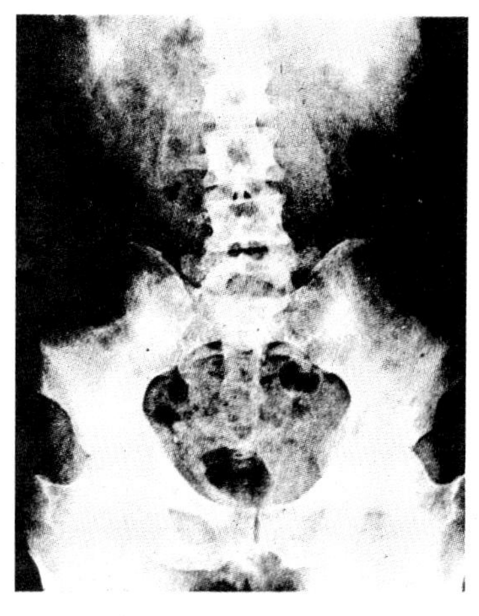

X-ray of the lower spine and pelvis

Palmer's techniques were greeted with ridicule by doctors at the time but it has since been discovered that some cases of deafness caused by circulatory problems can be remedied by manipulation. Professor Paul Bechgaard of the University of Aarhus in Denmark described a case in *Nordisk Medicin* June 1963, in which a 54 year old man suffering from lumbago and a long-standing hearing defect was given manipulation. A marked improvement in his hearing

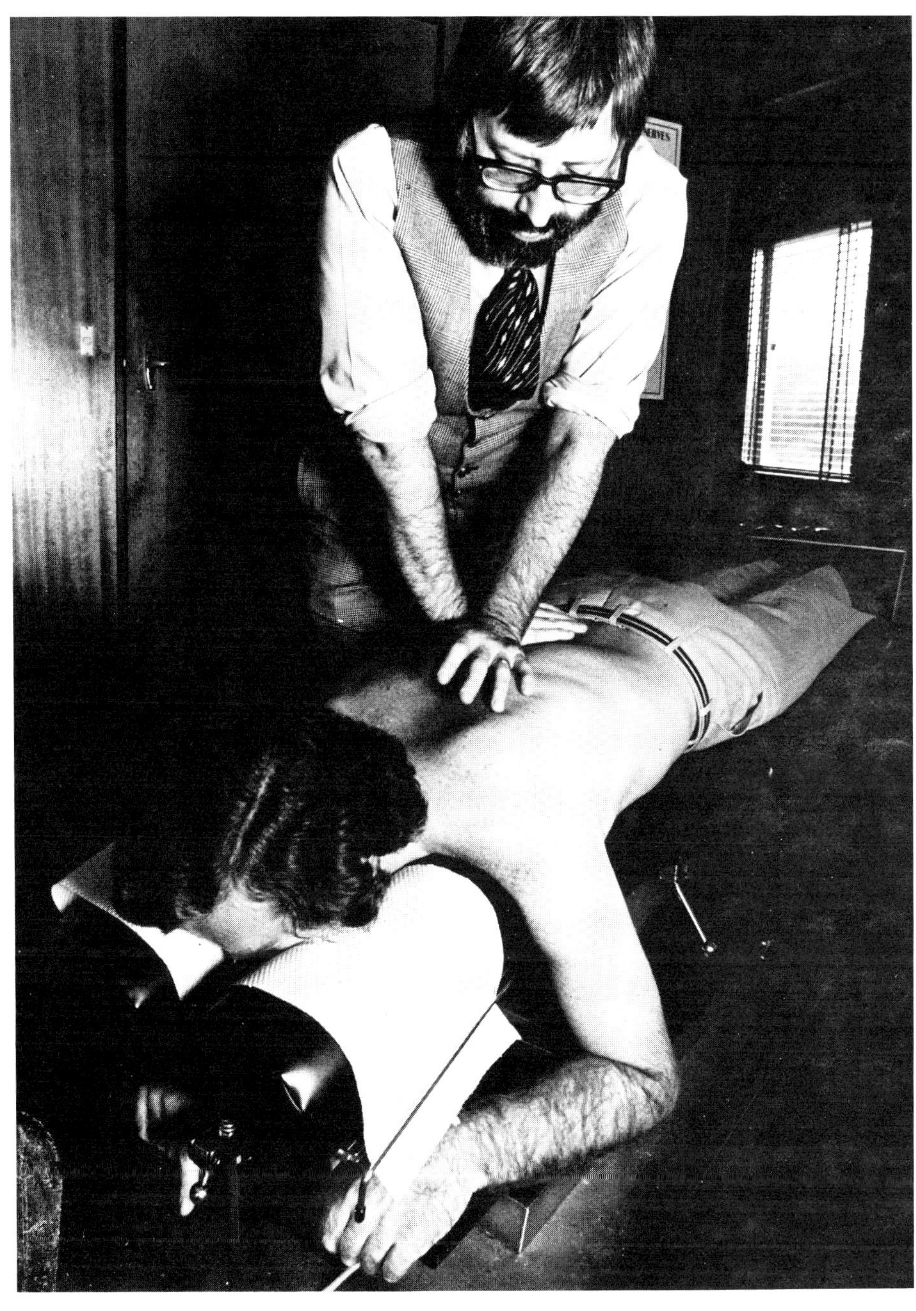

Careful manipulation is a key part of chiropractic technique

ability resulted and it was found that the blood supply to the 'organ of Corti' in the ear had been impaired by irritation of nerves leading from the upper spine.

The Spinal Column and Chiropractic

The spinal cord passes through a series of vertebrae which are stacked in the vertical column of the 'back-bone'. At various intervals nerve connections branch off to other parts of the body and it is at these linkage points that stress and pain may occur. The *cervical* (neck) region has eight pairs of spinal nerves; the *thoracic* (chest), twelve pairs, and the *lumbar* (loin) or lower back, five pairs. The nerves from these regions branch into the head, torso, arms and legs which explains, for example, why lower back manipulation can relieve pain in the 'pinched' sciatic nerve felt in the leg.

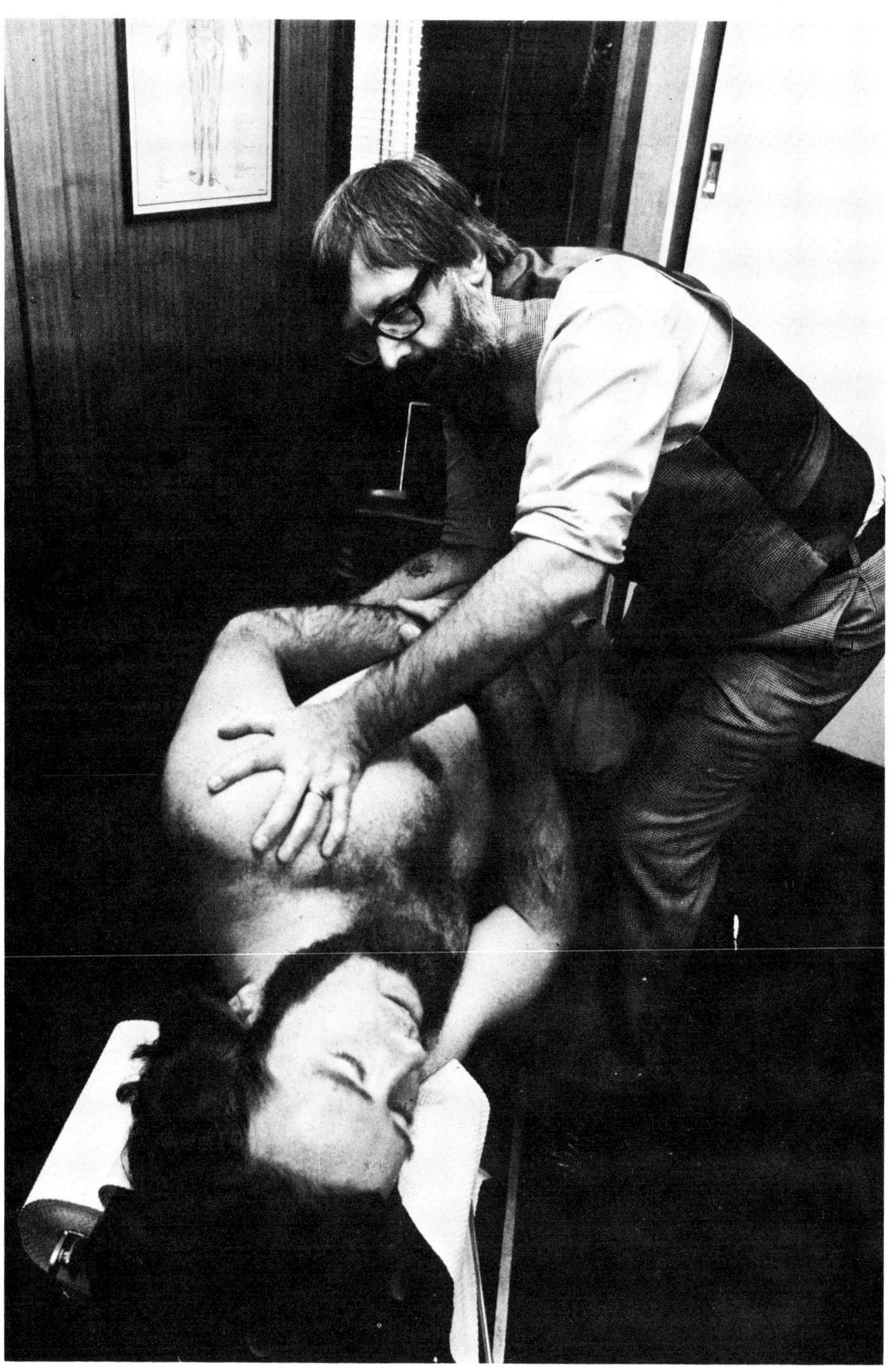

Chiropractic technique demonstrated by Dr Jonn Mumford

Like some practitioners of the Alexander Technique, many chiropractors feel that man's body structure is inherently unsuitable for the strains of vertical posture; his framework is not sufficiently evolved to sustain it. The length of time a baby takes to learn to walk exemplifies this : most animals are able to walk soon after birth.

The sheer weight of gravity exerts a noticeable downward thrust on several organs in the body, including the intestines, arteries and veins, – producing hernias and circulatory problems. Many of these stresses impinge on the spinal column.

The spinal vertebrae are separated by cartilage layers which allow easy and smooth movement o the bones and also act as shock absorbers. Man's erect posture brings about the possibility of displacements of the vertebrae in the spinal column and other distortions or curvature (scoliosis). A chiropractor diagnoses such abnormalities by examining the spinal pattern in the back, often in conjunction with an X-ray.

Chiropractic techniques still remain controversial despite widespread popular acceptance. Dr Neville Ussher of the Santa Barbara Clinic in California reported in the *Annals of Internal Medicine* that after 15 years research using only chiropractic manipulation he had been able to cure a number of disorders, including occipital and facial neuralgia, bronchial asthma, circulatory problems, chronic appendicitis, and various types of spasm.

Dr James Cyriax believes that chiropractic is most beneficial for back pain, lumbago and sciatica, which derive from problems with spinal discs, while he continues to doubt the value of the techniques for disorders in other organs. However he believes that the major obstacle to the acceptance of manipulation is the prejudice of a great number of doctors rather than any fault with the methods themselves. Writing in the *General Practitioner* Dr Cyriax notes:

The reason why manipulation, especially spinal, lies under a cloud today is not that it is ineffective – everyone knows of cases where it was dramatically successful – but that it is carried out by people of whom doctors disapprove. It is up to medical men not to deride their failures but to study their successes . . .

This view is supported by T.A. Vondarhaar, president of the Northern California College of Chiropractic who states:

Chiropractic has remained outside the mainstream of modern medicine because its major premise, that the body has inherent capacities for health, has simply been out of fashion in the United States and the Western world. The holistic view of health is regarded with suspicion by the medical establishment because it does not rely on technological intervention in the body . . . which can be measured and controlled.

The medical dispute aside, it is perhaps appropriate to heed the experience of commerce and industry, where lower back problems have resulted in hundreds of thousands of lost man hours. Andrew J. Sordoni, a former Secretary of Commerce in Pennsylvania and administrator of a number of companies with a $20 million payroll, has gone on record stating that chiropractic techniques are favourably regarded by many sections of the production industry – because of their practical effectiveness. In an article titled *Chiropractic and Industry* he noted:

Based on my experience, I firmly believe that chiropractic is the best method of coping with certain health and accident problems in industry. Many insurance companies are recognising the benefits of chiropractic techniques and are paying for them. This is most significant as is the fact that State Workmen's Compensation Acts are more and more recognising the need for chiropractic services. These bodies form their decisions and base their policies on statistics, not on sentiment.

DR JONN MUMFORD

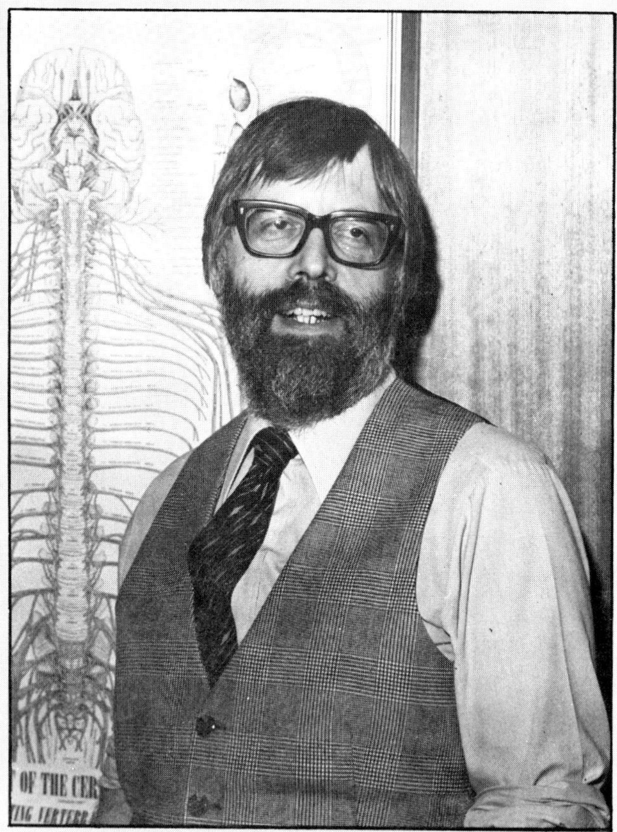

Well known chiropractor and writer Dr Jonn Mumford runs the Rose Bay Chiropractic Clinic and also lectures on anatomy and physiology at several alternative health-care centres. Medium in height, with a distinguished black and grey beard and heavy rimmed glasses, Jonn goes about his work with a mixture of professional seriousness and spontaneous good humour, as his mood takes him. Born in Windsor, Ontario in 1937, Jonn grew up in an unusual family environment. His father pursued a professional career in the Canadian army and consequently much of Jonn's early life was spent in one military camp or another. Mother, on the other hand, was a somewhat bohemian lady who buried herself in Egyptology and poetry when she wasn't throwing eccentric parties.

Jonn didn't see much of his parents in his early years though. Because he suffered from bad asthma he went to live in the southern United States with family friends located variously in Laredo, Texas; Tucson, Arizona and the small town of Beatty, Nevada. For four or five years he didn't go to school but hung out at hamburger stalls where was intrigued by trigger-happy Texas border patrol officers who seemed to fire their guns off whenever it pleased them. Beatty made a distinct impression on him, though, of quite a different kind. Here were ruddy coloured mountains, expansive deserts and a sense of space. From an early age Jonn was interested in metaphysics and the feeling of mystery underlying Nature.

After his father retired from the army Jonn moved back to Canada — this time to Vancouver. Here he completed high school and commenced an Arts degree at the University of British Columbia. He had specialised in psychology and English but found himself drawn to another interest: chiropractic. He had received successful chiropractic treatment for his asthma and found it extraordinary that pain could be relieved by manipulating the spinal column. Jonn still feels that chiropractic is 'special'. The healer has a personal relationship with the patient through his hands and with correct chiropractic treatment, healing is immediate!

Jonn enrolled to study chiropractic at Western States College in Portland, Oregon, but didn't complete his degrees until coming to Sydney in 1962, after travelling in India and Britain. He finally graduated with a diploma from the Sydney Chiropractic College in 1968 and gained his doctorate in 1976.

Jonn emphasises that chiropractic is now the second largest healing profession in the western world after allopathic medicine — a very special contribution to world health-care techniques by the Americans who invented and systematised it. He points out, however, that chiropractic is not a cure-all but is aimed predominantly at rectifying muscular and skeletal disorders. As such it is an important adjunct to orthodox medicine and is recognised by every medical fund in New South Wales. Chiropractic is expanding rapidly in both Australia and New Zealand, and around 250 000 Australians visited chiropractors in 1980.

Clearly, chiropractic is no longer regarded as being in any way a pseudo-medical practice. The Webb Committee reported to the Australian Government that financial support should be made available for chiropractic training and in New Zealand the recent Commission of Inquiry highlighted the fact that chiropractors have special manual therapy skills not generally found among medical practitioners and physiotherapists. The Inquiry praised the high level of training at Victoria's Preston Institute and recommended that New Zealand students should receive bursaries to attend. Jonn also pointed out that chiropractors are winning their fight against the AMA in America which has denied chiropractors ready access to medical pathology services and hospital facilities. In addition, the American National Safety Council has shown that as a method of treating industrially-caused back injuries, chiropractic is three times more effective than hospital treatment in terms of work-days lost and almost twice as effective as orthodox medical care.

Jonn feels strongly that in the 1980s chiropractic will come to be thought of as no longer 'alternative', and there will be developing bonds between chiropractors, orthodox general practitioners and orthopaedic surgeons. It is no longer feasible, he says, for chiropractic to remain outside the mainstream of contemporary health-care systems.

COLOUR THERAPY

We live in a world filled with colour – a visual universe of hues, pigments, shades and tints that can be found in every conceivable combination.

Colour therapy is a technique of restoring imbalances by means of applying coloured light to the body. The idea is an ancient one: it was used, for example, in the Healing Temples of Light and Colour at Heliopolis, the Egyptian centre for the worship of Atum-Ra. In more recent times colour therapy has owed a debt to the mystical thinkers Rudolph Steiner and C.W. Leadbeater who were interested in auric colours; Dinshah Ghadiali who wrote a definitive work on colour vibrations *(The Spectro-Chromemetry Encyclopaedia)* and contemporary theorist Faber Birren, author of *Color Psychology and Color Therapy*.

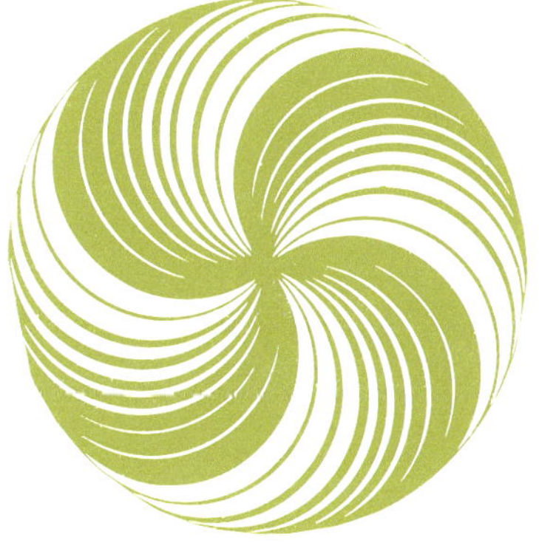

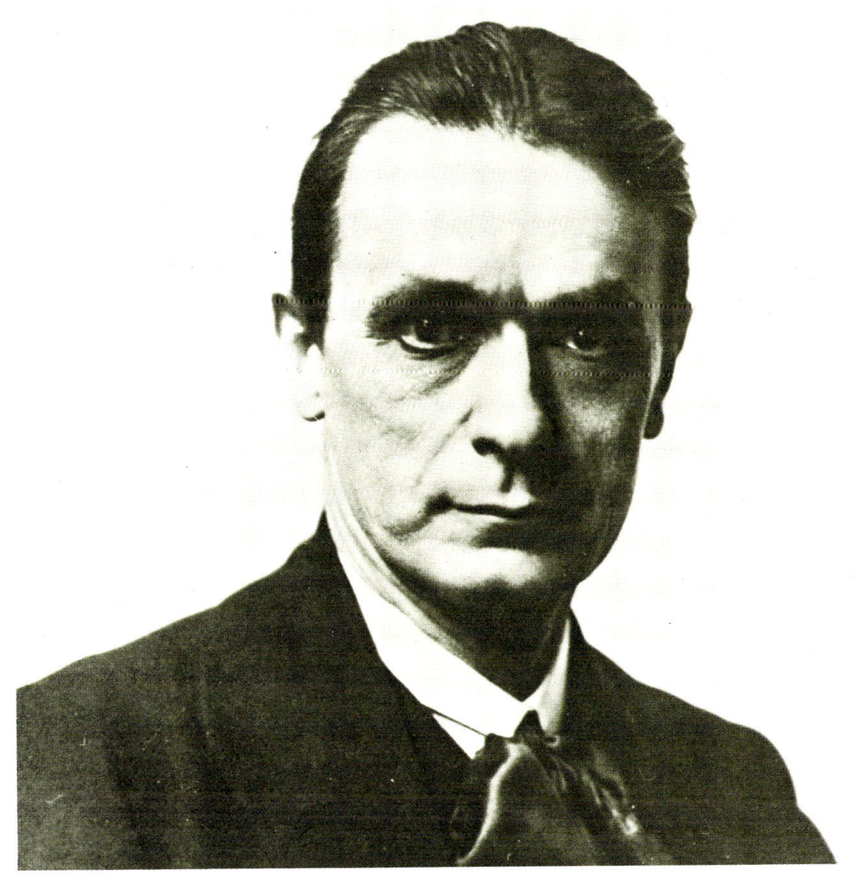

Rudolph Steiner: the mystic interpretation of colour

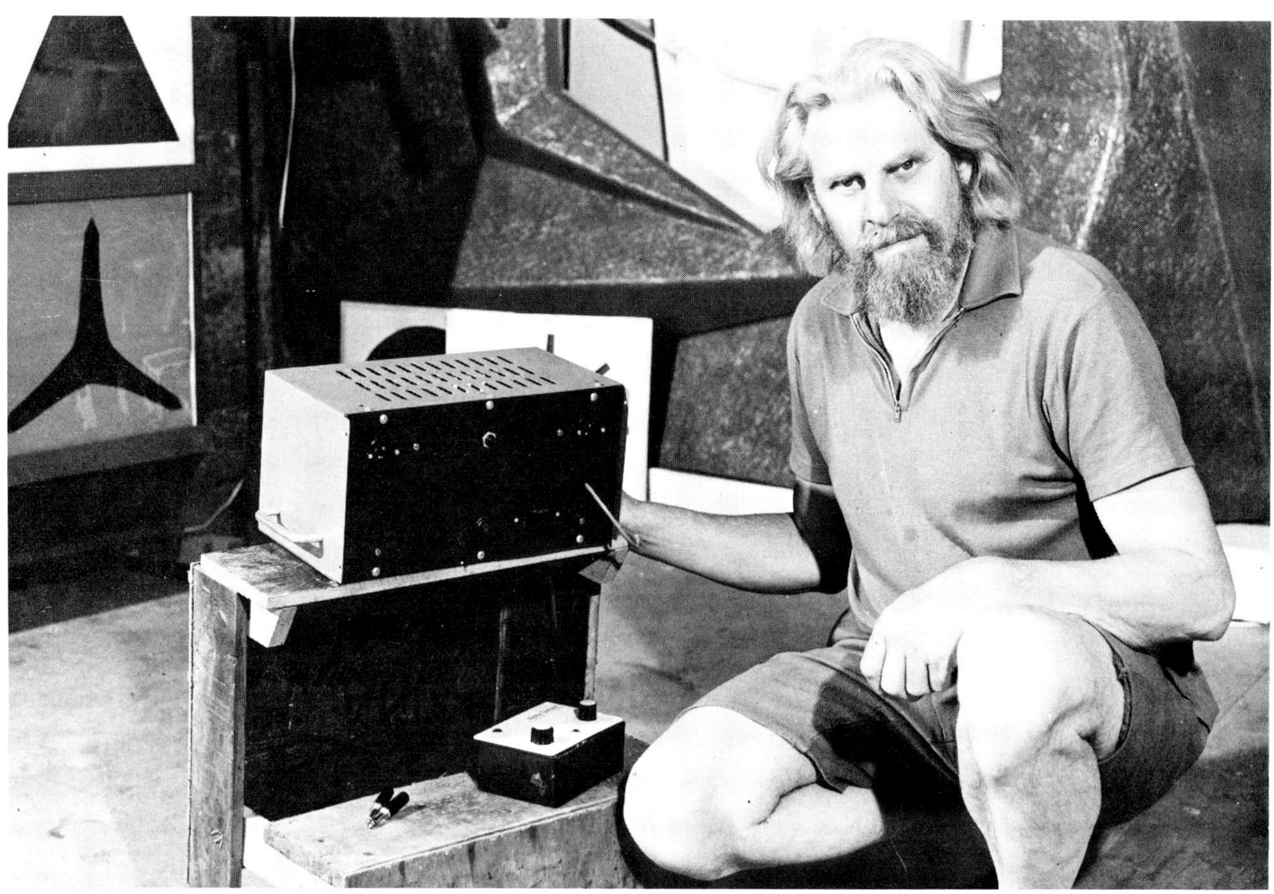

Theo Gimbel, a leading colour therapist

We know that colour influences us emotionally. Blue, for example, has a calming effect on most human beings and the English colour therapist Theo Gimbel, in a survey of 1100 people, discovered that it was by far the most popular colour. (It rated around 33% with red a poor second at 16%). Dr Andrew Stanway notes that in a study at the New England State Hospital in the United States, 25 members of staff with normal blood pressure were bathed in blue light for just under half an hour. A universal fall in blood pressure occurred. When red light was applied the blood pressures rose.

There are several techniques of colour therapy, some of them extremely simple, others more complex.

Dr Ghadiali used to treat his patients by shining light on them through coloured glass. The patients would also drink water irradiated by the same colours. Other therapists sometimes recommend the drinking of liquids from coloured containers or a diet which draws on food of specific pigments (e.g. red = beetroot, radishes).

In some colour therapy centres in Europe, patients are asked to wear white clothes and receive colour from a Colour-Form-Rhythm-Beamer, an instrument which radiates coloured light through apertures. Sessions last exactly 24 ¼ minutes and a patient may receive between one and four sessions a week. No more than three colours should be used during any given 24 hour period and one of these should be blue.

Australian colour therapist Fai Lloyd also recommends colour breathing exercises during which one visualises the colour with the opposite meaning from the colour of the thought form one wishes to destroy:

Holding the visualisation of the colour, see it as a radiant colour breath travelling rapidly upward beneath the outer skin, rising in a spiral about the body and ending above the head in a brilliant swirl of cleansing, transmuting colour. At the same time raise the arms above the head in a relaxing gesture. Then exhale gently feeling the colour breath pass out through the pores of the skin carrying all impurities with it.

Although colour analysis and applications vary from therapist to therapist some of the healing qualities and uses of different coloured light are summarised below:

Red Symbolic of heat, fire and anger and also the circulation of the blood. Used by some therapists to cure paralysis and any blood ailments.

Orange Symbolic of prosperity and sometimes pride. Used to increase the pulse rate, stimulate the milk-producing action of the breast after child-birth, dispel kidney and gall-stones and treat hernias and appendicitis.

Yellow Associated with joy and happiness, and also the intellect. This colour provides energy for the lymphatic system and is used to treat diabetes, indigestion, kidney and liver ailments, constipation and some eye and throat infections.

Green Usually applied in the emerald hue, this colour is used to treat nervous conditions, hay fever, ulcers, influenza, syphilis, malaria and colds. Therapists regard green as the colour of harmony.

Blue A cool colour, associated in some mystical systems with the throat chakra. Used to alleviate pain, reduce bleeding, heal burns and treat dysentery, colic, respiratory problems, skin aberrations and rheumatism.

Indigo A purifying colour associated with the pituitary gland and the energy centre in the forehead. Therapists use it to heal cataracts, migraines, deafness and skin disorders. It exerts a soothing effect on the eyes, ears and nervous system.

Violet Linked to the crown chakra and the pineal gland, which is often associated with psychic and spiritual power. It is applied in treating nervous and emotional disturbances, arthritis and in easing child-birth. With green and yellow it may be used to treat incipient skin cancer.

Note: the colour *magenta* is also used by some colour therapists, to treat heart conditions and mental problems.

THEO GIMBEL

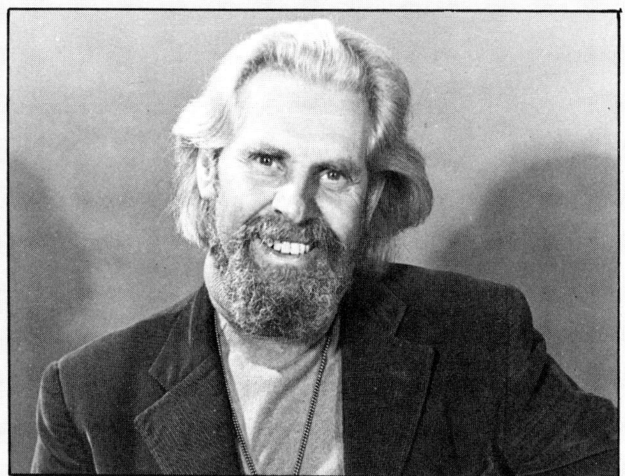

Few settings could be more suited to the practice of colour therapy than the beautiful Avon valley in Gloucester. Here among the soft green and brown shades of the Cotswold hills, Theo Gimbel devotes his life to healing with colour. From his home in Avening he treats and counsels patients, continues the research he has been conducting since 1956, and runs courses and conferences for teachers, nurses, doctors and all concerned with the effect our environment has on us. Colour, he teaches, is not simply an adornment to our lives but an environmental factor that can influence our physical and mental well-being.

Born in Bavaria in 1920, Theo Gimbel was brought up in Switzerland and educated at the Rudolph Steiner Schule in Basel. As a small boy he met Rudolph Steiner and the philosopher, who believed that colour could be used as a supplementary treatment for certain conditions, became a major influence in his life. He took a diploma in agriculture and worked as a farmer in France, Switzerland and Germany.

In 1949 he settled in England, became a British subject, and taught art and general subjects to mentally handicapped children at St. Christopher's School in Bristol. It was at this time that he became deeply interested in the way his pupils responded to colour. Although they were unable to read or write, he found that colour could be used to organise their daily routine.

Each child had its own colour which was used for the coat hanger, desk, bed and other items. In this way the children were always able to find their personal belongings. This helped their development and self-confidence.

By 1968 Theo Gimbel had become head of the art department and gained the Diploma of Curative Education. It was in that year that he decided to give all his time to the study of colour. He set up a centre at his home, naming it Hygeia Studios, after the Greek goddess of healing. In his work there he combines the therapeutic wisdom of the past with the findings of more recent research. He writes of the Greek and Egyptian temples and the colours they chose for their sanctuaries, which were believed to produce certain psychological responses, and of the Tibetan teachings that use colour in their meditations. The difference between the use of colour in the past and today, he explains, is that it is now possible to measure its effect on living substances. He refers to the Californian psychologists, Gerrard and Hessey, who found that while red light stimulates and raises blood pressure, blue light has a calming effect. This finding can be employed in the treatment of asthma. During an asthma attack the sufferer will experience relief if subjected to blue light. In his book *Healing with Colour* Theo Gimbel says that of all colours blue is the most healing, reducing blood pressure and relaxing the whole body. Orange, the colour of joy, acts as an anti-depressant, benefits the metabolic system and helps digestion. He uses turquoise to rest the nervous system and reduce inflammatory conditions.

In his counselling work Theo Gimbel asks patients to complete a questionnaire giving details of their favourite colour, music, food and hobbies and of past illnesses, together with a photograph and copy of their signature. Then follows a consultation, in which he uses a dowsing method to check any imbalance in the body. This is done with a chart of the human spine. With the chart in front of him, he slowly moves the middle finger about half an inch above it, from the base of the skull to the sacrum and coccyx, at the same time holding in his mind the name of the person, their age and sex. He says that there will be at least two, usually three, vertebrae out of true and this is perceived by a kind of tickling feeling as if an electric current were sparking from vertebrae to finger. When the diagnosis is completed he makes a colour report for the patient, advising which colours would be most helpful for them to wear. He also suggests appropriate music for them to either listen to, or play, advises on diet and, if they require it, provides an astrological report to indicate possibilities open to them in the future. He sees his work as a colour therapist as being supplementary to any other treatment they may be receiving.

Often in his counselling, he feels that the hobby of an individual should be their true vocation, but they lack the courage to make the change, and as a result become ill. He tells of a case of absent healing which concerned a young woman named Heidi who was seriously ill with meningitis. Hospital reports indicated that she would not recover. Through a meditation group the colour turquoise was 'sent' to her at nine-o-clock one evening. As he had known her, he also visualised her face and where she was. A week later a letter arrived from her asking if he had sent a colour just after nine the previous week, as she had experienced the feeling of being bathed in a bluish light. At that moment her high temperature dropped and she recovered. Theo Gimbel sees his work in all its many facets as being that of a guide who helps others find the road to self-healing.

COPPER EFFECTS

When Dutch settlers began to explore the Rhodesian hinterland they discovered that among the tribal people who lived there that rheumatic ailments were unknown. They explained to the Europeans that their copper ornaments had a beneficial healing effect. These days many Westerners – Alistair Cooke estimates up to 5 million Americans, for example – wear copper bangles and ornaments to alleviate bodily aches and pains. Is there any scientific reason why copper would have this effect?

The Australian researcher Professor W.R. Walker of the University of Newcastle discovered that the weight of copper bracelets worn to counter rheumatism decreased by around 40 mg a month. This did not appear to result from abrasion and Professor Walker felt that perhaps the copper dissolved in human perspiration. It is possible that the copper merges with a natural amino acid, enters the veins and thereby reaches the source of inflammation.

Lt Col. A. Forbes of Cheltenham in England has produced copper bracelets for many years to aid sufferers from rheumatism, and he has also developed copper-bearing straps to be worn by race horses and pet animals. Forbes notes that the pacer Black Prince became lame for no apparent medical reason but after copper inserts were fitted to his straps he went on to come second in the 1965 Epsom Derby.

Many people who work and live in humid or damp conditions have found the copper bands have kept discomfort away and have healed any existing condition. It seems that although the use of copper to aid rheumatism has come down to us as a tale from folklore, it does have some basis in scientific fact.

CUPPING

Cupping is a time-tested technique dating back to the times of the ancient Egyptians. It was later used by Alexander Tralianus who lived during the time of Emperor Justinian. Especially useful in treating some types of arthritis, rheumatism, boils, bronchitis and asthma, cupping is a means of getting the blood to rush up to the surface of the body through suction.

There are two types of cupping, wet and dry, and the latter is by far the most common. Thick glass or metal cups are taken and herbs or cotton wool are burnt inside them. After the burning is complete the warm cup is placed on the area of the skin where the problem has arisen, creating a partial vacuum as the cup cools. The skin is drawn up into the cup and blood courses through the small blood vessels. Cups are left in position for 5–10 minutes and the process may be repeated half a dozen times on different parts of the body.

In the 'wet' cup technique the same procedure is followed but shallow cuts are made in the raised skin. The cup is applied again, drawing blood into it.

Cupping may be applied over the spine, on the chest, above the solar plexus and along muscles. It is sometimes combined with modern acupuncture but is also known to be used on its own in Finland and some of the Greek islands.

DIET AND HEALTH

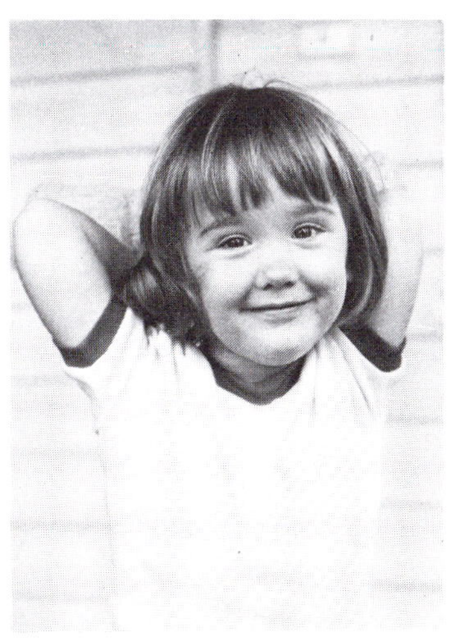

Hippocrates wrote: 'Let your medicines be your food and your food your medicines'. Naturopaths have long recognised the vital role of food constituents for health. Although dietary requirements vary according to sex, age, lifestyle and body type, everyone needs to be aware of the healthy balance of dietary constituents including intake of proteins, carbohydrates, fats, vitamins and minerals.

Protein

Proteins are extremely important nutrients and constitute around 20% of our body weight. Proteins build the body, help ward off infections and constitute the major component in muscles, organs and bones. All foods of both plant and animal origin contain some protein and the typical Western diet has included a blend of both. Animal protein in our diet comes from meat, eggs, fish, milk and cheese while plant protein can be found in grains, nuts, raw seeds, peas, beans and lentils. Plant foods are more easily digested than animal

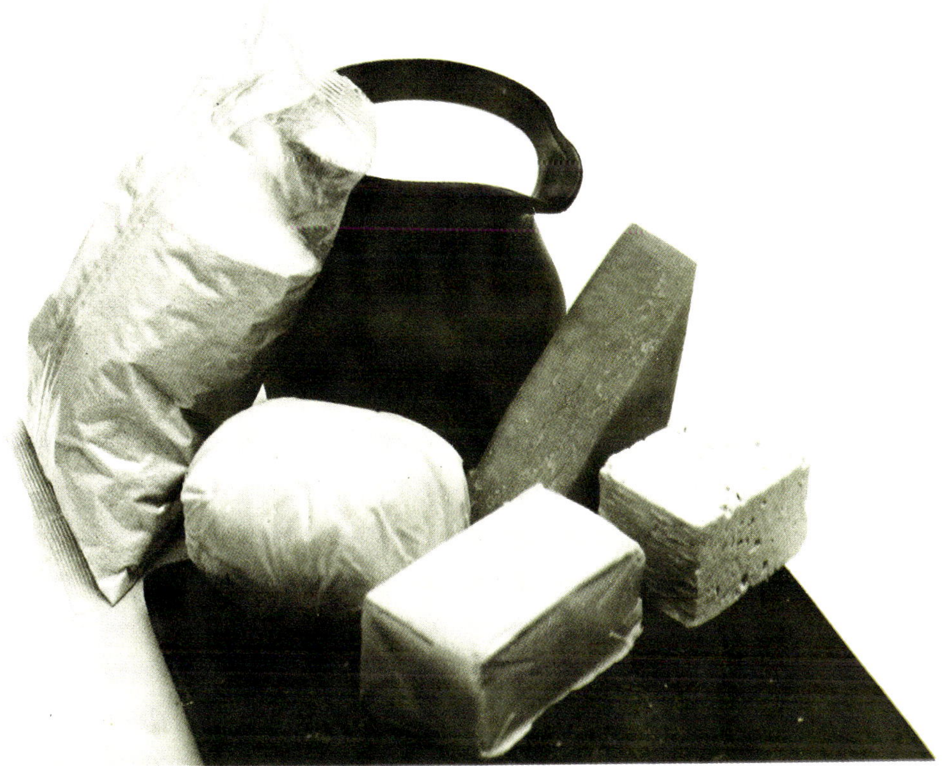

products which contain animal cholesterol and saturated fatty acids. Meat is a complete protein containing all of the essential amino acids necessary for the assimilation of proteins into the body but it also includes toxins and bacteria. Accordingly, vegetarians seek alternative sources of complementary proteins. There are several non-meat foods that include high concentrations of protein: gluten flour, nuts, soybeans and soybean milk, wheat germ, dried peas, sesame seeds, brewer's yeast, peanuts and cereals.

As nutrition author Nathaniel Altman points out in *Eating For Life*, a sense of balance is essential:

'*A deficiency of protein can cause anaemia, the inability to resist disease, loss of stamina, muscle deterioration, fatigue and difficulty in healing bruises and wounds. An excessive protein intake over a long period . . . can aggravate or potentiate certain chronic disease states*'.

Vegans – those who eat no animal, fish or dairy products at all – argue that animal foods contain vaccine and hormone additives which are harmful to the body and seek complementary proteins in other food supplements.

Carbohydrates

Found mainly in fresh fruit and vegetables, carbohydrates are transmitted to the bloodstream and become a vital source of energy. In the form of starches and sugars they are easily metabolised in the body and also assist in the breakdown and assimilation of proteins and fats. Refined sugar-cane crystals contain the highest percentage of carbohydrate (99%) but lack other nutritional qualities necessary for sustaining life. Accordingly, sugar is not usually regarded as a food per se, despite the fact that it is present in a wide variety of common food products. Significant quantities of natural carbohydrate can be found in such substances as barley, chestnuts, rice, sultanas, wheat, apples, pears, peaches, apricots, raisins, dates and whole rye grain.

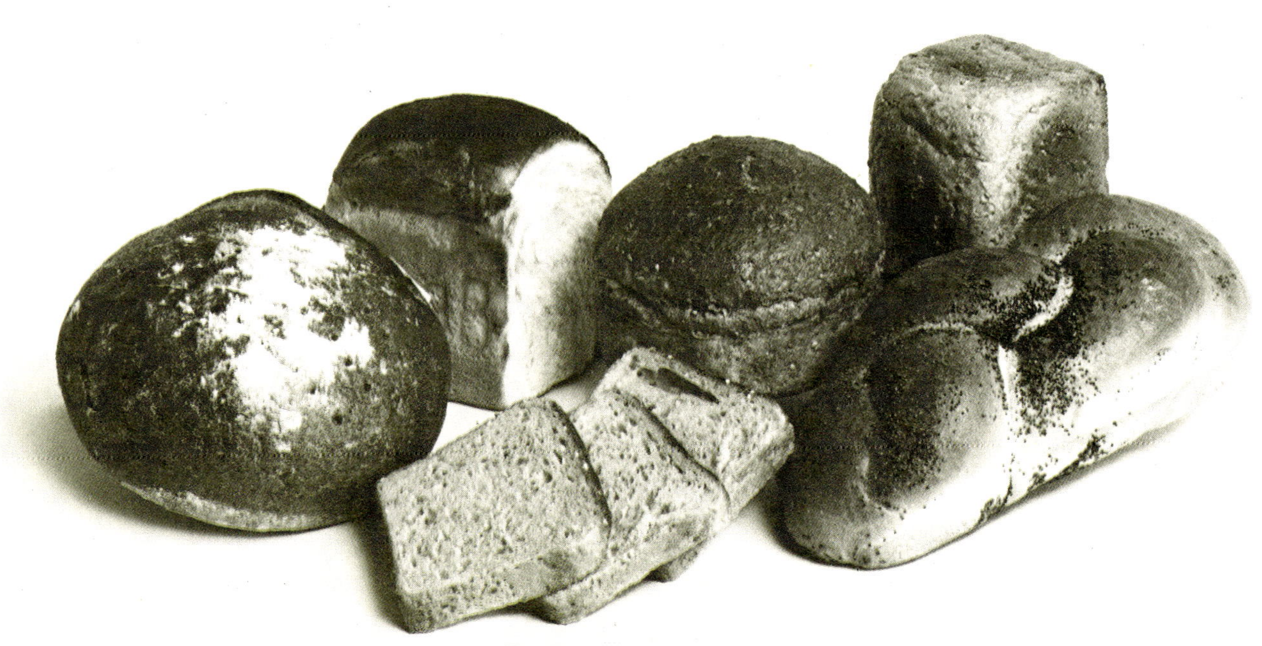

Foods which contain large quantities of processed carbohydrates have poor nutritional qualities and do not assist the body in fighting infection. Wholegrain breads are preferred, and it is unwise to combine excessive amounts of carbohydrate – rice, potatoes and bread – in the same meal, for digestive reasons. If an excess of carbohydrate is taken in, an increase in body-weight occurs. Animal products such as beef, fish, cheese, poultry and eggs are foods that head the low-carbohydrate category and for the vegetarian diet marrows, zucchinis, cabbage, lettuce, celery and spinach have negligible quantities of carbohydrate.

Fats

Fats and oils are harder to digest than other types of food but digestible fats are nevertheless essential nutrients in the diet. They represent an important form of food energy and are vital to the construction of soft fatty tissue which protects the bones, organs and muscles of the body. Fats provide considerably more calories (food energy) than proteins and carbohydrates, and also regulate the digestive function by slowing it down – easing the pangs of hunger!

The three essential unsaturated fatty acids sometimes known collectively as Vitamin F are necessary to keep the skin and tissues healthy and also have important functions associated with the blood, arteries, nerves and sex glands.

Polyunsaturated fatty acids are regarded as the most suitable for the body and derive from plant foods. They are the easiest to digest and generally produce a smaller accumulation of fat in the body than mono-unsaturated and saturated fatty acids.

An example of a high-density (saturated) animal fat is lard, while vegetable oils consist of a majority of unsaturated fatty acids. It is preferable to use vegetable oils that are extracted free from the influence of chemical solvents since this enables vitamins and minerals to be retained. Refined vegetable oils have few nutrients.

Fats are an essential part of the diet and except for blood-sugar are the most common source of stored energy in the body. There has been a tendency to downplay the role of fats in healthy diet but they have important roles to play – such as aiding the absorption of Vitamin D and assisting the entry of calcium to the bones and teeth. Nutritionalists recommend that refined or saturated fat intake should be minimalised and that, in general fats should represent not more than a third of the daily calorie count.

Vitamins

Proteins, carbohydrates and fats are not the only constituents necessary to maintain life. A series of experiments conducted in the 19th century involved feeding purified diets of these three constituents to a number of animals. They did not prosper, and developed opacity of the cornea, which is now known to derive from Vitamin A deficiency.

In 1911 the Polish scientist Casimir Funk suggested that there were various nitrogen compounds that were essential to life. He called them 'vitamines' (*vita* meaning 'life', couples with 'amine') but the name was later changed to 'vitamin' when it was discovered that not all essential food constituents contain nitrogen. Albert Szent-Gyorgyi and W.N. Haworth discovered and synthesised ascorbic acid, Vitamin C, in 1937 and subsequently considerable

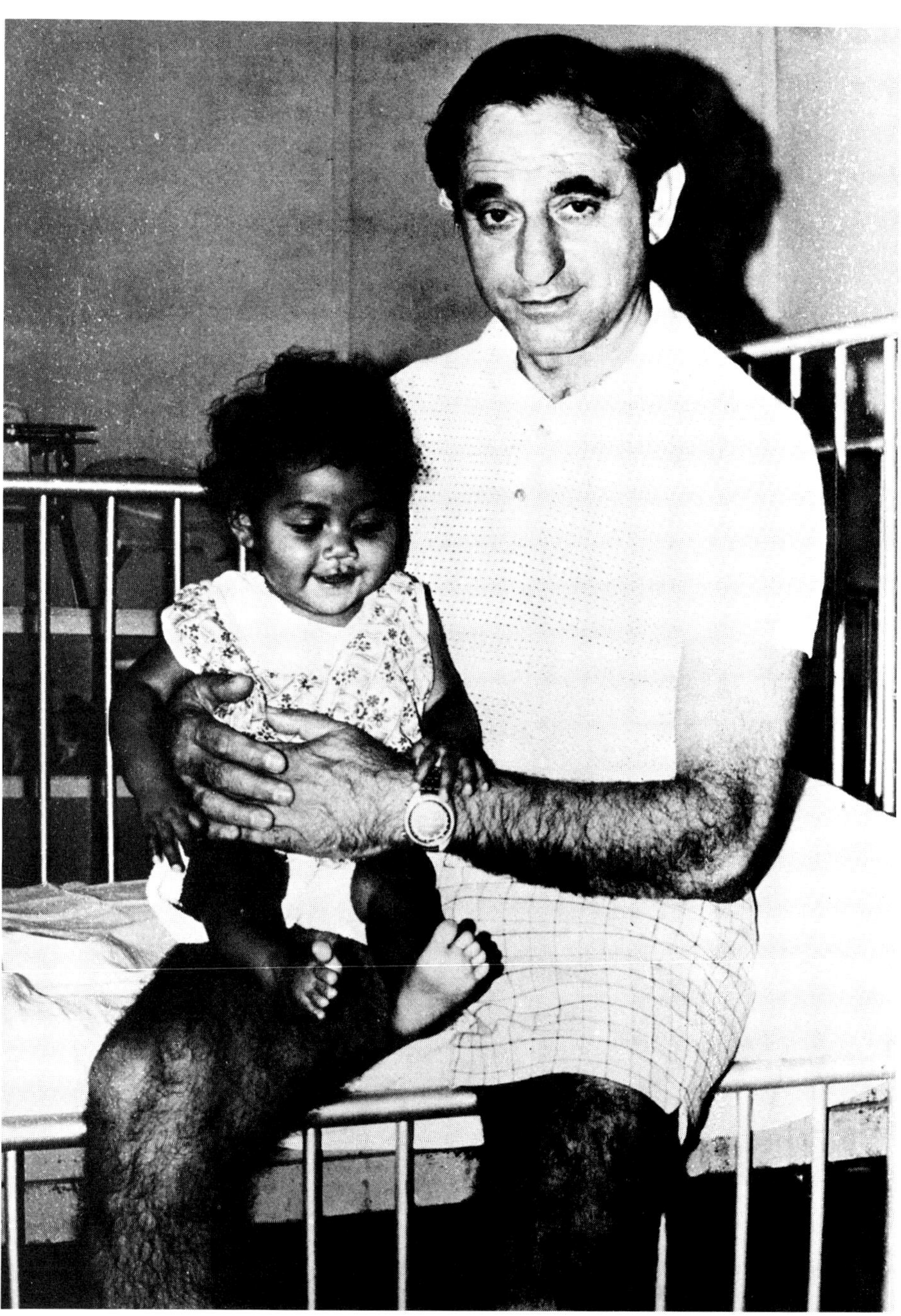

Dr Archie Kalokerinos: Vitamin C for health

research involving vitamin and mineral nutrients has been carried out. Dr William Kaufman discovered that high doses of nicotinamide, a B vitamin, were effective against arthritis, while Drs Abram Hoffer and Humphrey Osmond announced in Canada in 1952 that mega-doses of vitamin C and nicotinamide in combination with high protein diet, could aid schizophrenia. Meanwhile in Australia Dr Archie Kalokerinos has done extensive research to prove that the 'sudden infant-death syndrome' (or 'cot-death') could be eliminated by giving all sick infants large intravenous doses of Vitamin C.

In 1968 the double Nobel Prize winner Dr Linus Pauling used the term 'orthomolecular psychiatry' to describe the maintenance of mental health by varying the concentrations of vital body constituents like vitamins, thereby laying the groundwork for much contemporary nutritional therapy. Dr Pauling is also a strong supporter of Vitamin C against disease and has endorsed the work of biochemist Irwin Stone in highlighting the role of Vitamin C in combatting cancer, heart disease, mental illness, diabetes and arthritis.

In terms of normal dietary supplements, megavitamin therapy has developed as a means of adding high dosage of vitamins, either singly or in a combination, to the normal food intake. Examples of high-potency, megavitamins* include:

Vitamin B1 (Thiamine) in 100 mg tablets. Vitamin B1 plays an essential role in the utilisation of carbohydrate type foods. Severe deficiencies cause beri-beri which can prove fatal. When using high dosages of Vitamin B1 it is essential to ensure adequate amounts of other B group vitamins and Vitamin C.

Vitamin B2 (Riboflavin) in 25 mg tablets. Vitamin B2 is essential for the utilisation of carbohydrate type foods along with other B group vitamins. It also assists in the absorption of iron from the digestive tract. It is usually used in conjunction with other B group vitamins.

Vitamin B3 (Niacinamide) in 250 mg tablets. Vitamin B3 is essential for the utilisation of carbohydrate type foods. Chronic alcoholism and liver disorders can reduce the ability of the body to store Vitamin B3. Severe deficiencies can cause Pellagra and may prove fatal if not treated. Niacinamide is exactly the same as Nicotinamide and is the naturally occurring form of Vitamin B3. It is better tolerated by the body than niacin or nicotinic acid which can cause unpleasant hot flushes in large doses. To be most effective it should be used together with other B group vitamins and Vitamin C.

Vitamin B5 (Pantothenic Acid) in 200 mg tablets. Pantothenic acid is associated with the utilisation of carbohydrate, fat and protein foods. It is involved in the production of fatty acids, the usage of choline and the formation of blood. It is a very important vitamin. In stress conditions it is often used in conjunction with Vitamin C.

Vitamin B6 (Pyridoxine) in 75 mg tablets. Vitamin B6 plays an essential role in the use of proteins and in the synthesis of non-essential amino acids. It is also involved in fat metabolism and blood formation as well as in the production of amino acids needed for the transmission of nerve impulses. In experimental rats a deficiency of Vitamin B6 has produced increased loss of Vitamin C. Vitamin B6 is often used in conjunction with magnesium.

Vitamin B12 (Cyanocobalamin) in 100 mcg tablets. Vitamin B12 is involved in the metabolism of proteins, particularly the amino acids Methionine and Tyrosine. Vitamin B12 is found almost exclusively in animal foods and vegetarians who do not eat milk, cheese, and eggs may develop Vitamin B12 deficiency. Certain drugs such as Phenytoin can also bring about a B12 deficiency.

Para Amino Benzoic Acid in 300 mg tablets. This is a B group vitamin which has a favourable influence on the synthesis of folic acid in the intestines. It is used in the treatment of white patches on the skin (Vitiligo) and as a sunscreen agent in some suntan creams.

*Information supplied by Vitamin Supplies Pty. Ltd., Chatswood, Sydney.

Vitamin P (Rutin) in 300 mg tablets. Rutin is a member of several substances collectively referred to as bioflavonoids. It assists in maintaining normal permeability of the capillaries. Rutin has complementary action to Vitamin C and is frequently found in foods with a high Vitamin C content. It is also found in herbs such as buckwheat.

Vitamin C in 1000 mg tablets. Vitamin C in large doses helps the body to produce anti-bodies and resist infection. It is essential for the assimilation of iron. Vitamin C is not stored in the body for any length of time. Where zinc deficiencies exist Vitamin C is lost more rapidly than normal.

Minerals

Increasing levels of pollution, the depletion of minerals in the soil and new techniques of agriculture are certainly affecting the quality of the food we eat. Research on the mineral constituent of food has been carried out by Professor H.A. Schroeder who came to the conclusion that mineral trace elements are even more important to health than vitamins. He discovered, for example, that modern nutrition includes excessive intake of cadmium leading to high blood pressure and that chromium deficiency can promote diabetes. Research carried out by the Australian health pioneer Maurice Blackmore led to the formulation of 'celloid minerals' which closely resemble the compounds present in living cells, related to the cure of symptoms. Since a deficiency of essential organic minerals in the body can lead to a breakdown in health, the celloid minerals were developed so that in precise and controlled dosages they could help restore health. They include Sodium Phosphate, Sodium Sulphate, Potassium Chloride, Potassium Sulphate, Calcium Sulphate, Calcium Phosphate, Calcium Fluoride, Magnesium Phosphate, Iron Phosphate and Silica. The physiological role of each mineral is described below*:

Calcium

Calcium is usually linked with bone but actually enters into the construction of every tissue. The colloidals, calcium phosphate and calcium fluoride, provide firmness and elasticity to most cells and tissues. The five best food sources of calcium are *figs, dates, almonds, fish and milk.*

Sodium

This has been called the 'youth' mineral, as it is the key element in the body and is important in the digestion of foods and the viscosity of the blood. It also aids in keeping calcium in solution so that it can reach all the tissues. As a phosphate, it is used for digestion and normal blood viscosity and, as a sulphate, to control the distribution of water in the system and to stimulate the liver and pancreas. The five richest food sources are *dried figs, spinach, dates, lentils and beans.*

Potassium

Potassium is a main healing element in the body and occurs as the colloidal compounds with phosphorus, sulphur and chlorine. With phosphorus, it is the main constituent of the grey nerve fibres and, combined with chlorine, it is the glandular element. Combined with sulphur, it is the oxygen transfer element in cells which suspends their decomposition. The richest sources of potassium in foods are *olives, beans, peas, lentils and raisins.*

Magnesium

Magnesium is available as magnesium phosphate and, as such, is the main constituent of white nerve fibres. This makes the combination most important for nerve problems and magnesium is Nature's own anti-spasmodic. The five richest sources of magnesium are *almonds, barley, figs, dates and walnuts.*

Iron

Iron is essential for the formation of haemoglobin in the blood. Thus it is important in the healing of injuries to the soft tissues and where inflammation and fevers are present. The Celloid* formula is in the form of iron phosphate. The five richest sources of iron are *spinach, lentils, strawberries, lettuce and figs.*

Silicon

This is a constituent of bone, tissue, organ and nerve sheath, hair, nails and skin. Sometimes called 'Nature's scalpel', it is used for the removal of accumulated morbid waste matter and for arthritic nodules and spurs. The five richest sources are *oats, barley, dates, dried figs and strawberries.*

Phosphorus

Phosphorus is a constituent of bones, teeth, blood, brain, hair and nervous tissue. It is a great general tonic for the nervous system and the Celloid formulas included as the phosphates of iron, potassium, sodium, magnesium and calcium. The five foods highest in phosphorus are *almonds, beans, lentils, whole wheat and peas.*

Chlorine

Celloids supply chlorine in the form of potassium chloride, which is very important to efficient glandular function, particularly the liver. The best sources of chlorine in foods are *fish, lentils, cabbage, coconut and spinach.*

Sulphur

The sulphates are great blood cleansers and are important to the processes of digestion and assimilation because of their effect upon the bile and pancreatic fluids. The best dietary sources of sulphur are *carrots, dried figs and dates, spinach and cabbage.* The Celloids* provide sulphur as calcium sulphate, sodium sulphate and potassium sulphate.

Another type of mineral therapy involves the so-called 'orotates' or mineral carriers. The vitamin B13, orotic acid, is present in our bodies and forms a bond with certain minerals carrying them through the digestive system to the blood vessels, heart and nervous system. Dr Hans Nieper of the Silbersee Clinic in West Germany has done extensive research on the orotates and several are now available commercially through health food stores. Magnesium orotate has been found to assist people suffering from high cholesterol levels and hardened arteries, calcium orotate provides relief to those suffering from lower back pain and 'slipped discs', while potassium orotate is prescribed for patients suffering from such heart conditions as inflammation of the heart and myocardial necroses. Zinc orotate is also available, and may be used effectively by those who suffer from skin disorders, prostate problems and loss of appetite.

Overall, minerals are playing an increasing role in nutritional therapy and alongside vitamins and megavitamins provide valuable supplements for the modern, often depleted, diet.

*'Celloid' is a registered name of Blackmore's Naturopathic Organisation to describe colloidal mineral formulations. Information supplied by *Nature and Health Journal.*

XANDRIA WILLIAMS

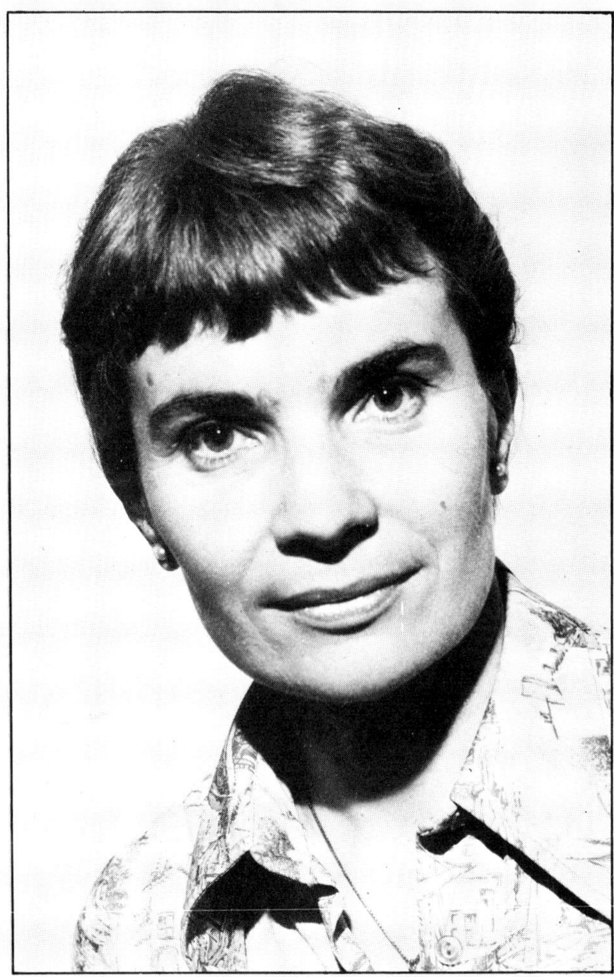

Originally Xandria Williams trained professionally in chemistry and geology and only later switched her emphasis to diet and nutrition. Her life has involved several major transitions and her story is a fascinating one.

Born in Dublin on the Leo/Virgo cusp, Xandria grew up in a High Church Anglican family. However her developing interest in science soon began to compete with her personal beliefs and by the time she had reached her early twenties she had reverted to atheism. After studies at Imperial College, London – always a highly competitive college, especially for female students – she had become convinced that man was essentially a molecular rather than a spiritual being. For four years after her graduation she embarked on overseas travel working and continuing her studies – this time for a Masters degree in Chemistry at Otago University in Dunedin. Returning to London she completed a D.I.C. and while living the life of an impoverished student discovered that she could stay alive very well by eating soya beans instead of steak . . . and it was a lot cheaper! Meanwhile she became interested in protein biochemistry and protein foods for the Third World and was horrified by her research into food additives – clearly these were areas for future investigation. However at this stage Xandria was still primarily a geochemist involved in geological surveys for mining organisations. Her work took her to Western Australia in 1968 and she conducted field research in many areas including Kalgoorlie and the Pilbara. Based just outside Perth at MonaVale, she grew her own food and continued her personal interest in healthy dietary practice.

Around this time she came into contact with Anthroposophy. An elderly couple who followed Rudolph Steiner's teachings and were also involved in organic gardening took an interest in her one acre plot and taught her how to cope with the unfamiliar conditions. Xandria was given anthroposophical literature to read and recalls that its 'scientific' components simply had to be shelved. However in Steiner she found evidence of a logical and profoundly esoteric mind which would continue to influence her in the years to come.

Moving to Sydney, she continued to consult in mineral exploration but began to feel she would like to run her own enterprise. The exploitative nature of mineral development was beginning to get to her and she felt she would somehow like to combine a scientific background with an activity involving health care. The idea of opening a health-food shop was suddenly born. After investigations reasonably close to home she found a suitable shop site in Cremorne and stocked it with health food products. Xandria then employed a woman to run it and continued with her own geochemical consulting. Gradually however she began to phase out of this and to spend more time at the shop. The upper level became a venue for nutritional counselling and she seemed to have found an activity that blended personal interest and financial survival.

Then just as things seemed settled, a new development occurred! Xandria met an anthroposophist from South Africa who was distributing the special homeopathic medicines *Wala* and *Weleda*. He needed someone in his factory to advise and write on nutrition and keep a 'moral' overview on his health-food distribution network. Although initially unwilling to go to South Africa, Xandria went over to help him and agreed to stay for a year. The politics of the country, and its racial tensions in particular, soon disturbed her and she began to think in terms of restarting in Sydney.

Finally she did return, having in the meantime begun studies in homeopathy and anthroposophical medicine. Back in Sydney she started the Demeter Bakery, producing bread from biodynamically grown grains, plus cookies and other related products. Eventually she found it wasn't sufficiently stimulating on its own, so, as a parallel activity she began to lecture in biochemistry and nutrition at the Sydney Chiropractic College at Ashfield . . . She also extended her own studies into the medical sciences, then bought back the health food store she had started, and reopened her naturopathic and nutritional clinic in the premises above.

Later she started lecturing in the same subjects at the NSW College of Natural Therapies (located at St Leonards) where she also studied and graduated in naturopathy. She is now Head of the Nutrition Faculty. She also lectures at the NSW College of Applied (Orthomolecular) Nutrition.

Communicating knowledge both to students and patients remains important to her, and she has been engaged in many free, open discussion groups on naturopathic and nutritional topics. Xandria feels that there is still much unwarranted bias against holistic medicine, especially from scientists and doctors who refuse to heed the evidence of nutritional and vitamin research. She feels similarly that orthomolecular methods have sound scientific data to support them, but that most (though fortunately not all) doctors and psychiatrists are continuing to resist the new lines of thought.

Xandria continues to exercise a strong influence on the local holistic health movement. She is a regular contributor to *Nature and Health Journal* and other magazines, and participates in professional and public meetings involving new issues in health care and nutrition. She is currently NSW President of the Australian Natural Therapies Association, a professional organisation which aims to raise the standards of natural therapists, provide postgraduate training, and provide the public with a list of registered member practitioners.

Meanwhile, in her premises at Cremorne she has endeavoured to create a true 'health centre'. The shop stocks the normal things you would expect in a health food store but there is also the dispensary where a wide range of remedies are available: homeopathic medicines, dried herbs, herbal tinctures and a large number of therapeutic products. And if all this isn't enough, she also runs lecture courses in the evenings to pass information on to her patients and customers.

LEN MASON

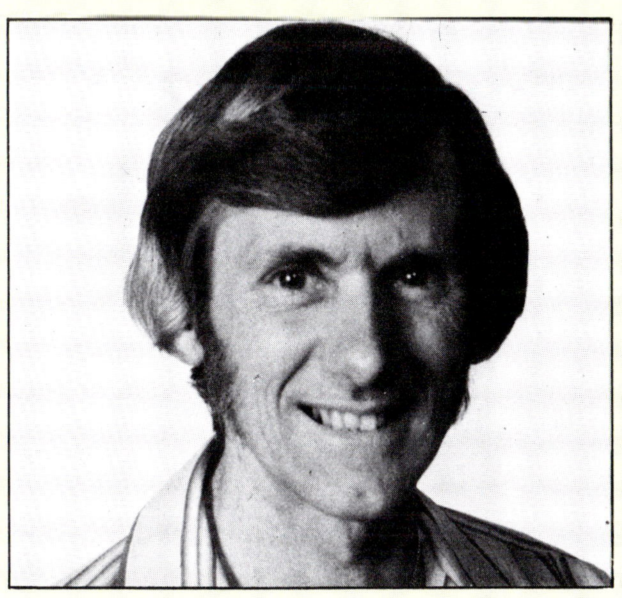

Len Mason is a gentle, quiet-voiced man in his forties. He looks you straight in the eye, and you get the feeling of undivided attention – that he concentrates solely on the matter in hand.

He has been a practising naturopath for about twelve years, after spending much of his early life searching.

He studied under Ray Powell and Sam Ashe, working day and night to memorise and learn all he could about natural healing. Len Mason believes that in those two years they covered more ground than the average modern student would in twice that time. Nevertheless, he is a little diffident about the shortness of his training.

Eventually, he set out on his own to help people. 'At first I thought I knew it all', he smiles quietly. 'I soon found it took more than a little knowledge, a lot of enthusiasm, and a wish to help.' He found that, for him, the necessary ingredient was love. Len believes that all people are linked by their humanity and their godlike qualities. So he, too, is linked to every person who comes to him for help. This means that healing is an extension of himself, and also of those whom he heals. He feels he is part of the whole, and therefore cannot be either greater or smaller than any other person.

As a naturopath, his approach encompasses the whole person and a wide range of therapies, including nutrition, osteopathy, herbalism, and massage for the treatment of a wide range of health problems. He also uses homeopathy when necessary.

Back problems are very common, and some people are referred to him by medical doctors. Other common complaints include digestive, bowel, and respiratory disorders.

Len Mason is oriented strongly toward nutrition. He says he sees a lot of deficiencies of calcium and vitamins C and E, caused through inadequate diet or by high requirements for individual nutrients in some people. He recommends that people cut down or eliminate meat from their diets, and include large amounts of fresh fruits and vegetables. Exercise is also important.

In New Zealand, therapists who are not medical practitioners cannot claim to cure people, but Len does say that most people can be helped .

Usually, only three or four visits are required. After that, the person will have improved or it will be clear that other kinds of treatment are required. Len does not believe in having people return again and again to achieve little or no improvement. 'If it doesn't help quite quickly, there is no reason to believe that more of the same will work.'

With his multi-therapy approach, it is often hard to tell just what element has brought about an improvement in a particular person. But, as he says, it does not really matter. The important thing is that people get well, or at least feel better.

Len's wife helps with massage in their treatment rooms under their home in Mount Albert, Auckland. With the help of a woman assistant, they work as a team, trying to bring relief to the sick and hope to the hopeless.

ENCOUNTER THERAPY

Historically encounter therapy grew out of humanistic psychology in the 1960s and embraces the work of such figures as Wilhelm Reich, Fritz Perls, Abraham Maslow and Carl Rogers.

Following Maslow's emphasis on the healthy 'self-actualised' person, encounter therapy seeks to uncover processes whereby a person can rediscover what pleasure, joy and self-fulfilment are all about.

In an encounter group there are usually between ten and fifteen people who sit in a circle on the floor. Often there is no specified leader. An encounter session may last for a few hours or extend into days and even weeks on end.

People taking part in an encounter group try to 'reach' and perceive each other in real ways and experience genuine inner feelings. Such therapy depends on developing honest relationships with the others involved and expressing such feelings verbally or physically.

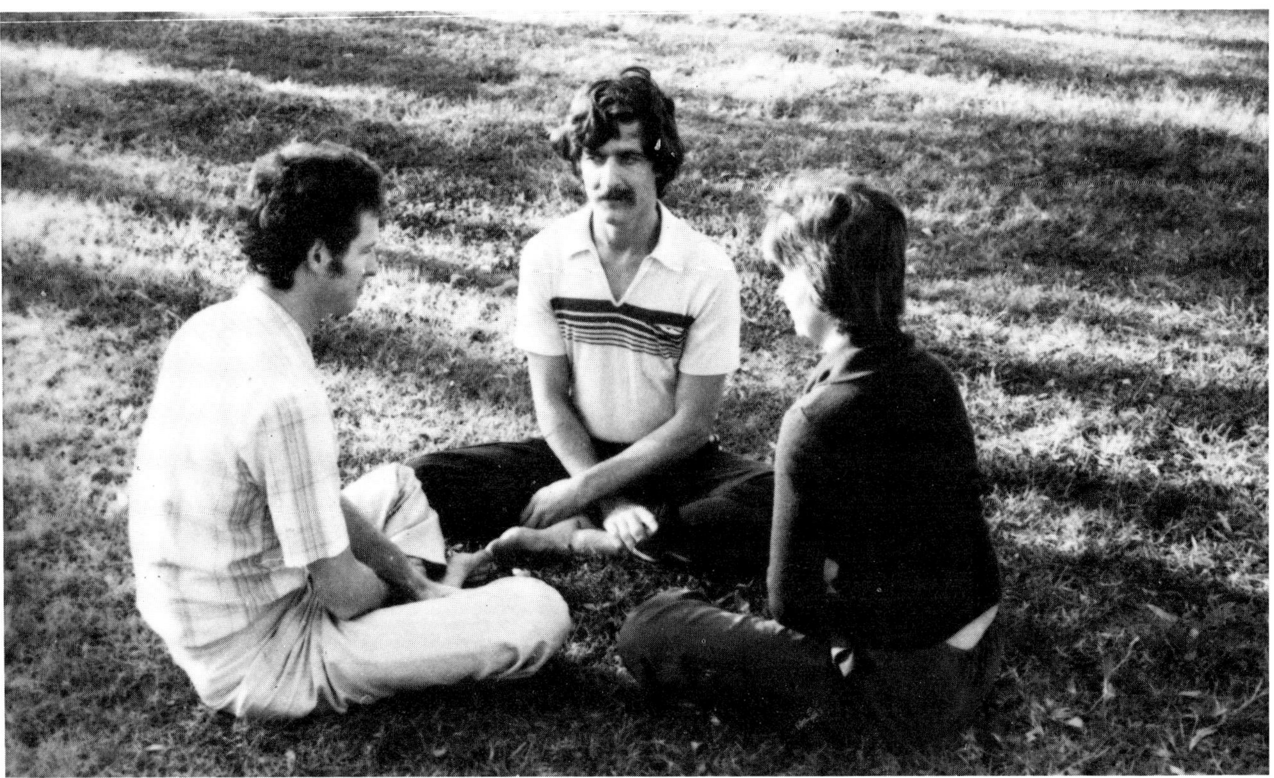

Encounter – reaching other people

In the approach adopted by Carl Rogers, members of the encounter group initially interact loosely waiting for information on what to expect and how to act. A sense of frustration often develops as the group comes to realise that it has to determine its *own* direction. Often members resist expressing themselves personally but then ease out of this by beginning to discuss events and situations that occurred in the past: ('When I was attending another group like this last year we found . . . ')

Rogers discovered that it is common for the first encounter exchanges to be negative ('I don't find you appeal to me'; 'Your manner of talking irritates me'; 'You are very superficial . . . ') but this is because deep positive feelings are harder to express than negative sentiments. Usually, however, providing the group passes through this phase without fragmenting, personally meaningful material begins to come through. A sense of trust emerges. In his book *Carl Rogers on Encounter Groups* (1970) the author recalls an exchange from an encounter group which shows immediate responses to highly personal admissions:

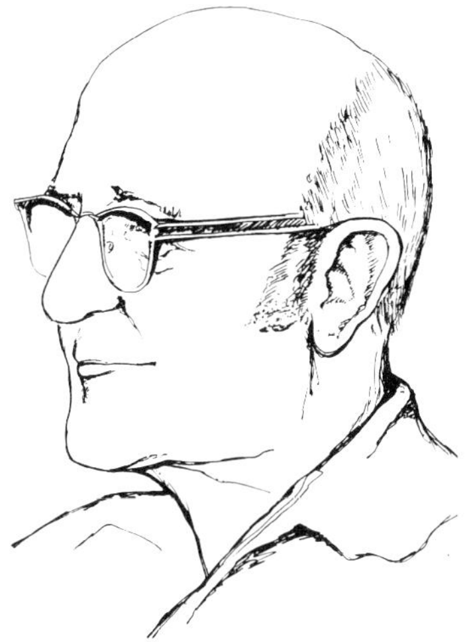

Carl Rogers

George: 'I think some of you know why I'm here, what I was charged with . . . Well, I raped my sister. That's the only problem I have at home and I've overcome that, I think'. (Rather long pause)
Freda: 'Oooh, that's weird!'
Mary: 'People have problems, Freda. I mean ya know . . .'
Freda: 'Yeah, I know but *yeOUW*!!!'
Facilitator: (to Freda) 'You know about these problems but they still are weird to you?'
George: 'You see what I mean, it's embarrassing to talk about it'.

As sensitive and important recall rises to the surface the members of the group begin to respond by seeking to help the people who have deep inner problems. In this way encounter group activity has a notable therapeutic quality. People come to accept themselves and learn new ways of being in order to heal imbalances. Defences are increasingly denied as the group continues, and often members quite ruthlessly insist that a person should open up completely to inner feelings. Any negative impulses tend to be followed by expressions 'of support, of positive feelings and closeness' and many participants later talk of encounter therapy as the most honest and moving experience of their lives.

However encounter is not without its dangers. Some people have not been able to cope with the probing effects of encounter and have lapsed into psychosis or depression. On the whole, though, encounter does help people to help each other. Those skilled in working with small groups can often guide the integrative, self-healing directions which encounter produces and use the context to bring about deeply felt personal experiences in those who are participating.

FASTING

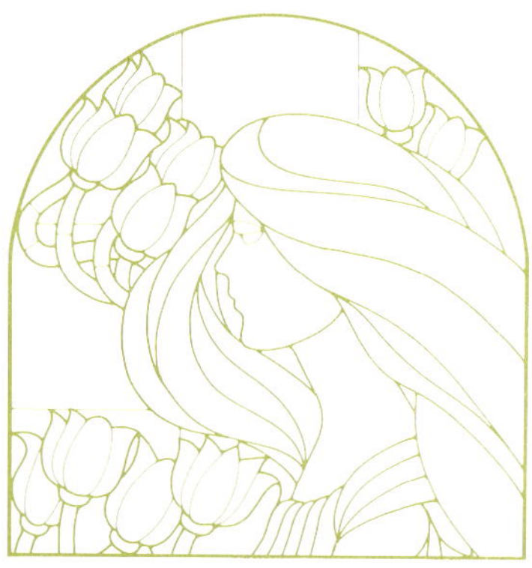

Fasting is not the same as starvation and the difference needs to be borne in mind. During a fast (Old English: *faestan*, 'to abstain') food intake is eliminated but water may be taken. The body draws on its reserves, which are contained in food stocks in the body cells and also glycogen in the liver, protein in the blood and fat deposits which have been stored. Starvation pushes a person beyond this situation into a state of extreme hunger and is destructive, whereas fasting can lead subsequently to a drop in blood pressure and cholesterol levels, the cleansing of such organs as the stomach and gall bladder and the rejuvenation of body tissues and cells. Accumulated waste matter in the bowels, lungs and kidneys is eliminated, digestion improves and body weight becomes normalised.

Fasting causes a dramatic change in body weight. The body consists of five-eighths water, so that a person weighing 160 pounds contains 100 pounds of water. The other components include protein (29 pounds); fat (25 pounds) and smaller quantities of minerals, carbohydrates and vitamins. When a person undergoing a fast stops eating there is a sodium reduction (sodium retains water in the body) and large quantities of water are discharged from the body. The first day of a fast may produce a loss of three or four pounds in body weight.

Some people are frightened to fast but in fact nature supports the body during this period. In his work *Man, the Unknown*, famous geneticist Dr Alexis Carrel notes:

Privation of food at first brings a sensation of hunger, occasionally some nervous stimulation . . . but it also determines certain hidden phenomena which are more important. The sugar of the liver and the fat of the subcutaneous deposits are mobilised, and also the proteins of the muscles and glands. All the organs sacrifice their own substances in order to maintain blood, heart and brain in a normal condition. Fasting purifies and profoundly modifies our tissues.

Fasting rests the digestive processes and reduces the amount of energy that has to be expended by the body in its normal process of fighting diseases and discharging waste materials. Consequently fasts are relaxing and calming, and after the first day or two the 'pangs of hunger' disappear. Historically fasting has been used as an aid to meditation and mental and spiritual growth. Pythagoras, Socrates and Plato fasted to retain intellectual acuity; Moses, Daniel and Jesus fasted as a spiritual purification, and it is still a current practice with many Jews, Moslems, Hindus and Buddhists.

Fasting has also regained its importance with many people following alternative lifestyle patterns. Dr David Phillips has written of a spiritual fast that he undertook in 1967. For the first three days his fast was 'physiologically devoted to an intestinal house-cleaning' and he spent the days relaxing, but after that time meditation occupied his mind more and more, producing an 'out-of-the-body' state.

Three or four times each day, I would feel extreme lightness in the body, followed by the sensation of all one's senses being apart from the body. There I was, lying prone on the bed, yet I was also aware of what was going on about me, as though I could 'see' the garden, the house beyond, the traffic on the street and even my own family, some miles away.

There were occasions when I not only saw transpiring the present, but found my consciousness reverted to past experiences in a manner of 're-assessment'. I found myself again in certain situations of the past, but now those situations were re-enacted such that I was aware of how they should have been handled – in fact, I was visiting the other people involved, explaining to them so that we all learnt from those past experiences.

The fast was broken after a week or so, but even while taking juices and later fruit Dr Phillips was aware of thought forms surrounding other people and remained sensitively attuned to them.

There is widespread agreement that fasting should not be practised haphazardly but under the proper supervision of an experienced practitioner. For that reason summaries of fasting regimes are not given here. Most people fast for a week to ten days although fasting specialist Dr Allan Cott notes that the body is quite capable of sustaining a fast for a month, or longer. Fasts have been known to extend in excess of 100 days.

Fasting practitioners often make the point that fasting in itself is not a cure or panacea. It simply allows the body to build up its defence mechanisms against disease and is thus an important facet of preventative medicine. And fasting, as we have noted, also adds a new quality to human perception. Dr Herbert Shelton writes: 'The freedom and ease that one experiences during a period of abstinence from food often enables one to discover new and previously undreamed-of depths to the meaning of life.'

DR DAVID PHILLIPS

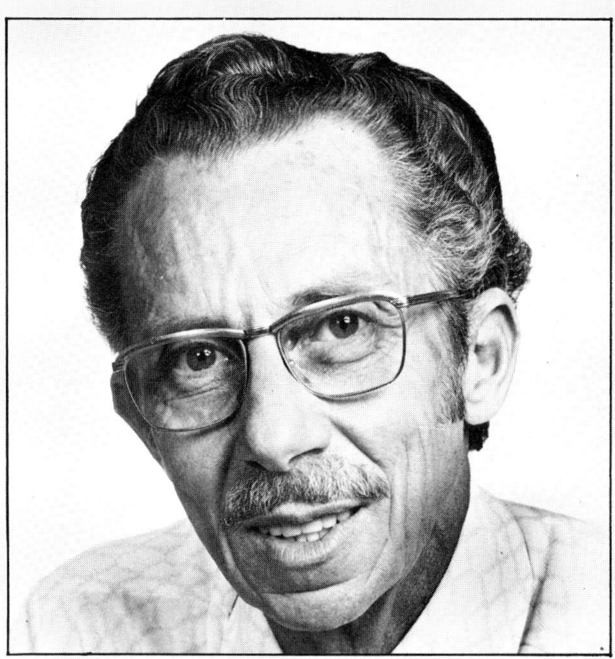

Dr David Phillips is unique among holistic health practitioners: quite aside from being an authority on nutrition, health foods and fasting he is also a widely travelled lecturer and author, marketing executive and numerologist. David was born in Sydney on 12 February 1934, and numerological analysis of these events confirmed that his personal direction would combine business enterprises with a humanitarian philosophy and extensive academic studies. David's life patterns have since borne these factors out.

The son of an electrical engineer, David pursued a similar course at the University of Technology (later the University of New South Wales), graduating after five years of study. He left to work in the car industry but found that there were too many rogues and absolutely no colleagues with any New Age awareness! For a while he undertook postgraduate work in psycho-electronics, evaluating the links between music and the emotions, and in particular studying the new systems then emerging for creating favourable light and sound atmospheres for retailers and shoppers and in factories. Soon, however, his old hankering for the car industry grew too strong and he established what was then one of the earliest car rental companies in the country – predating Budget and Hertz by several years. He would retire from this business only nine years later.

Meanwhile in 1965 David had started studying naturopathy and natural hygiene with Alex Burton and, as is so often the case, a dramatic personal incident confirmed his interest in alternative healing.

A close friend, still only in her late 20s, had been suffering from breast cancer and had had two tumors removed by orthodox surgery. Then, disappointingly, a third tumor formed which extended into the glands of the left arm. Doctors felt that she would have to have an arm and the left breast amputated. Instead she adopted a quite different course of treatment, and thankfully it worked. The method was disciplined fasting, under the watchful eye of an expert practitioner. The fasting lasted for a month and during the period she not only lost the tumor altogether but also an accumulation of mucous in the sinuses which had been affecting her breathing. Gone also was the recurrent asthma she had been suffering from for years.

The emotional impact of this recovery was profound for David Phillips. In February 1968 he undertook a major fast also, and as a side result developed extensive paranormal faculties while enhancing his powers of intuition. David also felt far healthier and happier as a vegetarian, which he had been since 1965, and he also instinctually began a period of celibacy which lasted for three years. The impact of these practices was enormous. He felt totally free and able to achieve anything he pursued.

In 1968 David began to discuss with local producers various means of distributing organically grown foods and a new company, Hygienic Food Supplies, was born soon afterwards. Later this interest took him overseas – to Africa, Europe and the Americas, from Canada in the North to Argentina in the south – in order to bring into Australia imported supplies of organic food.

Alongside these time-absorbing activities David continued to plunge himself into his studies, pursuing a blend of naturopathy and nutritional science. In order to complete a 6-month clinical experience requirement for his PhD (which he completed in 1971) he undertook to supervise fasts at the Shangri La Natural Health Institute at Benita Springs, Florida, and it was there that he also met his future wife Ann with whom he would later co-author the successful *Soil to Psyche Recipe Book.*

Apart from his working activities with Hygienic Food Supplies, David is also Managing Director of Publishers Distributors, promoting books on health, ecology and metaphysics, and is owner of The Pythagorean Press. In his spare time, David Phillips lectures and counsels in nutrition, health, numerology and metaphysics. His hobbies are singing, swimming and yoga, all of which relate to his love of fitness and his joy of living.

David anticipates that he will retire from the executive direction of Hygienic Foods in December 1983, completing a personal numerological cycle, and concentrate instead on teaching. He has already become a prolific author with such works to his credit as *From Soil to Psyche, A Guidebook to Nutritional Factors in Edible Foods* and a recent work on numerology, *Secrets of the Inner Self*. He plans new books on reincarnation, holistic lifestyle and nutrition and, with the Rixons, has been active in bringing the work of American mystic Ken Keyes to the attention of the Australian public per medium of such gatherings as the Morpeth Mind, Body and Healing Festival.

THE FLOWER REMEDIES OF DR BACH

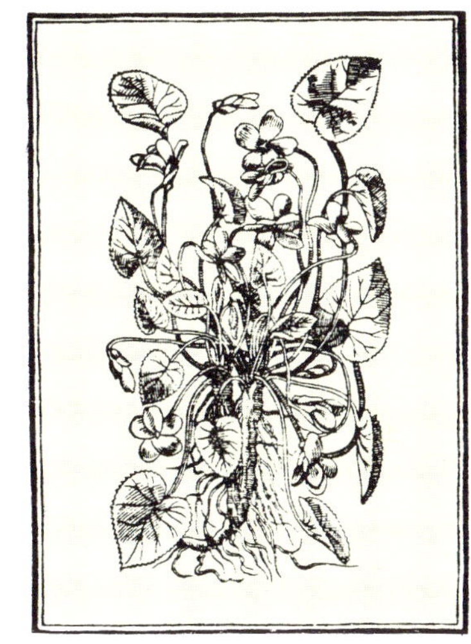

Dr Edward Bach (1886-1936) studied at Birmingham University and University College Hospital, London. Having graduated as a physician he set up a consulting practice near Harley Street but became rapidly disillusioned with orthodox medicine. He began to see that with his patients it was not the disease symptom that was the problem but the negative mental condition underlying it. Dr Bach turned for a time to bacteriology and gained some eminence in the field but he still found that he was not penetrating deeply enough. Disease seemed to have a psychosomatic origin. He felt it was 'our fears, our cares, our anxieties and such like, that open the path to the invasion of illness'.

Then he learnt of the work of German physician Samuel Hahnemann (1755-1843), the founder of homeopathy, who had said 'The patient is the most important factor in his healing'. Bach was impressed by Hahnemann's *The Organon of Medicine* and went to work at the Royal London Homeopathic Hospital. He came increasingly to adopt the view that patients had to be treated not in terms of their physical ailments but their emotional condition. Bach now looked for remedies to restore peace of mind to his patients and turned to Nature for his guidance. In *Heal Thyself* he wrote:

'Among the types of remedies that will be used will be those obtained from the most beautiful plants and herbs to be found in the pharmacy of Nature, such as have been divinely enriched with healing powers for the mind and body of man'.

In 1930 he abandoned his practice in London and went to live in the countryside where he now began to search the fields and meadows for flowers which might contain medicinal healing agents. Bach found to his surprise that if he held his hand over a flowering plant he began to feel that he was acquiring its properties and altering his mood. Sometimes the properties were positive, other times negative. Over a seven year period Dr Bach isolated 38 flowers that appeared to have qualities that could benefit a range of emotional afflictions such as fear, loneliness, exhaustion, impatience, intolerance and restlessness. Many of the flowers grew wild in the fields, blooming in bright sunlight. Bach would take the heads of the flowers and place them upon the surface of water contained in a glass bowl. Here they would remain for three hours, absorbing the sunlight and – importantly – transferring some of their life force into the water. Bach then removed the flowers and gathered the water for subsequent use. In the case of blossoms growing on trees another method applied. These flowers would be placed

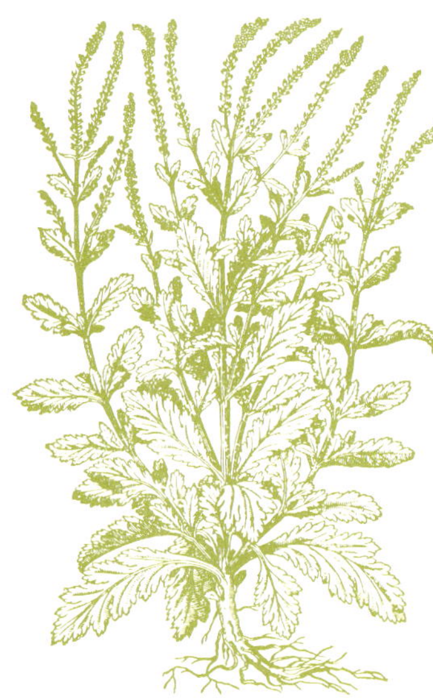

Vervain – one of Dr Bach's 'Twelve Healers'

in a sterile saucepan, covered with water, and gently boiled for 30 minutes. They were then similarly removed and the water bottled, often with the addition of a small quantity of brandy acting as a preservative.

In his classic work *The Twelve Healers,* Dr Bach noted that quite small quantities could be taken, with water or milk, and that none of his healing agents could cause any harm to the patient:

'In urgent cases the doses may be given every few minutes, until there is an improvement; in severe cases about half-hourly; and in long-standing cases every two or three hours, or more often or less as the patient feels the need'.

Dr Bach placed his 38 remedies under seven headings and asterisked the original plants that he had discovered (the 'twelve healers'):

For fear: Rock Rose; Mimulus*; Cherry Plum; Aspen, Red Chestnut

For uncertainty: Cerato*; Scleranthus*; Gentian*; Gorse; Hornbeam; Wild Oat

For insufficient interest in present circumstances: Clematis*; Honeysuckle; Wild Rose; Olive; White Chestnut; Mustard; Chestnut Bud

For loneliness: Water Violet*; Impatiens*; Heather

For those over-sensitive to influences and ideas: Agrimony*; Centaury*; Walnut; Holly

For despondency or despair: Larch; Pine; Elm; Sweet Chestnut; Star of Bethlehem; Willow; Oak; Crab Apple

For over-care for the welfare of others: Chicory*; Vervain*; Vine; Beech; Rock Water

(Note: these remedies are not interchangeable and more detailed listings and explanations of usages can be found in Dr Bach's *The Twelve Healers.*)

RON BARNES

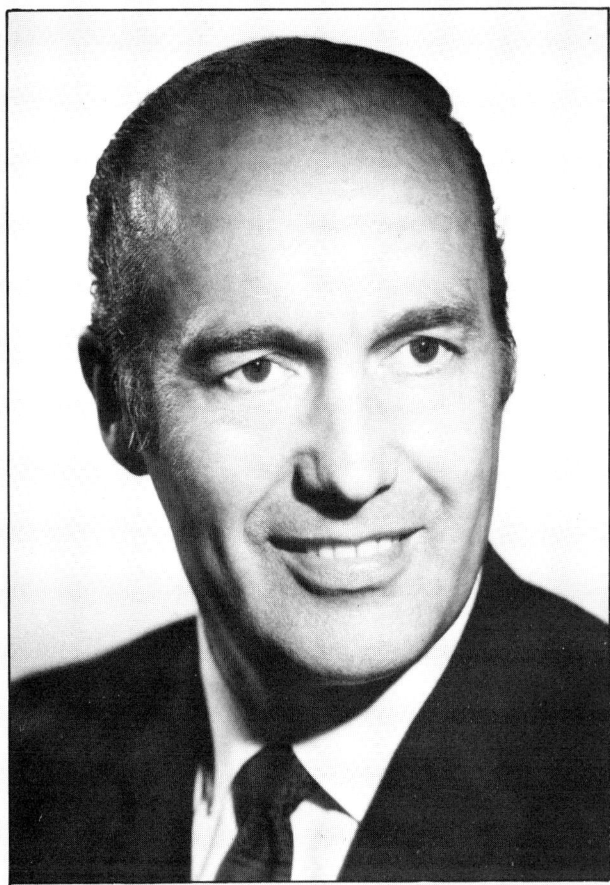

Ron Barnes used to be a chartered accountant, but for the last eight years he has been practising as a naturopath and osteopath, with a special interest in Bach Flower remedies, a system of natural therapy developed by Dr Edward Bach in the 1930s.

Bach Flower remedies, with their very small amounts of active ingredients, are not unlike homeopathic remedies. However, their method of preparation and especially the basic philosophy behind them are quite different. Homeopaths treat symptoms, while Bach Flowers are used according to emotions and personality types.

In common with many of today's doctors, Edward Bach believed that illness is not caused only by physical things. He believed that worry, fear, impatience, and other emotions deplete the body's ability to resist disease. His medical activities confirmed his opinions, so much so that he gave up his practice and spent the last seven years of his life looking for answers among the wild-flowers of the countryside. He believed he found these answers in 38 plants and pure water from natural rock springs.

In following Dr Bach, Ron Barnes prepares plants in two ways. For those whose flowers bloom during the late spring and the summer, the flowers are floated in rain or spring water in a clear glass bowl and are exposed to the strong rays of the sun for several hours. The boiling method for plants that are at their peak at other times of the year, involves boiling the plants in spring water. Brandy is added to the sun-drenched or boiled liquids which are then diluted several times before being prescribed.

Ron Barnes says the amounts of plant substances left in the final prescription are minute but, he says, they work, and are an important part of his Epsom, Auckland practice.

Although Doctor Bach suggested that his remedies should be taken individually rather than in combination, and most practitioners continue to do this, Ron says that he has found them to be very effective in combinations. He usually includes more than one Bach Flower remedy in each prescription. He says he does not feel he is going against Doctor Bach in this because he sees the remedies as part of a total programme that he suggests to people who consult him. The programme may also include herbs, vitamins, or other methods of healing. Diet is always involved.

Ron enjoys his work and cannot now imagine himself doing anything else. He says that is probably because of the Romany blood in his veins. Many old Gypsy remedies were told to him as a child 'but children do not always take much notice. I now wish I had'. But perhaps some of those old cures are still stored in the back of his memory because, he says, he sometimes finds he knows an answer and cannot remember exactly where he got it from.

In common with many natural therapists, Ron Barnes finds that many of the people who consult him also need a sympathetic listener or help with family or other problems. He says he does what he can and does not resent being called upon for advice. Because, like Doctor Bach, he also believes that emotions and illness are linked.

Ron Barnes sees Bach Flower remedies as part of a total programme of healing. He does not use them as a therapy on their own. He sees himself as still learning in all the areas in which he practises, and as by no means the only, or even the best, in his field.

JOHN RAMSELL AND NICKIE MURRAY

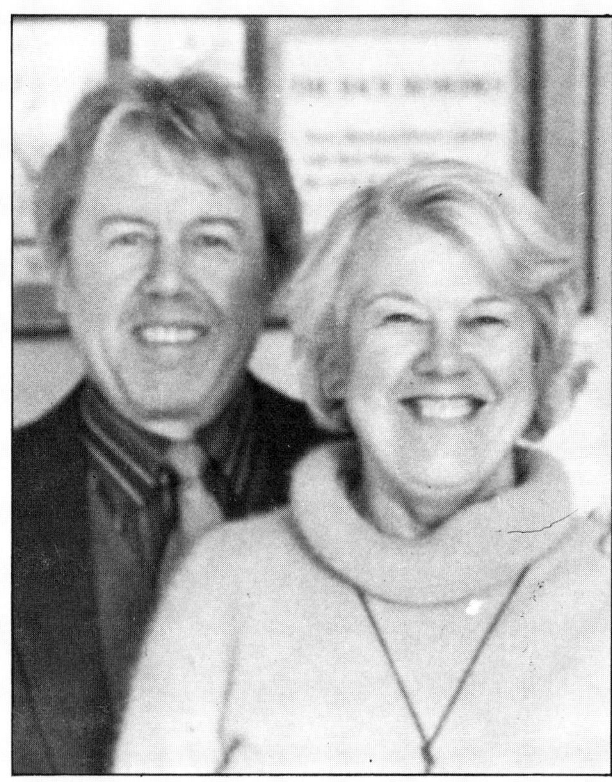

The Edward Bach Centre, Mount Vernon, at Sotwell, is an unpretentious, red brick house tucked away off a winding Oxfordshire lane, near Wallingford. This is where Nickie Murray and her brother John Ramsell carry on the work begun by the remarkable Welsh physician, Dr Edward Bach, discoverer of the flower remedies that bear his name.

The coincidence that brought them to Mount Vernon might almost have been pre-ordained. Both came from a family background immersed in healing and homeopathy. Nickie had been a spiritual healer for twenty years. One day, quite unexpectedly, she received a parcel through the post. It contained a set of the Bach flower remedies and a copy of the book *Medical Discoveries of Edward Bach, Physician* by Nora Weeks. They had been sent to her by someone who knew of her healing work. She was fascinated by the book and her very first use of the remedies increased her interest in them. She decided to get in touch with Nora Weeks, a former radiologist, who had given up her vocation in order to become the co-worker of Dr Bach. Now, after his death, she was continuing the work he had developed at Mount Vernon. Nickie began helping her on a voluntary part-time basis and was later joined by her brother.

John Ramsell had been a variety artist, playing in music halls throughout Britain. When he looks back to those days, touring the country, meeting every type of individual, observing every kind of behaviour, he realises how much that taught him about human nature. Now when people come to Mount Vernon and ask his advice about health matters he is able to draw on that background. He recalls the teachings of Dr Bach that you should treat the individual himself, his fears, anxieties, griefs and depressions, rather than physical symptoms.

When Nora Weeks died in 1978 John Ramsell and Nickie Murray became joint curators of the Centre, both dedicated to maintaining it exactly as Edward Bach would have wished. The flowers they use come from the same locations that Dr Bach selected in the surrounding fields. As he did, they place the gathered flower heads on the surface of a glass bowl of water and leave them in the sunlight for three hours. When the heat of the sun has drawn the life-force of the flowers into the water, this is bottled and preserved. John's wife and Nickie's husband help them and the bottling and preserving is done by friends who live in the locality. All the work is carried out by this cooperative team. They receive between sixty and a hundred letters each day, from all over the world, ordering the remedies or asking for advice about them. Although they have never advertised or solicited custom the demand for them constantly increases, a tribute to their effectiveness and to word of mouth recommendation. Among the many who use the remedies are practitioners, including acupuncturists, chiropractors and homeopaths, who give them as a supplement to their own form of treatment. Always in demand is the famous *Rescue* remedy, a combination of five remedies which can be used as an emergency first aid in cases of shock, severe stress, or accident.

During the year John and Nickie visit a number of displays and festivals where they present the remedies, among them the Festival of Mind and Body at Olympia in London. They also send out news and information in a newsletter which they publish three times a year. Recently the Bach remedies were officially accepted for registration in the United States Homeopathic Pharmacopoeia, under a separate classification, a signal honour to Dr Bach and recognition of the contribution he has made to healing. John Ramsell hopes that this will lead to similar adoptions in other countries. Through the many books and articles that have been written about Dr Bach and his flower remedies, and their world-wide use, Mount Vernon has become something of a Mecca for those who know of him. Visitors arrive, some on a walking pilgrimage with rucksacks on their back, others by car, but all are welcomed by John and Nickie, although they do like prior notice. They are happy to discuss the remedies with their guests, give advice on their use and show the house with the furniture that Dr Bach built himself when he left his lucrative London practice to live at Mount Vernon in comparative obscurity. They are determined that the work he did and the remedies he gave to the world will not be forgotten.

GESTALT THERAPY

Popular expressions like 'Be here now' and 'Let it all hang out' reflect colloquially the techniques of self-awareness developed by Frederick ('Fritz') Perls in his system of Gestalt Therapy. Perls became a fashionable guru figure in the 1960s following his workshops at the Esalen Institute, Big Sur, but the origins of the Gestalt school go back much earlier.

The German word *gestalt* refers to a pattern of parts making up a whole and the underlying principle of Gestalt psychology is that an analysis of parts does not lead to an understanding of the whole. Parts by themselves have no meaning.

Building on the pioneering work of Max Wertheimer, Wolfgang Kohler and Kurt Koffka, Perls noted that gestalt theory applied to the personality and to basic human needs:

Every organ, the senses, movements, thoughts, subordinate themselves to (an) emerging need and are quick to change loyalty and function as soon as that need is satisfied and then retreat into the background . . . All the parts of the organism identify themselves temporarily with the emergent gestalt

Born in Berlin in 1893, Perls struggled through his youth and school years but went on to receive an M.D. in psychiatry. Then he moved to Vienna where he met Wilhelm Reich and returned to Germany in 1936 to deliver a paper at the Psychoanalytic Congress, attended by the 'founding father' himself: Sigmund Freud. However quite early on in his professional career, Perls realised that Freud's concept of Eros (sex) and Thanatos (destructiveness) as the twin motivating forces of human existence was incomplete. He came to reject the idea of rigidly classifying instincts and analysing a patient's *past* – and chose instead to focus on the *here and now*. For people to be whole, or balanced, they needed to recognise bodily yearnings and impulses instead of disguising them. In fact, life was a series of gestalts that emerged one after the other – a variety of needs requiring satisfaction. Perls developed Gestalt Therapy to allow people to recognise their projections and disguises as *real feelings* and subsequently to be able to fulfil themselves.

After breaking with the psychoanalytic movement, Fritz Perls emigrated to tbe United States in 1946 and established the New York Institute for Gestalt Therapy in 1952. He moved to California in 1959. His friend, psychologist Wilson Van Dusen explains how, at the time, Perls' views were revolutionary:

We were all basically retrospective, strongly retrospective, in both our analysis and therapies. We wouldn't conceive of understanding a patient without an

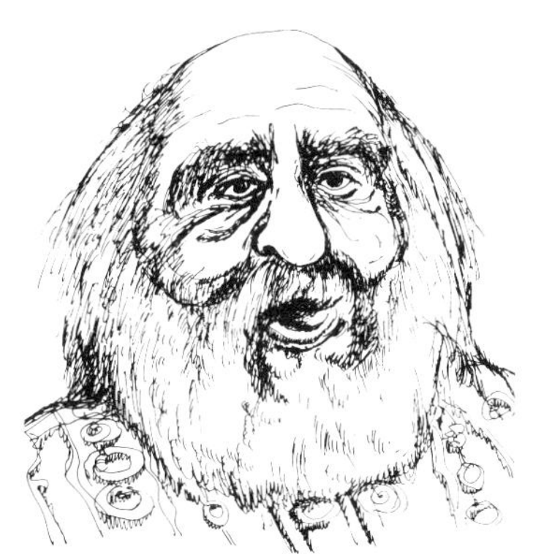

Fritz Perls – father of Gestalt Therapy

extensive history. And for a man just to walk into a room and describe people's behaviour so accurately added a whole new dimension. This is where I considered Fritz very great. His incomparable capacity to observe . . .

Fritz Perls had been strongly influenced by Reich's idea that the body reflected internal psychological processes. The person *here and now* showed everything through his being and behaviour – there was no need to delve into *analysis*: 'Nothing is ever really repressed', he wrote. 'All relevant gestalten are emerging, they are on the surface, they are obvious like the emperor's nakedness . . . '

As a therapist, Perls was often extremely curt and blunt, cutting through the niceties of social interaction to the person behind the image. At Esalen he would give demonstrations of Gestalt Therapy before over a hundred people. Sitting on a stage, he would invite members of the audience to participate with him in role-play. He had two chairs beside him. One was the so-called 'hot seat' which the participant sat in, engaging in dialogue with Perls. The other chair was there to help the person switch roles and enact different parts, engaging in the self-questioning process. Frequently volunteers showed up their weaknesses and limitations but there was, after all, a lesson to be learnt.

Perls was wary of the 'fun generation' who came just for entertainment and his dialogues were always brutally honest. For some these were moments of revelation and awe, for others shattering experiences. Fritz Perls' publisher, Arthur Ceppos, recalls:

I think that Fritz's greatest contribution was his horror at how ridiculous man permits himself to become; and by becoming aware of how ridiculous he is, he can emerge into an identity that is no longer ridiculous, but is relatively free. This is the whole secret behind Fritz's hot seat. He would show people how they made fools of themselves . . .

Essentially Perls believed with the existentialists that each person lived in his own universe and had to take the responsibility for his own behaviour and growth. The well known Gestalt Therapy prayer goes as follows:

I do my thing, and you do your thing,
I am not in this world to live up to your expectations
And you are not in this world to live up to mine.
You are you and I am I,
And if by chance we find each other, it's beautiful.
If not, it can't be helped.

Self-awareness and experience are crucial to Gestalt Therapy; be aware of what you are experiencing – *how* you experience your existence *now* . . . pay particular attention to the ways in which you sabotage your own attempts at sustained awareness . . . are these ways in which you habitually prevent yourself from fully contacting the world and your own experience . . . ?

Extending his scope from here-and-now interactions through dialogue and self-recognition, Perls also placed considerable emphasis on dreams. Here were messages that could help people understand the unfinished situations they were carrying around with them. In *Gestalt Therapy Verbatim* he wrote:

In Gestalt Therapy we don't interpret dreams. We do something more interesting with them. Instead of analysing and further cutting up the dream, we want to bring it back to life. And the way to bring it back to life is to re-live the dream as if it were happening now. Instead of telling the dream as if it were a story in the past, act it out in the present, so that it becomes a part of yourself, so that you are really involved.

Perls suggested dreams be written down with their various details as completely as possible. Then a dialogue or encounter between the different component parts or figures could be held. As the encounter process continued, a new integration was arrived at.

Perls described the dream as 'an excellent opportunity to find the holes in the personality . . . if you understand the meaning of each time you identify with some bit of a dream, each time you translate an *it* into an *I*, you increase in vitality and in your potential'.

At Esalen, Fritz Perls worked alongside other therapists like Will Schutz and Bernard Gunther, and became a central figure in encounter therapy. Later, in 1969 he established The Gestalt Institute of Canada on Vancouver Island but did not live to see its development. He died six months after founding it, in March 1970.

URSULA FAUSSET

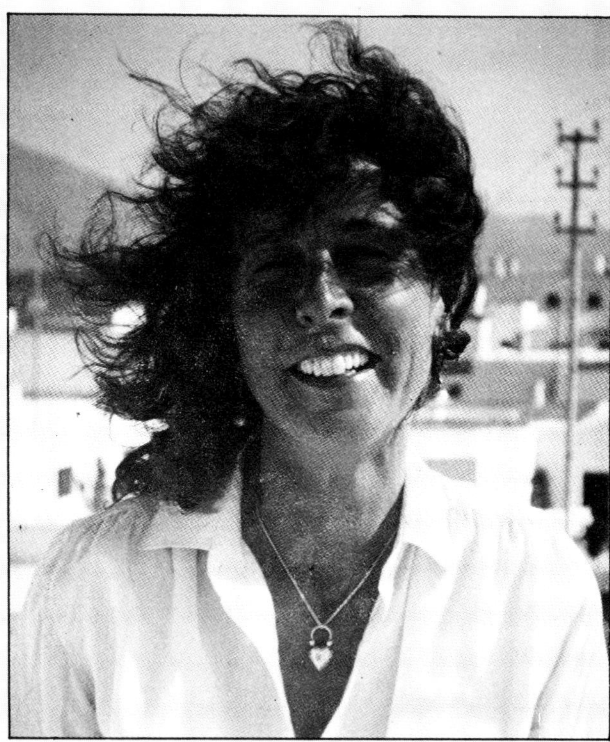

'Many of those who come to see me have allowed their lives to become a prison. I try to help them find their own key, so that they can let themselves out.' Ursula Fausset is well equipped to give such help. A leading gestalt therapist and gestalt consultant for professionals, she has been facilitating groups since 1971, specialising in gestalt since 1973 and leading groups throughout Britain and Europe. She was for a period a staff member of the Gestalt and Humanistic Institute in Tampa, Florida and was the first British representative of the European Gestalt Training Service. After she had completed her training in marriage counselling and applied behavioural science, she concentrated her work on couples and families. She also sees individual clients and works with groups numbering between eight and fourteen.

Previously, Ursula Fausset had been a professional painter, had her own pottery studio and was also an art teacher. She began to realise that she was more interested in the people she taught than the art she taught them, and became an art therapist in a hospital. Her involvement in gestalt therapy began when she attended an encounter group whose leader had been at the Esalen Institute, in California, the Mecca of the Human Potential movement. She knew at once that this was the work she wanted to do. She sees gestalt as a powerful method of helping people to grow, a speeding-up process of life. She emphasises that it is a way of living, far too valuable to be confined to those who have been labelled 'sick'.

Each one of us, she says, has within the potential to enrich our creativity, our capacity to love and our authenticity as human beings. She works with people to help them rid themselves of old, rigid patterns, relics of injunctions that have been imposed by parents, society and 'authority'. Eventually, she says, I see them become their *own* authority and the unique human beings they really are. Men, in particular, she finds, are victims of imposed injunctions – 'do not cry', 'do not be vulnerable', 'keep a stiff upper lip'. So much feeling is held back in this way that there is often little energy left for living in the 'here and now'. Much of her work is concerned with helping her clients to become aware of their habitual patterns of behaviour, 'the games people play', games which may once have been necessary but no longer work for them. She encourages those in her groups to take risks, and take responsibility for themselves.

Many who come to her feel that their negative aspects are unique and when they find that their fears and anxieties are universal they experience great relief. Others feel that they are not living a full life, that 'there must be more'. Because so many have lost contact with the child in them and are no longer able to be spontaneous, she uses fun and laughter whenever possible. This worked with a concert guitarist who suffered from tension that affected her performance. She was a perfectionist, unable to relax in her playing. 'Play as badly as you can' it was suggested to her. At first she looked puzzled, then entered into the spirit of the game and played her worst. At once she burst into laughter and for the first time experienced true relaxation. A lover of dancing herself, Ursula encourages it as a means of expression and an outlet for feelings. She uses art, too, and in their paintings group members often reveal aspects of themselves in what they draw.

Of particular importance to her is the environment in which she works. The ideal is a large, bright room, uncluttered with furniture or other objects, with large comfortable cushions on the floor for the participants and ample space for free movement. To those who come she suggests, in preparation, that as well as a notebook they bring an 'adventurous spirit' and that before entering the room they 'leave their shoes and their concepts outside'. She employs a holistic approach in her work, an integration of body, mind and feeling. 'Don't merely listen to what a person says, but see what their body is doing as they say it.' A woman, for example, might be talking lovingly of her mother but her clenched fists give a different message. Among those who have come to her, she tells of a woman who suffered from every neurosis in the psychiatric lexicon. She even confessed that her vocation was 'mental patient'. Over a lengthy period, Ursula Fausset worked with her and gave her the support she needed. Slowly and displaying a willingness to break out of her lifelong conditioning to take risks, she began to accept responsibility for her life. She discovered that she mattered and that she was lovable. Today she is a senior social worker, herself practising gestalt therapy. Perhaps there is little wonder, with results like these, that Ursula Fausset finds her work deeply satisfying.

HERBS

Herbal medicines are as old as recorded history and were the major means of restoring good health prior to the era of modern chemicals and synthetic drugs. Now that it is clear that many of the new medicines have negative side-effects there has been a resurgence of interest in herbalism as a form of natural healing.

Many ancient cultures had an extensive knowledge of herbs and made use of these soft, fragrant plants in medicine or for flavouring food. The Chinese *Pen Tsao* (3000BC) lists around 1000 herbal remedies and we know that cloves, myrrh, coriander, mint, garlic and indigo were used in ancient Egypt. A Sumerian herbal has been discovered dating from 2200 B.C. and a tradition of medicinal herbalism also developed in Greece. The earliest

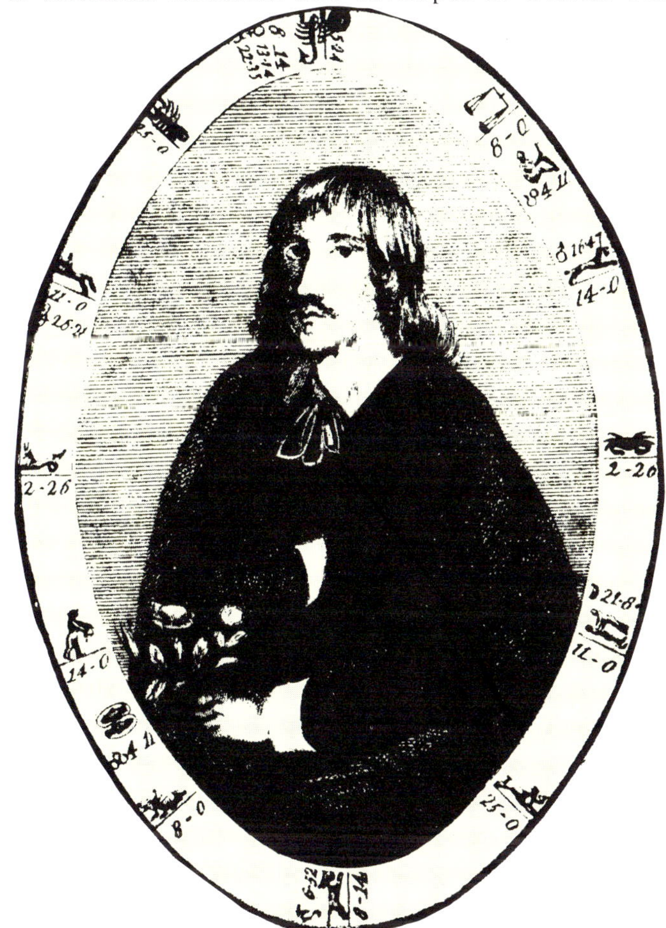

Nicholas Culpeper, the noted English herbalist

European writer on plants, Theophrastos, compiled *Historia Plantarum* in the 4th century B.C. and Dioscorides wrote a treatise on medicinal plants, *De Materia Medica*, in the first century A.D. Herbal knowledge came to Britain during the Roman occupation, declined in the Dark Ages but revived again with the growth of religious orders. The monasteries became centres of medical information and practical knowledge of herbs developed with the fostering of herb gardens.

Several famous herbals date from the 16th and 17th centuries. The first herbal in English was the *Grete Herball* (1526) followed by John Gerard's *The Herball, or general Historie of Plants* (1597) and Nicholas Culpeper's *The English Physician Enlarged* (1653). Culpeper combined astrology, magic and

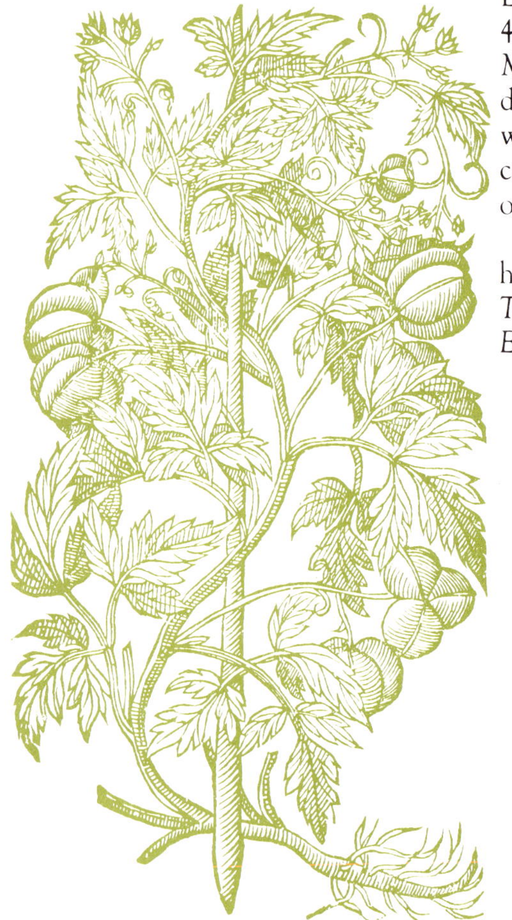

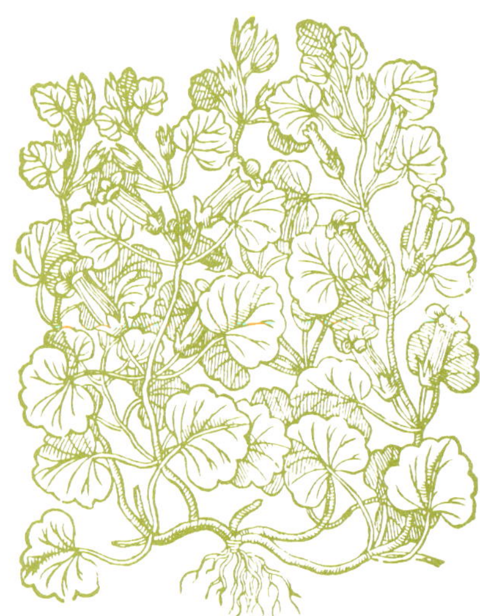

Illustrations from Gerard's Herball

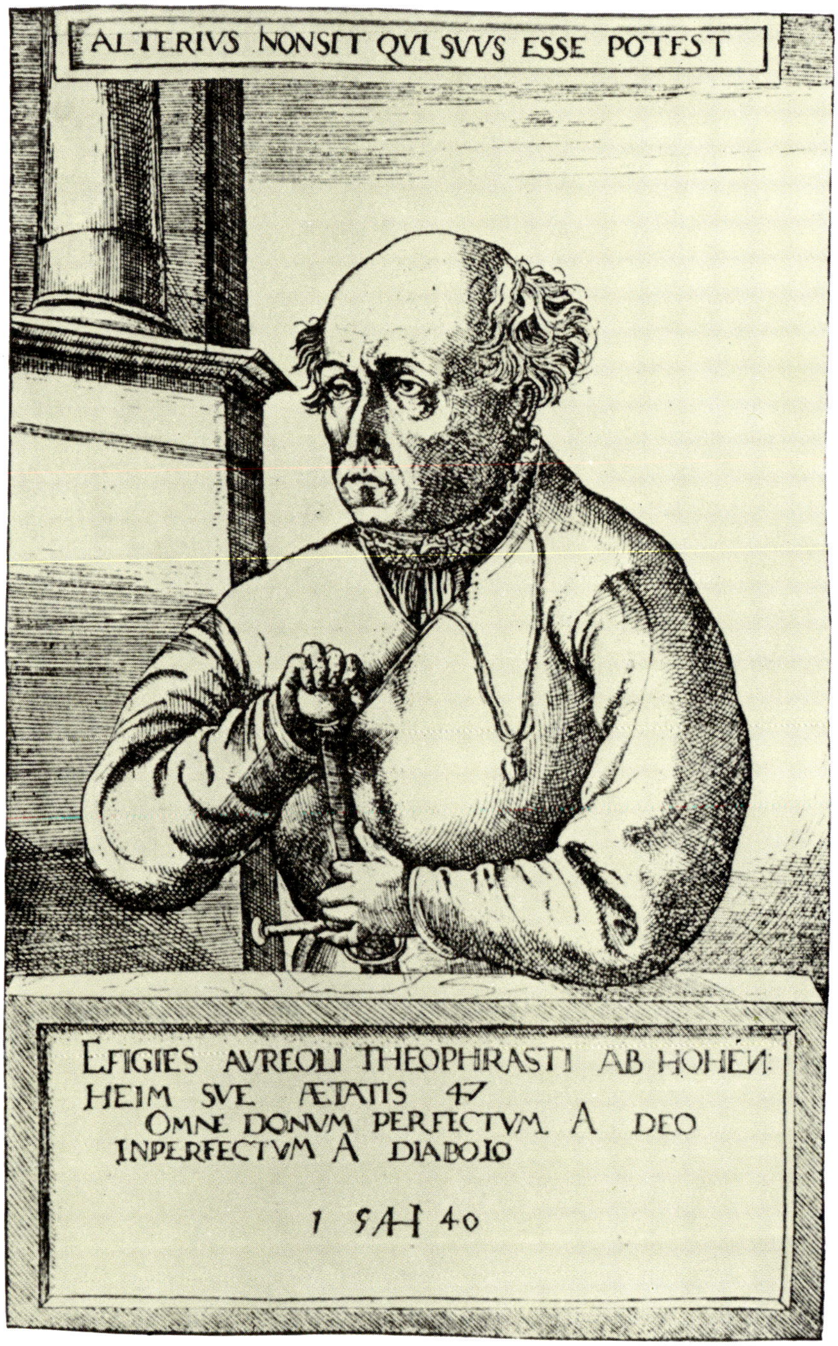

Paracelsus, medieval herbalist and alchemist

folklore and represented the more mystical approach to herbalism. This eclectic tendency also characterised the writings of Paracelsus who popularised the so-called Doctrine of Signatures. According to this philosophy the appearance of a plant was said to relate to its usage, e.g. yellow flowers or roots for jaundice. In medieval herbalism the mystical domain was never far away and a quaint herbal formula dating from around 1600 describes how a herbal oil could be used to see the fairies:

Take one pint of virgin olive oil and wash it with rose water and marigold water until it is white. The roses and the marigolds are to be gathered towards the east and the water thereof to be made of pure spring water. Put the washed oil into a vial glass and add hollyhock buds, marigold flowers, wild thyme tops and flowers, young hazel buds and the grass of a fairy throne. The thyme must be gathered near the side of a hill where fairies used to be. Set the glass in the sun for three days so that the ingredients can become incorporated. Then put it away for use . . .

Despite the mystical aura of herbalism during this period the herbalists assembled a vast knowledge of plant species and it is worth noting that at least a third of all modern pharmaceuticals today derive from, or are synthetic replicas of, plant substances.

Herbs can be used in many ways. They can be taken in teas or infusions, or applied in fomentations, ointments, plasters and poultices. They are effective for treating an extremely wide range of ailments including ulcers, nervous conditions, bronchial catarrh, colds, boils, cramps, blood disorders, toothache, kidney disorders, colic, asthma, rheumatism, rashes, urinary problems and arthritis.

Herbal medicine was popularised in the United States by such figures as Samuel Thompson (1769–1843) and Dr Benedict Lust who opened the first health food store in that country in 1896. Today herbalism has become an important part of the holistic healing movement and its medicinal applications have been systematically compiled in a wide variety of books and journals.

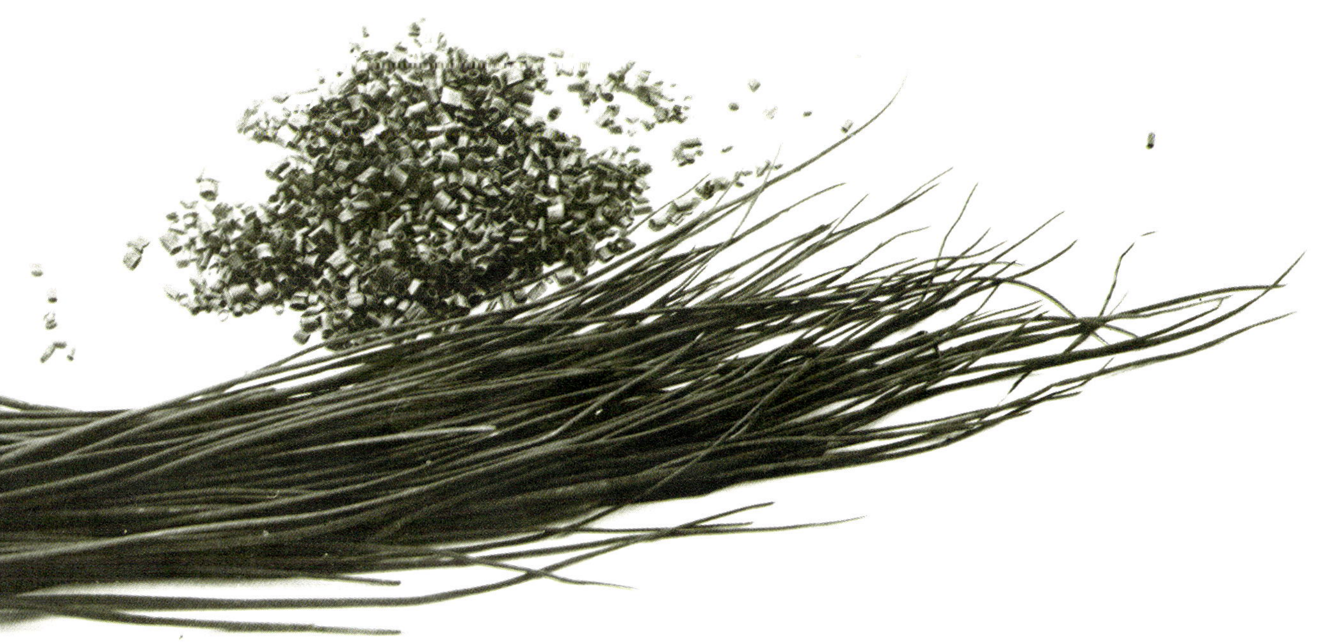

Herbs can be used to strengthen the natural functions of the body and modern herbalists seek to return the body to its normal state of balance. While early herbalists tended to use herbs individually, a tendency has developed for herbs to be used in combinations although some herbalists still prefer 'simples'. Californian herbalist Michael Tierra notes, however, that combinations of herbs with similar or complementary properties can be very useful. In an article titled *The Way of Herbs* he quotes as an example a combination of *uva-ursi/bearberry* (4 parts); *cleavers/bedstraw* (4 parts); *licorice root* (2 parts) and *ginger root* (1 part) that has the attraction of being a diuretic formula which is astringent, blood purifying and pleasant to taste. The ginger is added to stimulate the herbal function and the remedy is useful for bladder and kidney infections.

Modern herbalists tend to avoid herbs which might provide negative side-effects and on the whole herbal treatments are cheap, making them a very feasible practical alternative to expensive, orthodox medical care. Herbal prescriptions also have the advantage that they are individually prepared after a detailed assessment of the patient's lifestyle, diet and exercise patterns. Synthetic drugs, by contrast, are standardised and constant and usually aim to suppress symptoms. A herbalist is more intent on treating the patient rather than the specific disease, and will therefore recommend use of specially selected herbal medicines appropriate to individual circumstances. This point notwithstanding, certain herbs have been found to have generally applicable qualities. The following is a listing of herbs that are commonly used in medicinal treatments:

COMMON AILMENTS AND HERBAL REMEDIES	
ACNE	Burdock, English walnut, valerian
ASTHMA	Coltsfoot, comfrey, fennel, garden thyme, ground ivy, gum plant, mullein, sloe, willow herb, valerian
BLOOD PRESSURE	European mistletoe, garlic, hawthorn, onion, parsley, rue
BOILS	Chamomile, marjoram, marshmallow root, linseed, thyme
BRONCHITIS	Coltsfoot, comfrey, gum plant, liquorice
BURNS	Burdock, coltsfoot, comfrey, onion
COLDS	Catnip, chamomile, coltsfoot, ginger, peppermint, thyme
CONSTIPATION	Barberry bark, blackthorn, liquorice, senna, slippery elm
CRAMPS	Cayenne, fennel, rosemary, rue, wild yam, wormwood
DIARRHOEA	Blackberry root, cinnamon fern, oak bark, silverweed
DYSPEPSIA	Caraway, chamomile, dandelion, peppermint
ECZEMA	Internal: burdock root; external: chickweed
FEVER	Foenugreek, slippery elm, sorrel
GOUT	Celery seed, hyssop, juniper, meadowsweet, nettle
HEADACHE	Chamomile, hops, willow, wood betony
INFLUENZA	Garlic, yarrow
INSOMNIA	Aniseed, hops, lime flowers, valerian
MENSTRUATION	Chamomile, lady's mantle, mistletoe, sorrel, St John's wort
MENOPAUSAL DEPRESSION	Rosemary, St John's wort
NASAL CONGESTION	Foenugreek
NAUSEA	Caraway, chamomile, clove, lemon balm, peppermint

NERVOUS COMPLAINTS	Sage, peppermint, rosemary
NEURALGIA	Hops, passion flower, wild marjoram, willow, wormwood
OBESITY	Chickweed, fennel, ground ivy, willow
RHEUMATISM	Black cohosh, borage, celery seed, juniper, meadowsweet, wood betony, rosemary (external) wintergreen oil (external)
SORE THROAT	Sage, stinging nettle gargle
SPRAINS	Arnica, comfrey
STINGS	Burdock, garlic, goosegrass, horseradish
TOOTHACHE	Elder, yarrow leaves
ULCERS (STOMACH)	Chamomile, lemon balm, liquorice, peppermint
VOMITING	Chamomile, lemon balm, peppermint
WOUNDS	Comfrey

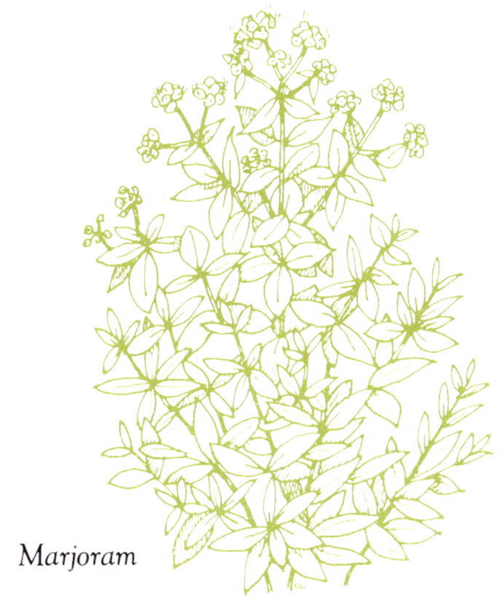
Marjoram

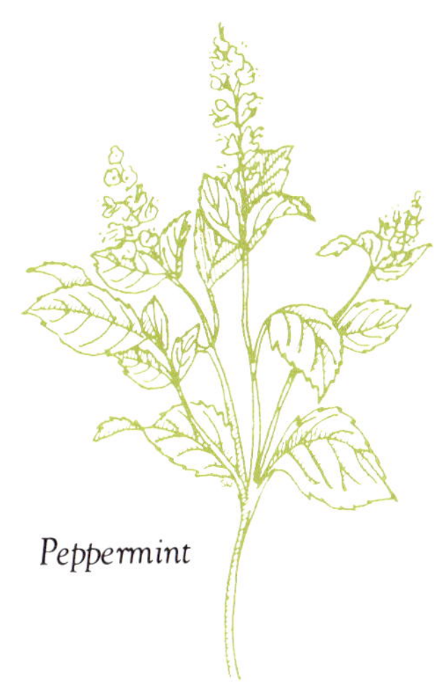
Peppermint

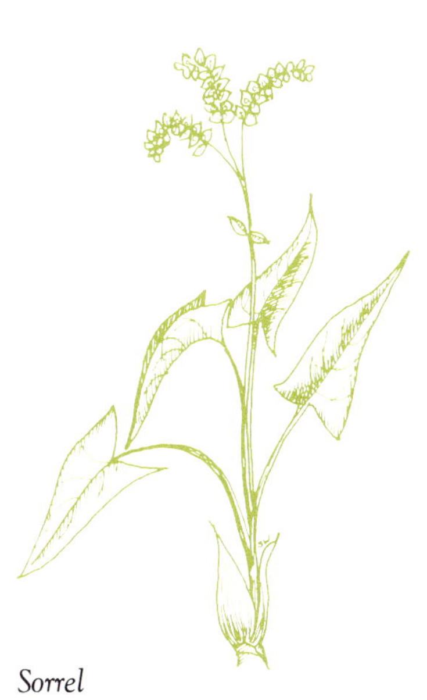
Sorrel

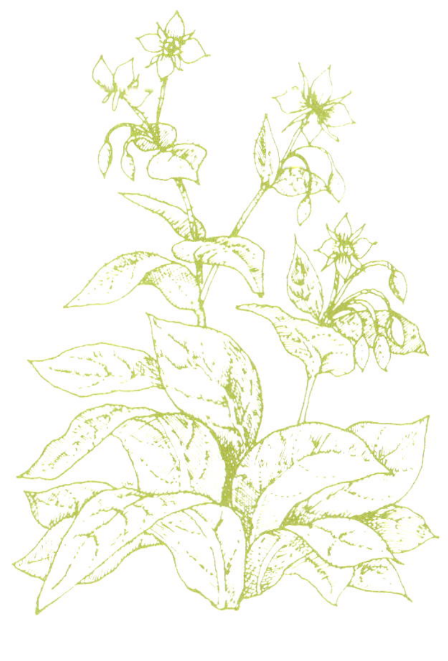
Borage

BETH HARVEY HELEN KING DERRIAN TURNER KATHY WOOD

From left to right: *Helen King, Derrian Turner, Kathy Wood, Beth Harvey*

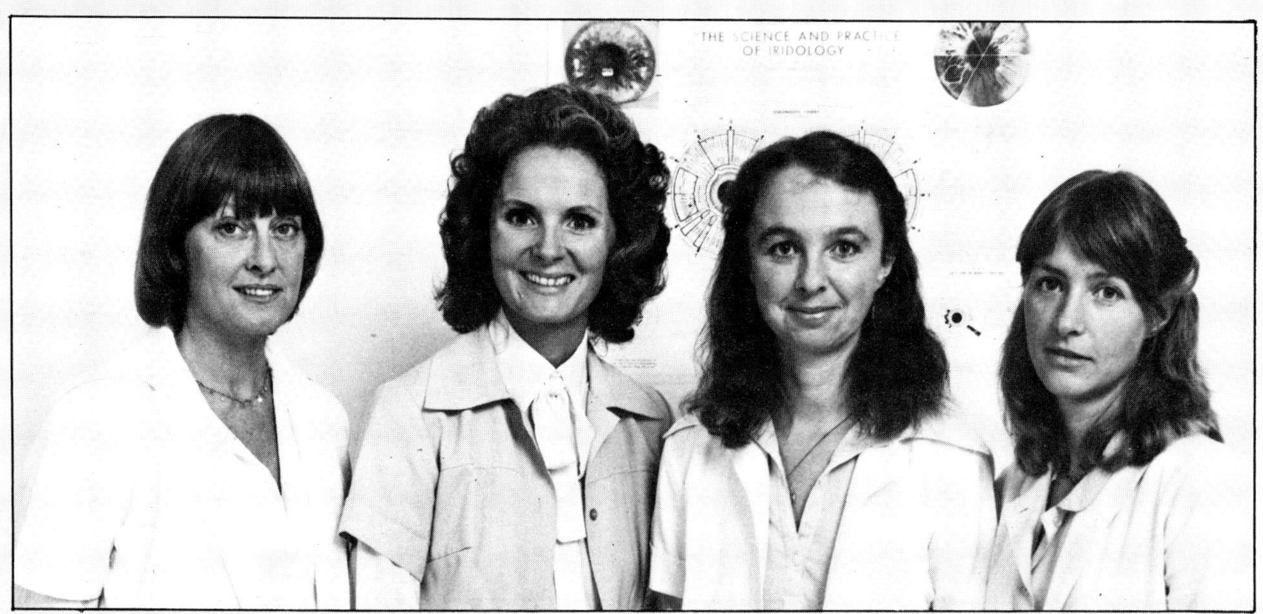

Tucked alongside commercial buildings in busy Crows Nest on Sydney's lower North Shore is a renovated cottage that has been transformed into offices. Inside, each room has an abundance of healthy indoor plants and interesting wall charts, and the atmosphere feels good. This is the Alexander Street Herbal Centre, a thoroughly democratic and so far commercially successful enterprise run by four women in their early 30s. The Centre, 'an equal rights partnership', opened in October 1980 and patients can be treated by more than one of the herbalists should the need arise. Derrian Turner, Kathy Wood, Beth Harvey and Helen King each have their respective interests and specialisations like iridology, reflexology, relaxation techniques, but each is broad enough in terms of training to substitute for a partner should the need arise. Although one could form the view that the Herbal Centre is a feminist enterprise, this is not the underlying raison d'être. The Centre is open four days a week and most of the partners work three days each, sharing in the secretarial and administrative responsibilities. The common philosophy at the Centre is that for holistic treatment to be effective, each of the partners should have a balanced and relaxed attitude to life and that the work component should not be allowed to become a chore. The Centre is closed on Wednesdays to provide a mid-week break and allow each partner to pursue other activities that are also important.

Two of the herbalists, Derrian Turner and Beth Harvey, are English, and Kathy Wood and Helen King are Australian. Each has had personal reasons for pursuing holistic healing:

Helen King began her career as a commercial artist and spent seven years in fashion graphics for newspaper advertising. Then she moved to the country, 35 miles outside Tamworth, and grew herbs. One of her two children suffered from croup and bronchitis and Helen gave her 'simples' (one plant for each treatment) although she did not have the herbal knowledge she now possesses. Helen felt she should take her daughter to a doctor in Sydney but a course of anti-biotics proved unsatisfactory. They then went to see a naturopath and her daughter 'became a real child again'. Helen subsequently took up studies at a leading herbal college and met her present colleagues from the Centre.

Kathy Wood worked in a health food shop part-time even while still at school and then studied social work at University. Ironically she found that this area did not provide her with enough contact with people so with a friend she established a health-food restaurant in Bondi called *The Zen Inn* and ran it for eight years. She now maintains a little farm in the picturesque mountain township of Bilpin and grows herbs.

Beth Harvey came to Australia in 1972. She had trained as a nurse after leaving school and worked briefly before emigrating. Several years ago she had been virtually crippled by a bone graft — a painful fusion of several vertebrae in her lower back. After enduring the pain for some time she decided to help herself — and got into herbalism. Beth's father is a biochemist and she feels that she was drawn to understanding the natural healing agents available through natural chemicals and herbal medicine. She has recovered from her back ailment and since coming from England has been pleased by the increasing acceptance of herbalism in Australia.

Derrian Turner had worked in Europe and Hong Kong as a model but was plagued by a long-term spinal complaint which manifested painfully through the sciatic nerve. She spent years exploring physiotherapy and chiropractic and a doctor in Hong Kong advised her that she might require a bone graft between her vertebrae.

After she had come to Australia and ended her unhappy marriage she found that her spinal problems had an emotional basis, not a physical one, and similarly disappeared. She came to the view that social and environmental factors are often crucial in understanding the nature of apparently physical complaints. A consideration of these aspects is also part of treatment at the Herbal Centre.

Why herbs rather than drugs? The natural advantage of herbs is that they normalise and strengthen metabolic processes rather than suppress symptoms. The naturopathic method is to treat the *cause* of a complaint thereby alleviating the symptoms, and the effect is long-term. The herbs dispensed at the Centre are non-toxic and reasonably priced (a six-week supply may cost as little as $3.50) and the herbs produce an internal balancing in the body if properly used.

JENNY DOUGLAS

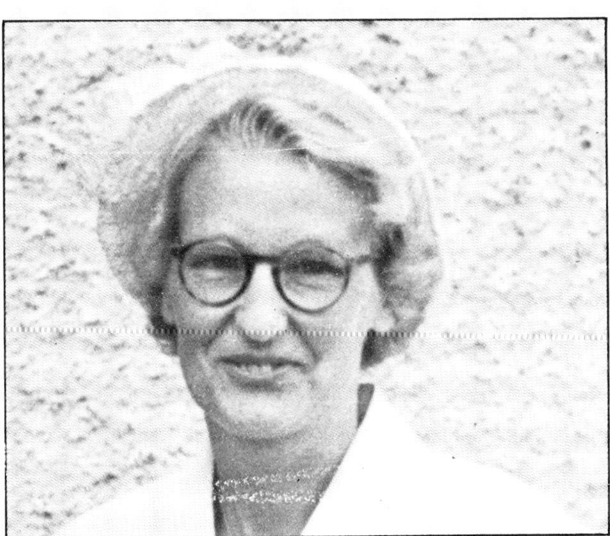

Jenny Douglas learnt her craft from her father, William Theophilus Anderton, one of the pioneers of natural medicine in New Zealand. 'He was really quite a remarkable man. He had this flair for picking what was wrong with people.' This is something Jenny also has — a talent for knowing what is wrong and also for dealing with people as whole human beings rather than through their illnesses alone.

Jenny's craft is perhaps the oldest of the physical forms of healing. Long before history began, human beings were treating illness by using the herbs that grew around them. A great deal of this knowledge has been passed down through the centuries, much of it, as in Jenny's case, verbally, from generation to generation. And a lot of it has never been written down, though Jenny, a hardworking grandmother, is beginning to keep notes. She is aware that if she does not do this, much of her knowledge will die with her.

Helping people has always been an important part of the Anderton and Douglas families. Both families have, for several generations, been strongly political and active in the Labour Party. Jenny's grandfather once led a march of unemployed people on the poorhouse in Britain, demanding beds for them and saying that those inside the poorhouse were better off than the people outside.

Jenny's father was also interested in politics 'It is,' she says, 'only because of this caring attitude that you ever get involved in politics. Otherwise it's not worth it.' Her husband, Norman, is a well known elder politician. Her three sons are also interested in politics.

It was 1923 when Mr Anderton first opened his small shop in Symonds Street, Auckland. From there, he dispensed his remedies and gave freely of his knowledge. His daughter, Jenny, joined him there soon after she left school.

In those days, they used to make pills by hand, and many of the remedies were formulated especially for each person. Jenny still prepares prescriptions for people who come to her. She sees herbs, vitamins, and other natural therapies as a part of food rather than as things that are taken only to fix a problem. She takes her B vitamins and other supplements as part of her meals. She does not see them as separate from the food she eats.

Herbal and natural remedies support the body's efforts to overcome problems, building up the body as a whole, and not treating symptoms in isolation.

The business grew, and the Anderton remedies were sold through other shops. Today, the family business thrives and many of the original formulations are still sold under the Red Seal label.

Jenny works for the family business, turning her hand to anything that needs to be done, from answering the many letters she receives from people needing help, to lending a hand on the production line, filling bottles, labelling, packing pills. She still finds time to talk to many groups who are interested in herbs. She sees this as quite important because 'in a group of 100, there may be just one or two who will really have the feel for it. It is these who will carry on the skills and the knowledge'.

But it is toward her daughter, Sue, that many of Jenny's energies are directed. Sue has the flair and the interest in learning, so Jenny is working with her, teaching and showing her the secrets of her craft, knowing that Sue will use them in the best way, and knowing, too, that the knowledge will not be lost.

'I know we must pass it on, and sometimes I have thought I might write a book. But I see so many books about it, and most of them are *so wrong*. I'm not sure I would want to be put in the same category as them.' The main thing is that Jenny is using her knowledge as well as passing it on.

HOMEOPATHY

Homeopathy was the brainchild of the brilliant doctor and scholar Samuel Christian Hahnemann (1755–1843) who was born in Meissen, Germany, and attended Leipzig University. Hahnemann was interested in translating medical texts from English, French and Italian and it was the *Treatise on Materia Medica* by Scottish physician William Cullen that led him towards what is now known as homeopathy. Cullen's text noted that the symptoms produced by quinine in a healthy body were similar to the symptoms it helped remove in illness. From this position Hahnemann conceived the notion that 'like could be used to treat like' in medical practice. It was not a totally new idea and in fact was mirrored in a statement by Hippocrates that 'fever is produced by what it suppresses and is suppressed by what it produces.'

The word 'homeopathy' derives from a Greek expression *homoion pathos* meaning *like* treatment of disease, or treating disease with the same substance; Hahnemann adopted another word 'allopathy' to describe the use of other, or *unlike* substances to remedy a complaint. The use of aspirin to relieve headaches is an example of this. Hahnemann first expressed his homeopathic ideas in an essay written in 1796 in which he rejected the concept of curing symptoms. From the start he took an organic view of the total man and was interested in the relationship of energy to matter. In this sense he preceded Wilhelm Reich, Rudolph Steiner and Carl Jung who would similarly ponder on the nature of a vital life-force. Hahnemann began to experiment along the lines of 'like curing like' by using potent poisons on himself, in small doses. He produced artificial disease in his body which he then eliminated with dilutions of the same substances. Included in his tests were aconite, strychnine and belladonna. Hahnemann continued to confound the medical establishment with his unorthodox approach. He had qualified as a doctor in 1779 so he could not be dismissed as a quack, and in 1810 he published a major work *The Organon of Medicine* . He followed it in 1828 with *Chronic Diseases,* which described the historical influence and recurrence of crippling major diseases over several centuries.

In essence homeopathy depends on the idea that the body contains its own healing properties and defence mechanisms and that these can be activated to eliminate illness. Hahnemann wrote 'All diseases are, in fact, diseases of the whole organism' and he considered them to be a sign that the vital force in the human organism was out of balance. In this sense pathological changes were a *result* of the alteration and imbalance, not a *cause* of it. Diseases expressed themselves through symptoms. 'When the physician has discovered all the observable symptoms of the disease that exist', he wrote, 'he has discovered the disease itself . . .' Hahnemann went on to classify disease states not in terms of dominant symptoms but in terms of the medicines that could be used to cure them.

A homeopathic doctor consequently records a very detailed list of the patient's total symptoms, many of which an orthodox, allopathic doctor would ignore. These symptoms are both physical and mental since homeopathy does not distinguish between mind and body in effecting a cure for the whole person. A homeopath does not look only for the most obvious symptoms of a complaint but also considers the accompanying emotional conditions: loss of weight, headache, debility, restless sleep, discomfort . . . and so on. Each treatment is accordingly highly individualised and homeopathic remedies are prescribed on this basis.

Homeopathy rejects the modern idea of a disease entity underlying the symptoms. Instead a symptom is regarded as the expression of the body's will to rid itself of disease. Hahnemann argued that the medicine which produced the identical symptoms in a healthy body would produce a curative effect in an ailing one because in small doses it stimulated the natural healing process. When this was demonstrated, the medicine could be said to be 'proved' for that particular set of symptoms. For example in a healthy person calomel produces diarrhoea, bloody and mucous stools, increased bile and salivation. A disease state showing these symptoms is treated homeopathically with a dilution of calomel.

In his writings Samuel Hahnemann posited three major rules: *Prescription by the Law of Similars; Minimum Dose* and *Single Remedy.* These have become the guidelines for homeopathic practice.

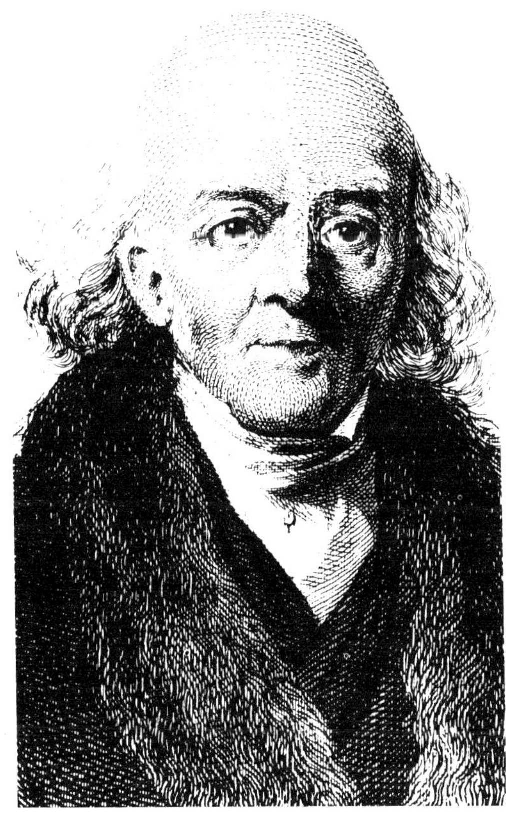

The founder of homeopathic medicine, Samuel Hahnemann

The Law of Similars

This is a reference to the idea of 'like treating like.' As we have noted, the homeopath records a detailed range of symptoms and treats the person rather than the disease. The symptoms are compared by the physician with a detailed listing of 'provings' and a remedy is prescribed on this basis. Hahnemann had noticed that medicines produced immediate effects on the organism, followed by later after-effects: *primary* and *secondary* symptoms respectively. A 'proving' is based on the initial response by the body to the medicine while the secondary effect is invariably quite the opposite and reflects the body's attempt to rid itself of disease. Consequently since the primary symptoms equate with the disease itself, the opposite effect produced by the organism neutralises or removes the disease. A 'primary symptom' remedy is therefore used to treat a set of symptoms where they arise in a sick person. Hahnemann managed to 'prove' around a hundred homeopathic remedies in his own lifetime.

The Minimum Dose

Because homeopathy initially aggravates the symptoms by adding to them (like to like), Hahnemann was obliged to reduce his medicinal doses considerably. He found that the primary symptoms lessened but the secondary responses, linked with the healing process, were unimpaired. The 'minimum dose' can be defined as the lowest potency required to provoke a reaction in the patient, and this in turn leads to an explanation of homeopathic 'dilutions'.

When a medicine is added to a solution of distilled water and alcohol in the ratio of one part medicine to nine parts water it is known as the 1x dilution, and in a 1 : 99 ratio as the 1c dilution. Remedies may involve dilutions up to 200x and beyond. The former are called 'low' dilutions and the latter 'high'. In everyday usage the strengths are usually around 6c and the medicines are taken every three or four hours until an improvement occurs. Dr A.C. Gordon Ross notes that in his own family medicine cabinet the following remedies were kept: tincture of *Arnica* for bruises; tincture of *Ledum* for stings; *Nux vomica* 6c, for stomach upsets; *Arsenicum album* 6c, for diarrhoeas; *Aconite* 6c, for early colds; *Gelsemium* 6c for influenzas. 'We became familiar with them and rarely required anything else. Sleeping pills, pep pills, tranquillizers, pills to reduce weight, pills for headaches, were quite unknown to us and we were the better for it.'

Dilutions are, nevertheless, one of the controversial aspects of homeopathy because Hahnemann believed that the 'higher' the dilution (i.e. the weaker), the stronger its medicinal effect, particularly where minerals were involved. The controversy arises where a homeopath uses a dilution beyond the 12c or 24x levels since these contradict the Avogadro Law. This states that the number of molecules in a gram/molecular weight of substance is 6.0225 x 10^{23}. Where a dilution is, say, 10^{-24} it is scientifically unlikely that any molecular trace of the original substance remains in the dilution. Accordingly critics have claimed that such treatments are only placebos. However systematic testing appears to challenge Avogadro's Law. In 1928 H. Junker added certain substances in 10^{-27} ratios to bacterial cultures and found they affected the growth of bacteria. Technically, nothing should have happened. J. Patterson and W. Boyd in Scotland changed the Schick test for diptheria from positive to negative by applying an alum-precipitated toxoid in a dilution

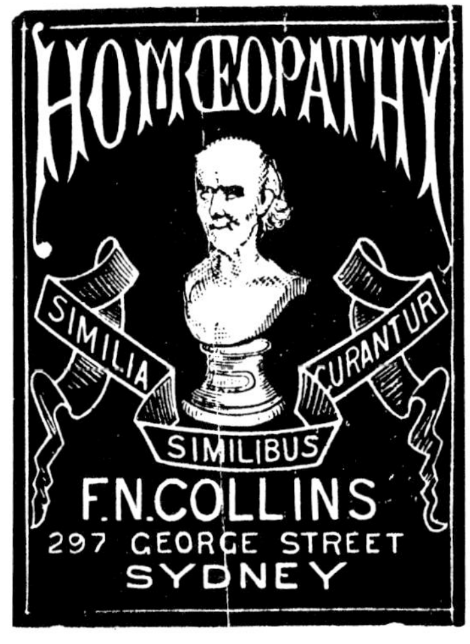

From an early homeopathic advertisement . . .

of 10^{-60}. Again, this shouldn't have happened. Other cases also exist in the scientific homeopathic literature.

The Single Remedy

A homeopath administers one remedy at a time since 'provings' are of one substance only. Even if one gave two substances apparently amounting to the manifested symptoms the cumulative effect could be quite different to the effects of the two substances individually. A chemical compound can only be used as a treatment if it has been 'proved' in its own right. Homeopaths use sodium carbonate and potassium sulphate among their many remedies.

In summary: *a homeopath prescribes a single substance in the minimum dose in conformity with the Law of Similars.*

Why has homeopathic medicine been so controversial? The answer seems to be that historically medical bodies have been caught up with power struggles, notions of authority and exclusiveness, and reasonably rigid concepts. Homeopathy was an 'alternative' during Hahnemann's lifetime and it remains so.

In the United States the American Institute of Homeopathy had been founded as early as 1844 but was immediately derided by the New York State Medical Society as a brand of quackery. In 1856 the AMA in that country banned discussion of homeopathic medical theory in journals and expelled members married to homeopathic practitioners. Most medical schools yielded to this pressure but the University of Michigan retained its curriculum. Nevertheless it proved to be a losing battle. Despite some homeopathic successes during the yellow fever epidemic in the South, the strength of the AMA and the growth of drug companies combined against Hahnemann's teachings. In 1910 homeopathic medicine was legally pronounced to be unprofessional and unscientific and eight years later there were only seven homeopathic institutes in the entire country. The Hahnemann Medical College of Philadelphia was obliged to switch from homeopathy to allopathy in the 1920s.

However in recent times a minor revival has been occurring in the United States, following a visit by leading Greek homeopath George Vithoulkas to a conference in California in 1978. It was agreed to establish a new foundation for maintaining homeopathic standards with schools of teaching in California and Athens. Many old-time homeopaths who had gone underground in the 1920s attended and there was new interest as well. The attitude of the AMA has not been noted.

In Britain, homeopathic medicine has had a less troubled existence because of its royal patronage. The Royal London Homeopathic Hospital was founded in 1850 and the late Sir John Weir, doyen of London homeopaths, was the personal physician to four monarchs including Queen Elizabeth. Homeopathy is recognised by the National Health Service although there are only around 300 registered members of the 'Faculty of Homeopathy'.

Quite aside from political and historical considerations, homeopathic medicine is philosophically opposed to the very tenets of allopathic medicine. As Richard Grossinger has written in *Planet Medicine*, from the homeopathic perspective allopathic doctors 'do not cure, they merely displace symptoms to ever less optimum channels of disease expression, each of which they consider to be a separate event because of its location in a new organ or region of the body. The disease meanwhile is driven deeper and deeper into the constitution because its mode of expression is cut off each time . . .' The American homeopath Constantine Hering (1800–1880) had discovered that when a sick person was treated by Hahnemann's methods, symptoms disappeared first from the vital areas of the body like the head and the heart and moved outwards to the extremities – the hands and toes. Many homeopaths today fear that since allopathic medicine tends to *suppress* symptoms through its techniques there will be an increasing rate of mental illness and heart disease . . . the reverse process taking place. In 1971 one third of the hospital beds in the United States were filled by mental patients.

And there is another side to this issue. Bacteriological research was one of the major forces overriding homeopathy at the turn of the century and consideration of a patient's *natural* resistance to disease was overshadowed. Now there is the distinct risk that some of the powerful new medicines have side-effects that have not been fully recognised. In its January 1969 issue *The Bulletin of Atomic Scientists* reported that more than 15% of all American hospital patients had iatronic illnesses, that is, caused by the medical treatment itself. Homeopaths are inclined to feel that this may represent the improper use of drugs by allopathic doctors who are concerned with treating obvious symptoms and ignoring the more minor manifestations of a personal illness. George Vithoulkas believes that modern medicine has often engaged itself in what he calls the 'false cure': 'Since allopathic drugs are never selected according to the Law of Similars they inevitably superimpose upon the organism a new drug disease which then must be counteracted by the organism'. Such charges do not please orthodox medical practitioners or their administrative bodies and although there are doctors who are medically trained in both allopathic methods and homeopathic treatments, any truce between the two traditions is unlikely to be an easy one. Despite its controversial history, homeopathy claims to be more specific in eliminating the symptoms of disease since it treats the total organism and not just isolated organs or body functions and rejects the notion of classifying disease categories. Some homeopaths even claim that 'there are no diseases . . . only sick people', and the debate continues.

PETER CHAPPELL

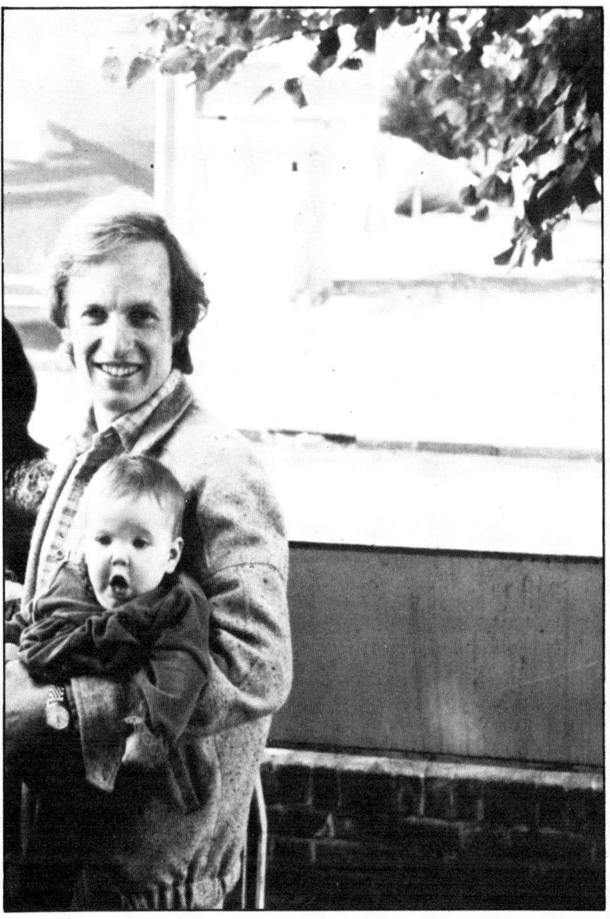

People come into the healing professions from every conceivable background. Before turning to homeopathy, Peter Chappell worked as an electronics engineer, moved into computer electronics and then began to question what he was doing with his life. At this period he became interested in Re-evaluation counselling, a method in which two people act reciprocally as counsellors for one another – each taking an equal time to give and receive attention. His interest in it grew and eventually he turned his home into a small counselling community run on cooperative lines. Counselling led him to investigate other therapeutic methods and he finally arrived at homeopathy. He met Thomas Vaughan, a man who had spent a lifetime in its study and practice, trained with him and then set up on his own.

When he talks of his work as a homeopathic practitioner, Peter Chappell emphasises the importance of listening and observing. His ability to do so himself is very apparent. Even talking to him one feels that he is picking up unsaid messages being transmitted with the spoken word. A rather different response to that of the ritual five minutes given by many GP's, followed by a scribbled prescription. One tries to listen, he says, to the general 'energy' behind what is being expressed. Is it anger, is it grief, or resentment, or sadness, or what? He tries to tune in to these things. By nature an optimist, in dealing with his patients he takes a positive view of them. He encourages them to get their lives to function better.

'Ill-health is so often the outcome of an unsatisfactory lifestyle.' In this context homeopathic medicine helps to 'get their energy moving'. He tells of one patient whose symptoms were related to her underlying anger. Homeopathically there are a number of remedies appropriate to this symptom, but it was the way she spoke of her husband, how she related to me and the world that helped him decide the most suitable remedy. 'What I would expect to come out of that treatment would be a more positive approach to life. I would regard that as a good prescription with a good result.' The situation is similar in the case of grief. So many people, he says, are unaware of the grief locked inside them. 'When I take the history of a patient, I may find that they lost their father as a child, or a brother or sister died, or perhaps a boy-friend jilted them. One begins to unravel a whole family history that has left its mark. You may be dealing with a person who has internalised their grief and it's a question of prescribing the right remedy for them to bring them out of the past and be alive in the present'.

In his consultations Peter Chappell will often go back several generations to trace the weaknesses that have most likely been transmitted. He has found that homeopathic remedies work for all races, colours and creeds, for the whole range of human ailments, from simply physical to disturbances of the psyche. Among his patients are those who come because orthodox medicine has failed them. Perhaps they have read an article about homeopathy, or heard a radio or television programme about it and decided to try it as a last resort

What of the comment that homeopathic medicine works through a placebo effect? Perhaps, he says, you should tell that to the cat I recently healed, or the many young children among my patients. I doubt if they have ever heard of a placebo but they still seem to regain their health!

Peter Chappell is active in many areas of homeopathy. He is a member of the Society of Homeopaths, which maintains a register of qualified practitioners and works to promote research into homeopathy. He is also associated with the College of Homeopathy which teaches the pure Hahnemannian principles of the method. A number of his patients have become students at the college. A recent venture he has introduced is a class for teaching people, especially parents, the basic principles so that in certain circumstances they can prescribe for themselves. He believes that homeopathy has a great potential for becoming a self-help system of medicine and is doing his part to bring it about. 'I aim to practise the pure form of homeopathy as taught by Hahnemann. It is over 175 years old and it works as well today as it ever did.' His underlying philosophy in all his work is an awareness of the holistic nature of the treatment he gives and of life itself.

HYPNOTHERAPY

Hypnotism is popularly known as 'mesmerism', and historically hypnosis derives originally from Anton Mesmer's theories of 'animal magnetism' conceived in the 18th century. Mesmer did not originate the concept of magnetism itself and references to it can be found in the works of Paracelsus, J.B. Van Helmont and Robert Fludd. However soon after Mesmer graduated in medicine from the University of Vienna in 1766 he began to use magnetism in his treatments. His first patient, Frauline Oesterline, was an epileptic. Mesmer attached three magnets to her stomach and both legs and was pleased when she claimed that painful subtle energies within her were subsiding to the lower part of her body. Her convulsive symptoms disappeared after six hours.

Later Mesmer went to Paris where he treated wealthy aristocrats in lavish consulting rooms. Mesmer wore a shirt of leather, lined with silk, to prevent his personal 'magnetic fluid' from escaping from his body. His patients meanwhile were asked to sit in a circle around a tub filled with water and iron filings. A number of iron rod conductors protruded from the tub and the patients were asked to hold these while also being bound by a cord in a continuous circle, to close the 'force'. Mesmer claimed that magnetism from the tub would transfer to the patients, alleviating illness. By 1784 Mesmer's colleague M. D'Eslon was combining induced trance as well. A report by the French scientist Jean Bailly is as follows:

The sick persons, arranged in great numbers, and in several rows around the baquet (tub), received the magnetism by means of the iron rods, which conveyed it to them from the baquet by the cords wound round their bodies, by the thumb which connected them with their neighbours and by the sounds of a pianoforte, or an agreeable voice, diffusing magnetism in the air. The patients were also directly magnetised by means of the finger and wand of the magnetiser, moved slowly before their faces, above or behind their heads, or on the diseased parts. The magnetiser acts also by fixing his eyes on the subjects; by the application of his hands on the region of the solar plexus, an application which sometimes continues for hours.

Meanwhile the patients present a very varied picture. Some are calm, tranquil and experience no effect. Others cough and spit, feel pains, heat or perspiration. Others again, are convulsed . . .

Mesmer and his followers claimed that a fluid or force radiated from the magnetiser to the subject but this view was disputed by Alexandre Bertrand, a young French physician. Bertrand made a study of induced trance and pub-

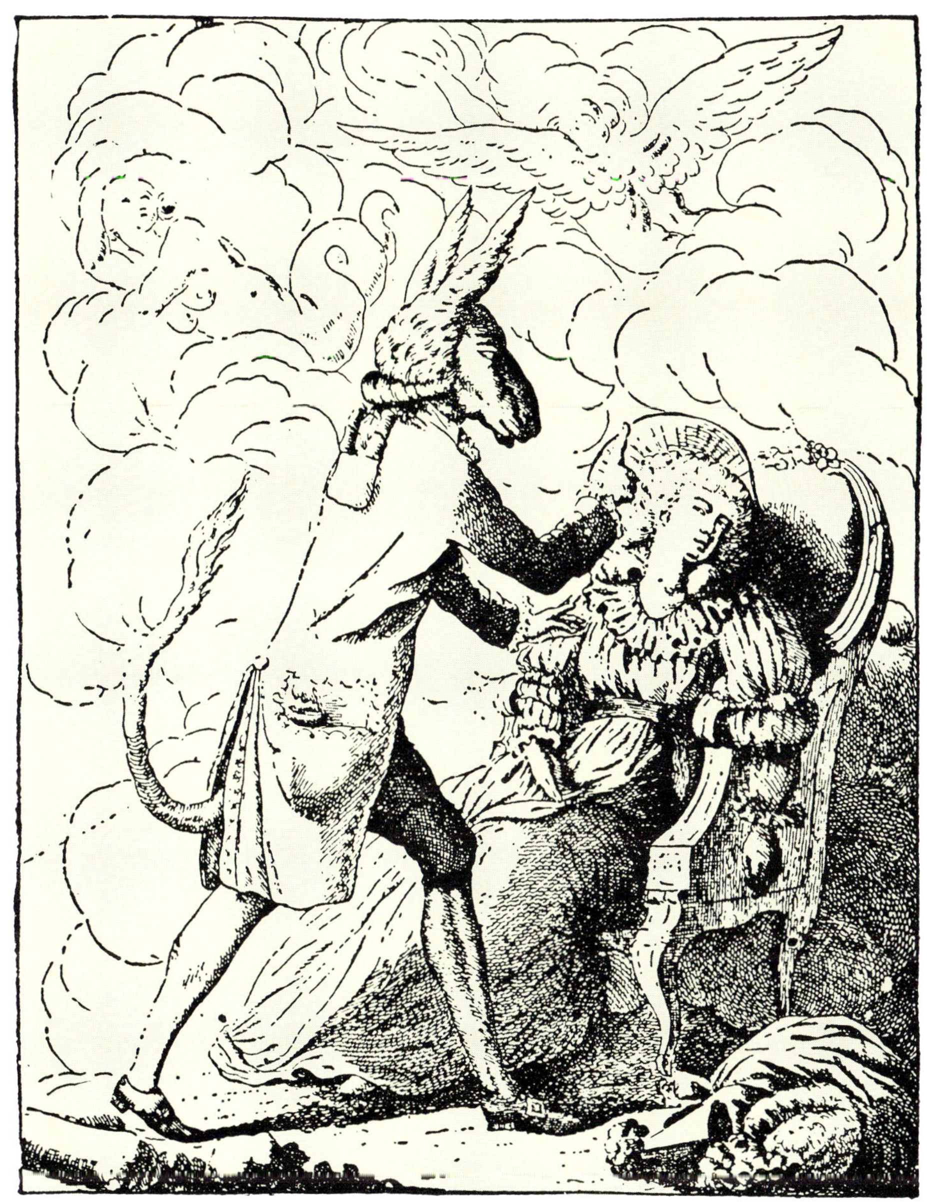

'Animal magnetism' was the precursor of modern hypnotherapy. This illustration is a caricature of Mesmer's techniques

lished two important works, *Traite du Somnabulisme* (1823) and *Du Magnetisme Animal en France* (1826). He believed that the cures resulting from treatment in trance states did not derive from animal magnetism but from the suggestions of the practitioner acting on the imagination of the patient whose suggestibility was increased.

Dr James Braid, a Scottish surgeon practising in Manchester, arrived independently at the same conclusions as Bertrand. Braid had observed a demonstration of 'animal magnetism' by the Swiss mesmerist Charles Lafontaine in 1841 but rejected the theories of Mesmer. Instead he put forward his own view – in a book titled *Neurypnology* published in 1843 – that the combined state of relaxation and enhanced awareness should be called *hypnotism*. He took the term from the Greek work *hypnos*, meaning 'sleep'.

Braid remained somewhat unorthodox himself, and included phrenology in his hypnotic treatments. He claimed that as the hypnotist placed his fingers on different parts of the scalp the patient passed from one emotion to another.

Despite these views, which are not accepted today, Dr Braid is credited with being the founder of medical hypnosis.

Braid's analysis of hypnotism was understandably limited and, in fact, such treatment has far wider ramifications. Hypnotism is not equivalent to sleep although hypnotic trance may be brought on by progressive relaxation. The range of hypnotic conditions is interesting. Some subjects can be induced to become hyperactive in trance, while a Russian study also discovered that 20 out of 25 hypnotised subjects in an experiment could perceive and remember spoken material presented during sleep without realising they were doing so.

Hypnosis is an altered state of consciousness which involves the patient in intensifying personal concentration and attentiveness, an enhancement of memory and increased suggestibility to cues from the therapist. Hypnotic states, as we have noted, are usually induced by relaxation although the

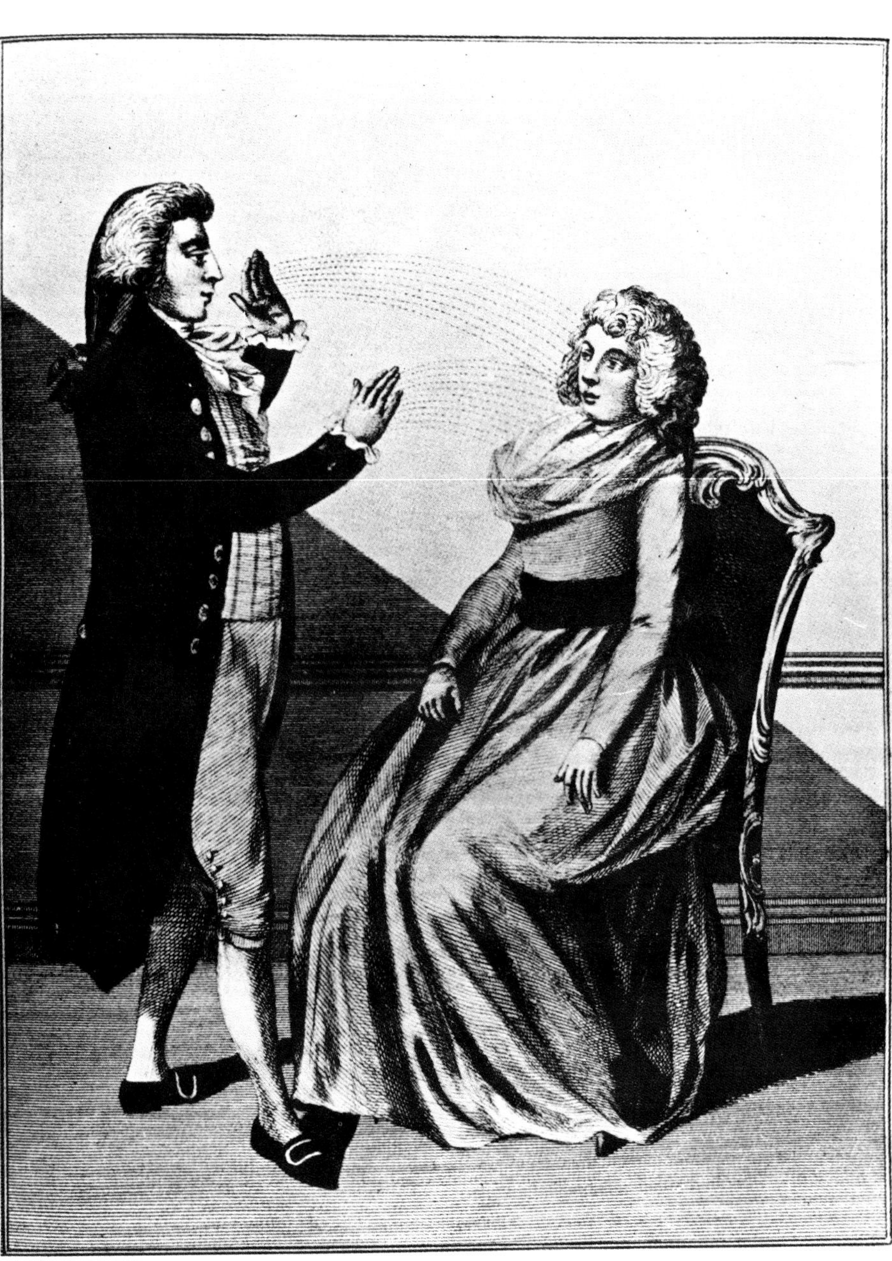

Originally hypnotism was regarded as a transfer of energy. This view has now been rejected

Balinese fire dancers and Whirling Dervishes, for example, use different methods for entering trance. The trance condition appears to be generally accompanied by high readings of alpha brainwaves, which are also characteristic of meditative states.

Mesmer's idea that the practitioner transfers 'waves of force' to the patient has now been rejected. The hypnotic situation does not involve *control* of one person by another as such. The hypnotist transfers the patient to a mental state where he can overcome blockages presented by his normal state of consciousness and explore the regions of his own mind.

Dr Milton Erickson confirms that the results of hypnosis do not derive from the therapist but from the patient himself:

. . . the hypnotised person remains the same person. His behaviour only is altered by the trance state but, even so, that altered behaviour derives from the life experience of the patient and not from the therapist . . . the therapist merely stimulates the patient into activity, often not knowing what that activity may be, and he then guides the patient and exercises clinical judgment in determining the amount of work to be done to achieve the desired results.'

Hypnotherapists emphasise that the reactivation of memories, for example, has positive value to the individual concerned and is certainly not dangerous. Raphael H. Rhodes notes: 'Hypnotism never harms the memory; rather, it strengthens it. Hypnosis achieves its results not by destroying mental channels but by reclaiming them.'

Modern Applications of Hypnotherapy

Hypnotherapy is often used to treat such problems as smoking and obesity. Very often the strategy involves replacing the pleasurable feelings associated with smoking and eating with disagreeable emotions in an effort to rid the patient of his habit. In the trance state, the patient is told that he will be increasingly less inclined to indulge his habit and controlling it will contribute to his self-esteem and feelings of happiness. Doctors Herbert and David Spiegel use the following variant in treating smoking through techniques of self-hypnosis:

'For my body, smoking is poison.'
'I need my body to live.'
'To the extent that I want to live,
I owe my body this respect and protection.'

Other conditions such as alcoholism, phobias, migraine and asthma can also be treated by hypnotherapy. Dr S.J. Van Pelt, who has been the President of the British Society of Medical Hypnotists, believes that hypnotism can be very effective in treating alcoholism providing there is a real desire to be cured. Van Pelt believes it is possible that alcoholism may be the result of a post-hypnotic suggestion self-given in an accidentally self-induced hypnotic state. Alcoholics are particularly good hypnotic subjects and are also victims of their own emotions. A typical case from Van Pelt's files concerns a married woman aged 45 who had begun to drink for social reasons. As her commitments increased she drank increasingly to cover up her nervousness. As she realised she was becoming dependent on alcohol she had an awful realisation that she might finish up in an asylum 'like her father' but this led her to drink even more heavily in order to bury her fears. Orthodox

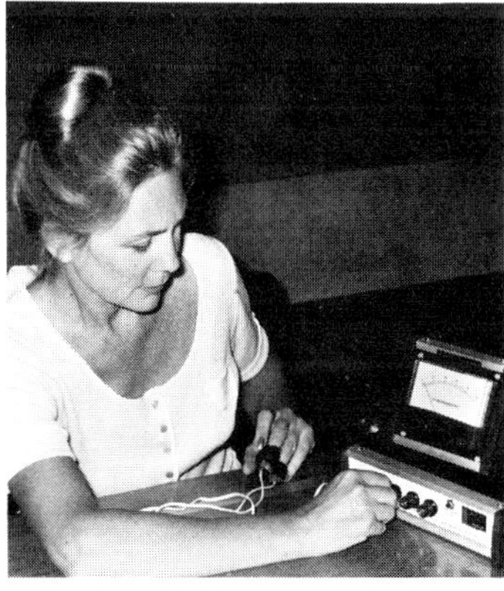

Australian hypnotherapist Natalie Matyuk demonstrating the use of biofeedback in treatment

medical treatment was of no avail but she responded perfectly to a few hypnotic sessions.

The Spiegels have preferred to develop techniques of self-hypnosis to avoid their patients becoming dependent on the therapist. Their instruction for asthma is as follows (from *Trance and Treatment)*:

As you feel yourself floating, imagine that the tubes in your lungs are slowly opening up, and cool, fresh air is entering them. As you feel yourself floating with these cool breezes coming into your lung, you develop a tingling numbness inside your lungs, and an opening of the bronchial tubes. By concentrating on this floating sense and on the feeling of a cool breeze in your lungs, you enable your lungs to open up. In this way you will find that each breath is a little deeper. Every time you take a new breath, you find that you're able to inhale a bit more deeply, and you feel your lungs opening up and getting wider and wider.

Who are the best hypnotic subjects?

It used to be thought that neurotics were especially suggestible, and women more hypnotisable than men, making them better subjects; however neither situation appears to be the case. Good hypnotic subjects usually perceive themselves as co-operative, trusting and emotive. They are capable of inward concentration and do not resist transferring from one spatial orientation to another. Poor subjects on the other hand are strongly rational, prefer to be in control than extend trust to someone else, are critical of new ideas and like to stay in their present spatial environment. The factor of sex does not pertain in hypnotism and it is generally considered that the claim that women make better subjects derives from the sexist judgment that women are more passive than men.

Hypnotism has had an extremely colourful history but is now regarded as a valuable medical technique. Those wishing to seek hypnotherapy treatment are advised to consult specialists trained in clinical methods.

NATALIE MATYUK

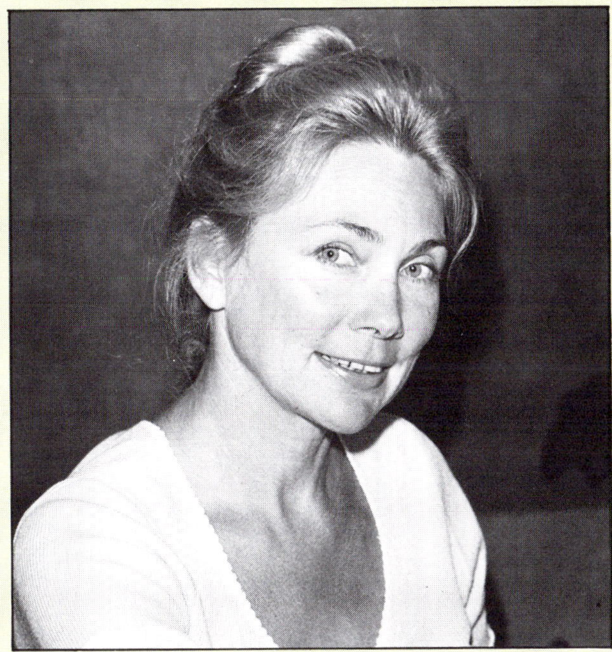

Born in Harbin, Manchuria, of Russian parents, Natalie Matyuk grew up with a passion for ballet. Strikingly attractive, with blue-grey eyes and long flowing blonde hair, Natalie could easily have been drawn to a career in film or theatre, but it was not to be. At the age of 18 she emigrated with her family to Australia and undertook university studies which culminated in a degree in applied chemistry with a double major in psychology. She then completed her Arts degree and is now practising as a clinical psychologist. When she was studying she found the traditional behaviourist frameworks of modern psychology rather limited. Her natural orientation was towards a more humanistic mode and she found herself drawn to the work of such figures as Abraham Maslow, Carl Rogers and the Gestalt Therapists. Following a series of family crises, including the death of her grandmother and her father, Natalie became deeply interested in the work of Elisabeth Kubler-Ross and attended her lectures; she also acquired a lasting fascination with Jung's frameworks of the unconscious mind.

During the last year of her Master's degree Natalie began to simultaneously pursue studies in hypnotherapy through the auspices of the Australian Society for Clinical and Experimental Hypnosis. Influenced by medical hynotherapists like Dr Howard Merrington and Richard Warburton, she now felt a strong urge to research in depth the potentialities of the psyche, especially in relation to mental health. However she found that often the formal medical approach to mental problems focused on symptoms rather than eliminating causes.

In recent times Natalie has been strongly influenced by the American Transpersonal Movement which emphasises holistic methods of healing and values well-being and the visionary aspects of human potential. In particular she has found strong affinity with the writings of Frances Vaughan who practises as a psychologist while also holding an academic post as Professor of Psychology at the Californian Institute of Transpersonal Psychology. Frances Vaughan has become well known for her perceptive works *Awakening Intuition* and *Beyond Ego*, and Natalie Matyuk has employed a comparable approach of heightening unconscious creative potentialities in her work as a hypnotherapist. In general she tries to develop the creative impulses in her patients and to encourage the healing process through self-expression. On one occasion a 56 year old woman studying to become a barrister came to her with excruciating writer's cramp that appeared to have a psychosomatic origin. Natalie helped to build her confidence and focus on her powers of creativity. In a single session the patient was cured of her cramp but also discovered that she could write beautiful poetry that for years had been trying to manifest!

Another case involved a shift-worker in his mid-30s who suffered from such extreme anxiety that his bowel movements were being affected disastrously. Orthodox medical examination had revealed no specific cause for the problem. Under hypnosis the subject revealed to Natalie Matyuk that he had a strong desire to paint although he did not do so in real life. Using guided imagery techniques, Natalie planted post-hypnotic suggestions that would encourage him to paint landscapes, and after three sessions the young man began to vigorously pursue his new interest. After a week the bowel problem had totally disappeared and the anxiety had vanished.

Natalie says that her therapy sessions are usually short and condensed, and she feels that many unscrupulous hypnotherapists have clouded the value of the techniques by being greedy and extending therapy unnecessarily. In her own practice Natalie employs biofeedback equipment and trains her patients in self-hypnosis techniques so that they can subsequently pursue their own course of self-development. Invariably she also asks them to try meditation and related consciousness-expanding techniques like Tai Chi and Yoga.

Natalie finds hypnotherapy especially valuable for treating migraines, high blood pressure, insomnia and other psychosomatic problems. She has also investigated the controversial domain of orthomolecular psychiatry, especially the use of mega-vitamins in treating schizophrenia, and believes that this is a new and valuable area of research.

While, in a sense, Natalie Matyuk has become something of a 'loner' among local hypnotherapists, she has found allies in the International Transpersonal Movement where the pursuit of holistic health methods has strong support. She now regards her main role as one combining both healing and teaching so that her subjects can be guided by hypnotherapy to explore the domains of higher consciousness.

IRIDOLOGY

It is often said that the eye is the mirror of the soul and in recent years the scientific practice of iris analysis, or iridology, has lent substantial weight to the view that the eye is a detailed map of personal health and well-being.

Modern iridology owes a great deal to the Hungarian doctor Ignatz von Peczeley who published his analysis of the iris in Germany in 1881. Peczeley believed that the iris was an indicator of organic disease and that specific afflicted organs could be highlighted in iris diagnosis. His work included charts correlating sections of the iris with various organs and life-systems in the body.

Shortly afterwards the Swedish homeopath Nils Lilequist published a complementary work titled *Diagnosis From The Eye* which annotated changes in iris pigmentation following the presence of such substances as quinine and iodine in the body.

Today iridology attracts a strong following in Europe where there are at least 10 000 practitioners, and there is increasing interest in the United States, Australia and the United Kingdom also.

Dr Bernard Jensen, whose iris diagrams are central to the subject, developed a complex system of dividing the iris into 96 components consisting of radial, circular and segmental sections. In many ways his iris diagrams resemble a clock, with specific areas of the body featured around the dial. As one looks at the left iris of another person, for example, one may highlight the neck area around 1 o'clock, the spleen at 4 o'clock, the kidneys between 6 and 7 and the thyroid near 10.

Generally speaking, iridologists divide the iris into three concentric circles. The innermost one corresponds to food preparation and absorption, the second one to organs of transport and utilisation and the outermost one to organs of structure and support.

In any iris, fibres radiate outwards from the pupil to the periphery. Dr Jensen introduced the concept of 'fine silk' and 'coarse burlap' to differentiate the relative textures of the iris and there are many other tell-tale signs of health reflected in the iris fibre patterns. Broadly, there are two main categories of iris signs. The first relate to changes of density in the fibres and are indicative of organic changes in the body. The second are changes in pigmentation and may relate to the presence of drugs, chemicals or toxic substances in the circulation systems.

Both Dr Jensen and another noted iridologist Theodore Kriege have isolated three primary iris colours: blue, grey and brown. When a person is in

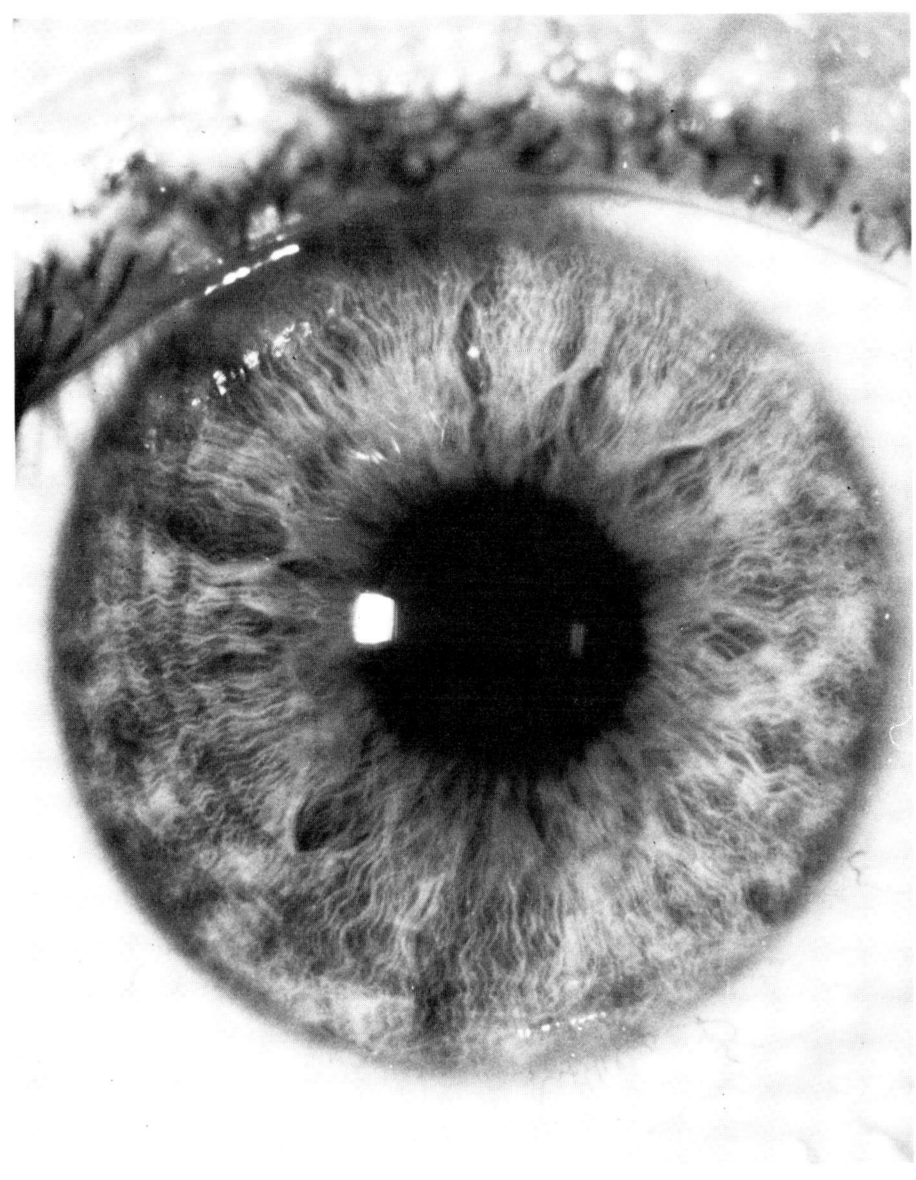

Probing the iris for its mysteries

a good state of health the colours of the iris are bright, clear and vibrant. Ill-health is reflected by dull iris coloration. Kriege believes that accentuated lines, flakes and clouds in the iris are problem areas and Australian iridologist Dorothy Hall has highlighted the negative presence of *radii solaris*, or dark incisive lines in the iris as a sign to watch for. A typical pattern of health decline in a person with blue eyes would show firstly an accentuation of white markings (acute) becoming yellow (subacute), transforming to grey (subchronic) and finally black (chronic). The sequence would be reversed as health was regained.

Why should the iris reflect all these changes? The American iridologist Dr Henry Lindlahr believes that the fine nerve filaments of the iris receive impressions from, and are linked with every organ and nerve system in the body. It is these connections which allow for specific correlations between sections of the iris and other parts of the human organism. Abnormal nerve impulses throw the nerve fibres out of alignment and capillary circulation activity causes alteration to the pigments in the surface layers of the iris.

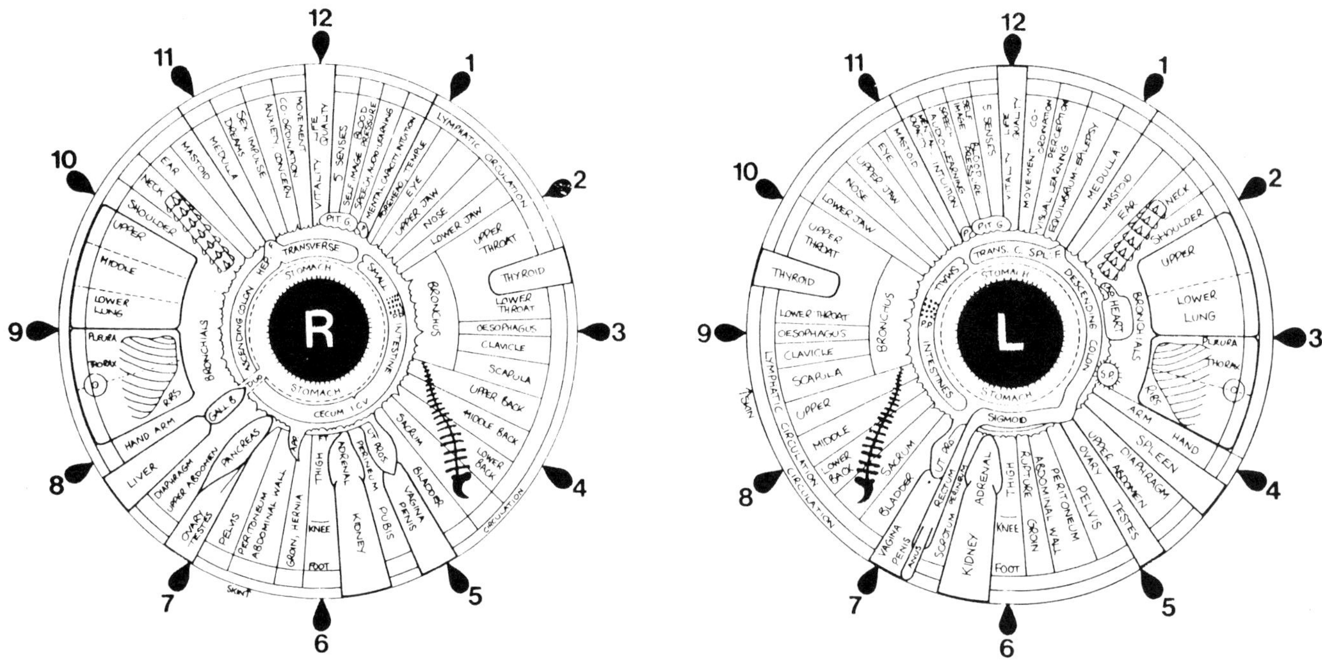

The Iris Map, right eye (looking at another person's right eye)
The Iris Map, left eye (looking at another person's left eye)

A Californian optometrist, Dr James Carter, maintained detailed health histories of his patients and observed changes in their irises over a two year period. Carter agrees with Lindlahr that the iris reflects body abnormalities. Since the iris is so closely connected with the brain, and also the circulation and nervous systems, and since the iris also absorbs and retains toxins, changes of colour are a very accurate guide to abnormalities. It is also evident that since the iris is linked to the sympathetic nervous system it responds to stress, and the fibres move their position accordingly.

Carter has come to the viewpoint that iridology is a particularly valuable predictive tool since it shows 'warning signs'. For example it is possible to warn of an impending heart attack by focusing examination of the iris on the areas associated with the organs likely to cause it. The blood circulation regions of the iris would also be important in such analysis.

Although the iris diagrams seem extremely complex the actual diagnosis by the iridologist is comparatively straightforward. Usually the practitioner uses a glass of between 4 and 10 times magnification and holds a pen-light at an angle to the iris in order to illuminate the fibre markings. Detailed diagnosis comes with practice but any person using a recognised iridology manual will be able to benefit to some degree by analysing his or her own fibre patterns.

Iridologists vary in the extent of their dependence on this technique. The eye has been compared with the mandala and as such described as a reflection of the whole person. Dorothy Hall is more cautious. 'Iridology', she notes, 'is not a complete system of medical, emotional, personality, and type analysis on its own. . . . It is a tool only, a screen from which to read off visually many things about a person'. All iridologists are agreed, though, that the iris offers a remarkably detailed and sensitive map of the body health and as such iridology is one of the most central natural therapies in alternative medicine.

DOROTHY HALL

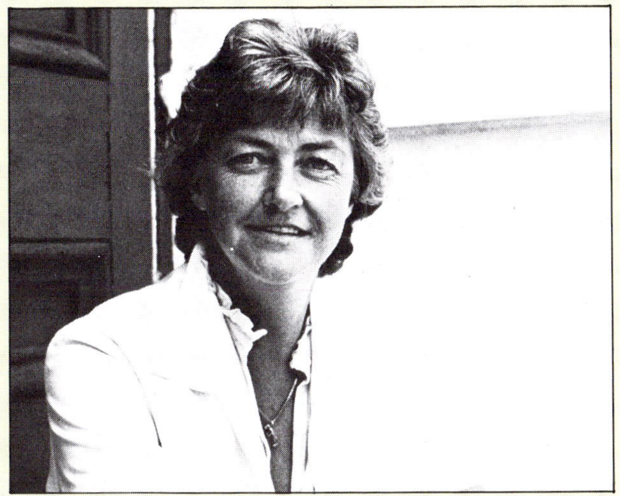

The College of Herbal Medicine, a crisply renovated late Victorian building, faces imposingly onto the otherwise dusty Darling Street in Sydney's inner suburb of Rozelle. Inside, by way of contrast, the appealing aroma of medicinal plants adds a special quality to the atmosphere.

Sydney-born Dorothy Hall has been teaching herbalism, naturopathy and iridology here for five years and at present has nine associates and between 160 and 180 students. She is also very busy consulting and treating patients. Many of the people who come to the College to train are from orthodox medical or scientific backgrounds – current doctors, nurses, biochemists and social workers who want to obtain an additional perspective on illness and different facets of healing. Invariably they gain a great deal from the learning process, as do the teachers and practitioners themselves. According to Dorothy Hall while she and her associates may outline naturopathic theories to the students and patients, they look to the latter to prove the theory through their symptoms and their growth back to health. Learning here is very much a two-way process.

Dorothy has been aware of, and surrounded by, the beneficial effects of nature as long as she can remember. Her grandfather was a government agronomist and she can recall growing and gathering herbs from an early age at the family home in Gordon, where the nursery had 4500 plants! Later, as people inquired about their uses, she found herself acquiring an increasing knowledge of their medicinal properties.

From the age of 19 she practised at home a herbalist, began to lecture, and undertook further training at the Double Bay College of Naturopathic Medicine. Later she would extend her studies at the Heilpraktilser Schaft and Schule in Munich and Dr Vogel's Clinic in Basel, but meanwhile in Sydney she lectured to naturopathic students and acupuncturists about new frontiers in healing.

One of the 'revived' sciences pioneered in Germany and Russia was iridology, a subject which is now locally synonymous with Dorothy Hall following her recent breakthroughs in this field. Dorothy believes that the eye, in her own words, is 'a map of the person'. The iris is a sensitive tuning tool which allows her to diagnose current traumas and illnesses existing in the body. Deeply felt emotional and organic malfunctions will eventually manifest in the patterns of the iris fibres, with resultant changes of colours and shapes.

While many alternative medicine therapies are eastern in orientation, iridology is primarily western in scope for the simple reason that it is easier to recognise colour shifts in a blue European eye than in the characteristically deep brown Asian one. Dorothy also believes that eastern and western medicine should not be mixed haphazardly, since the metabolism and diet of nationalities from different regions is quite distinct. Eastern peoples tend to have a metabolism built on sodium and potassium minerals while the western person draws more on calcium and magnesium. The hardest cases to treat are those of mixed metabolism, where the patient has a rich and varied cultural background!

Dorothy Hall feels strongly that she needs the patient to be present during her consultation. It isn't advisable, for example, to attempt diagnosis only from a photograph of the iris. At least half the time taken during any session is 'educative' – Dorothy endeavours after evaluating the patient's total living environment to 'explain the process whereby the body became ill'. She doesn't talk in terms of cures but believes rather that her purpose is to increase the efficiency of the traumatised part of the body. Where there is well-being there is no illness. There are of course occasions where patients may need further clinical help and Dorothy Hall freely admits that it is often beneficial to refer her patients to orthodox medical practitioners, especially when they have a complaint like acute appendicitis or a large cyst. Her naturopathic methods are intended to complement and work alongside western medicine not establish a sense of opposition.

Where does Dorothy Hall go from here? Following a recent visit to Egypt and the Middle East, Dorothy believes a vast new area of knowledge needs to be unfolded in terms of recording ancient medicinal techniques. With Dr Roy Hand, an Egyptologist who has worked in the Cairo and British museums, she hopes to unravel more completely the detailed healing knowledge of the ancient Egyptians, whose medical papyri she believes have frequently been wrongly translated. Quite apart from the remarkable range of herbal treatments practised by the Egyptians at such centres as Heliopolis and Alexandria, she also considers that they may have practised an early form of iridology. Recently in a museum Dorothy discovered two blue obsidian eyes from a sarcophagus and they had iridology-type fibre markings engraved on them! So there is much to discover. Some of Dorothy Hall's most important work probably still belongs to the future.

KIRLIAN DIAGNOSIS

Kirlian photographs are often strikingly beautiful and typical examples show a brightly coloured energy field or 'corona' surrounding the organism. In many cases the photograph is of a fingertip, palm impression or plant. The Kirlian process does not use a lens but records the electrical field surrounding the object placed on a photographic plate. In summary, the Kirlian 'camera' involves a flat metal plate with unexposed film positioned on top of it. The object is placed on the film and high voltage electricity at very low amperage is pulsed through the plate. The electricity passes through the film exposing it and when the latter is developed it shows the characteristic corona of light. An exposure time of between 0.3 and 0.5 seconds is usual although this varies according to the design of the Kirlian device.

The process was discovered accidentally by the Soviet electrician Semyon Kirlian who was called on one occasion to repair an instrument at a research institute. While he was there he happened to observe a person undergoing electrotherapy. He noticed tiny flashes of light between the electrodes and the skin and wondered if it would be possible to photograph these flashes. Kirlian burned himself in his own experiments but succeeded in producing an impression of luminescence around his fingers. For the next ten years Kirlian worked with his wife Valentina refining the process and developing new types of instruments. He claimed that his corona photographs produced information relating to the energy present in leaves, hands and fingers and noted that if photographs were taken immediately after a leaf was picked, for example, a clear and precise electrical field was depicted. Only an hour later, this field would be seen to diminish in subsequent photographs. The implication was that the 'life-force' was departing.

Dr Victor M. Inyushin, a biologist from the Kirov State University in Kazakhstan, believes that Kirlian photographs depict the so-called 'bioplasmic energy body' – a counterpart of the physical form, and reflects patterns of health and emotional states in human beings. Although there is some evidence for this view, it has its detractors also. Dr William Tiller of Stanford University concedes that some Kirlian patterns seem to parallel changes in emotional states and has put forward the view that this could result from changes in the skin's surface chemistry and electrical resistance which would influence the electrical field effect. However, it is a case of not reading too much into colour variations. In the *Journal of Applied Physics* (Issue 44, 1973) he wrote:

. . . we should not be at all surprised (or dismayed) to find a perfectly reasonable physical explanation for the generation of light and for the colour observations.

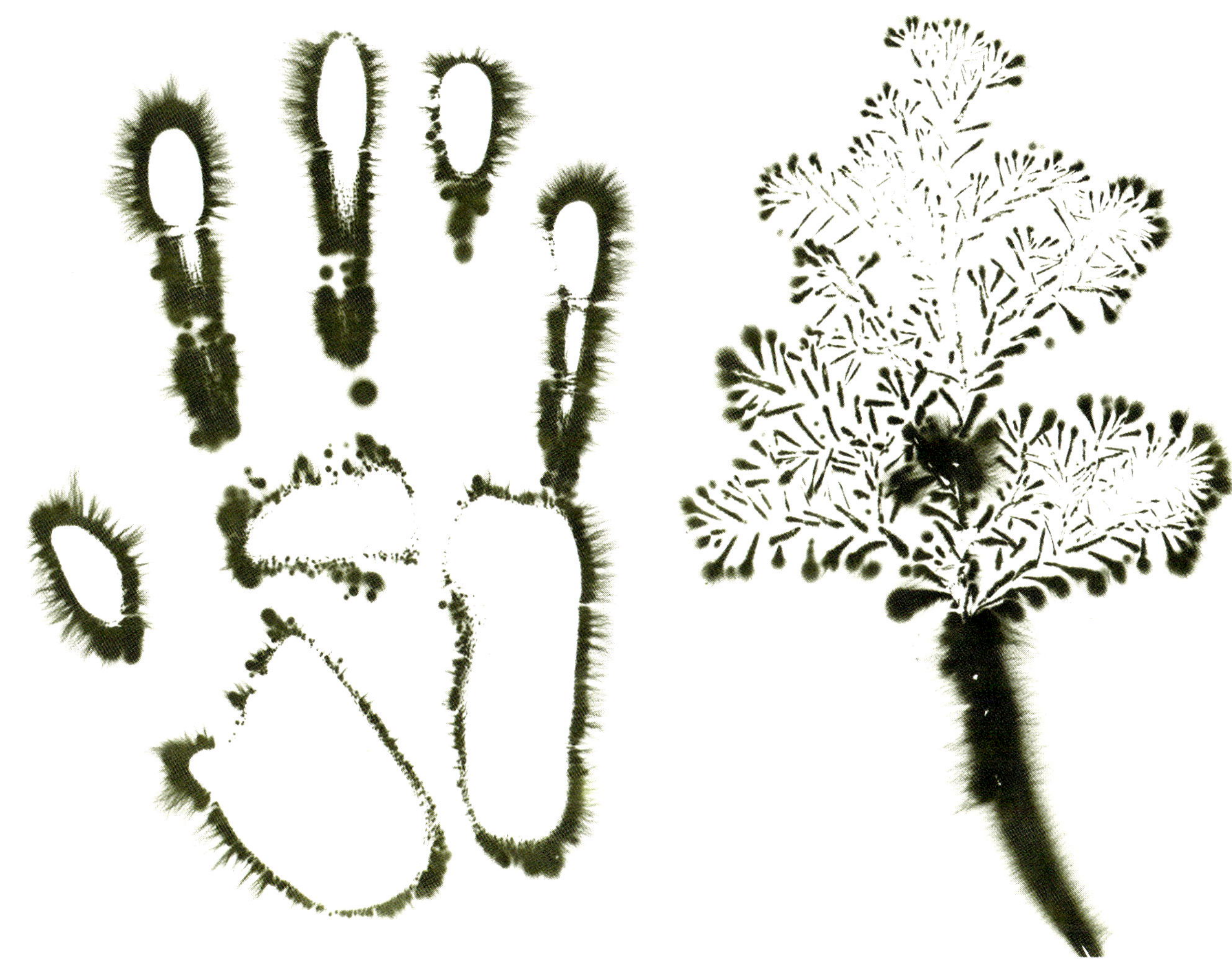

Kirlian photographs by Australian researcher Graydon Rixon

The important and difficult step is to prove that such observations are indeed directly correlated with energy changes in the living system, rather than just the random fluctuations associated with inadequate experimental techniques. This has not yet been proved one way or the other.

At UCLA Dr Thelma Moss began testing the possible links between health patterns and Kirlian photographs and conducted experiments with the psychic healer Olga Worrall. Dr Moss had noticed that if a leaf was scratched slightly and then photographed the wound was accentuated as a red blotch on the Kirlian photograph. In the experiments, when Olga Worrall passed her hand over a gashed leaf the blotch disappeared and the energy and colour of the original returned. Over a period about twenty 'green-thumb' healers were able to 'restore' brightness to damaged plants, but there were other subjects who had powers in quite the opposite direction. Their 'brown-thumbs' caused plants to wither and die and in some instances the Kirlian corona disappeared altogether!

Sometimes when a plant has its tip cut off, a phantom leaf effect appears on the photograph. The exposure must be taken within seconds of the severing and the effect does not occur consistently. Dr Moss finds a clear phantom image occurs only once in 400 cases although her colleague John Hubacher claims a 5% success rate. Hubacher, Kendall Johnson and Clark Dugger have all produced phantom images at UCLA and the effect has also been replicated by Viktor Adamenko in Sao Paulo, Brazil, and Robert Wagner at the Californian State University at Long Beach. The existence of an 'energy image' after removal of part of the plant tends to favour the hypothesis that living physical organisms are supported by an inter-related energy form, or 'bioplasmic body'. This aspect of Kirlian photography remains controversial but has suggestive implications for notions of the soul and human aura which have been central to religious and esoteric thought for centuries.

Thelma Moss is currently continuing her work on Kirlian analysis and health issues. During research on cancer tissues she conducted double-blind tests which demonstrated that Kirlian techniques could distinguish cancers from normal tissue and so had diagnostic value. Meanwhile tests have been held at the Heuristic Institute which appear to show visual energy changes in the fingers of cigarette smokers. Pictures were taken of the right index finger tips of all subjects after they had smoked for five minutes. A large red blotch with a kidney-like silhouette appeared on the fingertips of the smokers, above the fingernail. Non-smokers did not exhibit these effects.

Another researcher, James Kightlinger of the Shenango Valley Osteopathic Hospital at Farrell, Pennsylvania, has correlated Kirlian patterns with acupuncture meridians. After examining subjects with duodenal ulcers, carcinoma of the stomach, bronchitis and lung disease, he was interested to discover that they showed corona blockages in the acupuncture meridian areas of the feet and hands associated with the afflicted organs. In related research, David Sheinkin and Michael Schacter used Kirlian techniques to monitor the condition of schizophrenic and psychotic subjects and took photographs of the fingertips before and after treatment. Blurred images, red blotching and corona blockages were prevalent before psychiatric help but rehabilitated subjects showed the blue and white energy field associated with normal healthy people.

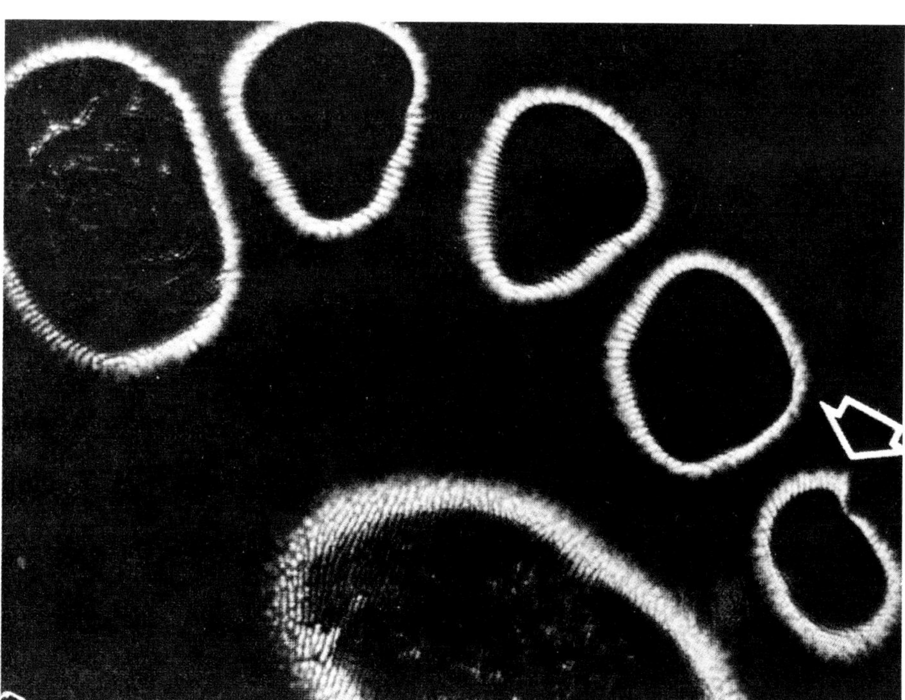

This Kirlian photograph shows an acupuncture connection between the small toe of the right foot and a defective kidney. From research conducted in the United States by James Kightlinger

Kirlian photographs remain controversial and researchers are still divided on the implications of what they actually depict. However there is no doubt that human Kirlian patterns do mirror changes in emotional states and perhaps reflect actual energy flow transitions. The evidence for the Soviet hypothesis of a 'bioplasmic body' seems to be increasing.

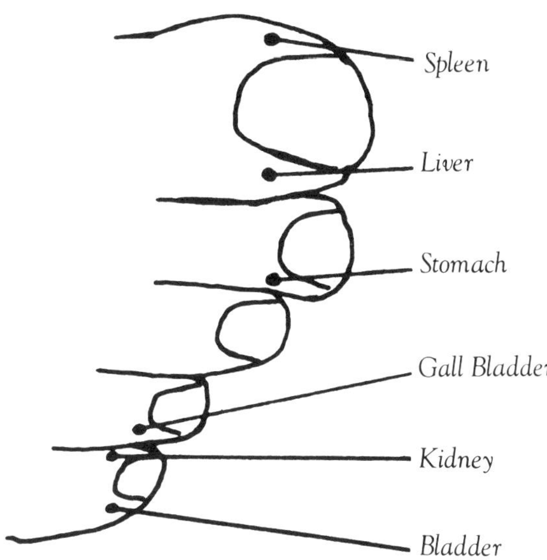

GRAYDON RIXON

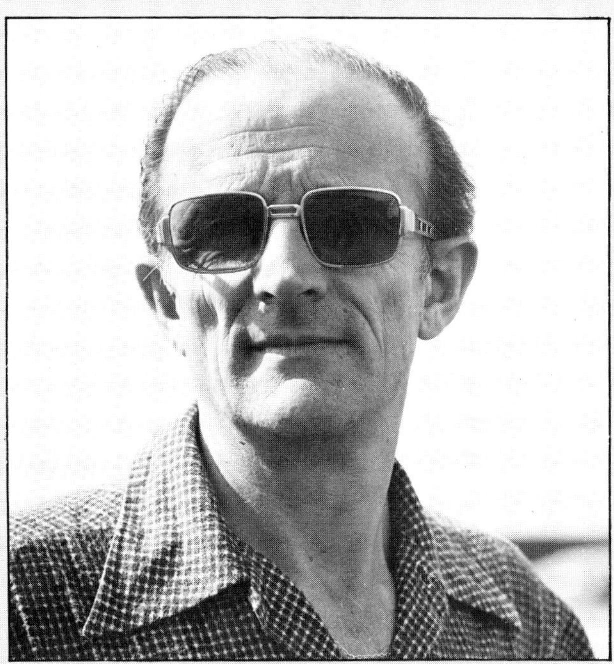

In recent years Graydon Rixon has become well known for his pioneering work in the field of Kirlian photography although he is also very interested in such areas as pyramid energy and the use of negative ions for health.

Originally trained in electronics and television maintenance, Graydon read Sheila Ostrander and Lynn Schroeder's book *Psychic Discoveries Behind the Iron Curtain* and realised that he had the practical knowledge to build his own Kirlian camera. Housed in the body of a portable tape recorder, his device included two glass sheets in an acrylic frame and between them transparent conductor liquid and an enclosing silver conductor wire. A horizontal glass section allowed 'photographs' of energy fields to be registered on photo-sensitive paper.

As with overseas Kirlian experiments Graydon has found that energy vortexes indicate the presence of life-force and, for example, in the case of detached, dying leaves, the energy fields can be seen gradually departing. With the human hand, energy fields are particularly noticeable streaming from the finger tips and they also align with major acupuncture points, thus indicating that Kirlian photography can assist considerably in our knowledge of medical and healing techniques.

Recently Graydon has been researching the effects various drugs have on Kirlian patterns. His initial experiments, which admittedly need further verification from other researchers, suggest that substances such as tobacco, alcohol, tea, coffee, valium and the psychedelics all register noticeable and detrimental effects on the energy body of the human organism. He has noticed with tobacco smokers, for example, that their Kirlian impressions show a marked reduction in 'life-force', while alcohol reveals a different pattern. Here the energy field seems to shrink into the body to combat the alcohol content and stays until it has been absorbed; the life-force then expands again to its normal position. With psychedelics like LSD and even the much milder intoxicant marijuana, the energy field which is normally closely aligned with the body image starts to displace itself and 'drift'. The implications of this are clear. Graydon claims that this drifting of the energy field is detrimental to health over an extended period of time and may be the cause of death in drug overdoses.

Aside from his Kirlian work, Graydon has been investigating the uses of pyramid frames for meditation and also the application of negative-ion producers to counter the effect of dust, carbon monoxide and other pollutants in the atmosphere. Graydon manufactures both products and has been particularly interested in any means of improving the psychic atmosphere of one's environment for meditative purposes.

For Graydon Rixon the spiritual side of his work is not something to be neglected or played down. He has found, in fact, that his research into parapsychology and energy fields has yielded significant results which complement his spiritual orientation. The son of a Baptist minister, Graydon went through the traumas of an unsuccessful marriage and then moved into a household where meditation was a regular practice. He found that his orthodox religious background was suddenly shown to be incomplete and he was keen to know more about altered states of consciousness. In 1970 he trained in the Mind Dynamics course – a system of active imagination techniques – and later taught it for 2 ½ years. Pursuing a western rather than eastern spiritual orientation he then discovered John Roger's Movement of Spiritual Inner Awareness and the Insight Training, which teaches its adherents to live with and accept the inherent beauty of all human beings. With a group of other people, Graydon and his second wife, Kharime, went through 50 hours of intensive work analysing behaviour reactions and 'unlocking energies' in a seminar conducted by John Roger himself. Since pursuing this approach Graydon now feels that he will use his Kirlian research to assist people who feel they are emotionally out of balance and searching for spiritual growth.

An active figure in Australia's New Age movement, Graydon, with Kharime and other friends and helpers, was recently involved in planning and implementing the third Mind, Body and Healing Festival at Morpeth in central New South Wales. A notable overseas visitor to this Festival was American Ken Keyes, whose work Graydon has been anxious to promote as a leading New Age philosophy. These festivals are now run by Loving Links, a non-profit organisation founded in 1979 by Graydon and Kharime. Loving Links supports the right of every person to follow his or her own spiritual path, linking all philosophies in harmony and supporting unconditional love as the eternal religious teaching.

Working for and helping people is the only path that gives Graydon Rixon personal satisfaction.

MACROBIOTICS

Macrobiotics is a term that was applied by Japanese philosopher George Ohsawa to the study of healthy, creative diet. Underlying the concept of macrobiotics is the traditional oriental distinction of *yin* and *yang*. *Yin* is the feminine, passive principle; *yang* masculine and active. In macrobiotics, foods are classified as being predominantly *yin* or *yang*.

YIN:
Grown in a hot climate
Generally acidic
Grown high above the ground
Fruits, leaves
Sweet and hot foods
Foods that are purple, blue or green
Foods that contain more water and perish quickly

YANG:
Grown in a cold climate
Generally alkaline
Grown below the ground
Roots, seeds
Salty and bitter foods
Foods that are red, yellow or orange
Foods that are dry and store well

Of course, many foods have both qualities and one has to consider the dominant aspects. Foods acquire many of their characteristics because of their patterns of growth. During the winter the energy in plants descends into the root system and at such times a plant is more *yang*. Plants such as carrots and turnips grow in late autumn and winter and store well, retaining their vitality. By contrast in the spring and beginning of summer the plant energy ascends and new green shoots appear. These plants contain more water, do not store for long periods, and are more *yin*.

Macrobiotics practitioners consider that illness arises when there is an excess of either *yin* or *yang* and that the diet should be balanced.

Cereal grains have a special place in macrobiotics because they combine seed and fruit (*yang* and *yin*) and span the complete vegetal cycle. They comprise 50–60% of the recommended macrobiotic diet and include whole wheat, barley, oats, brown rice, maize and rye. Fresh vegetables represent 20–30%

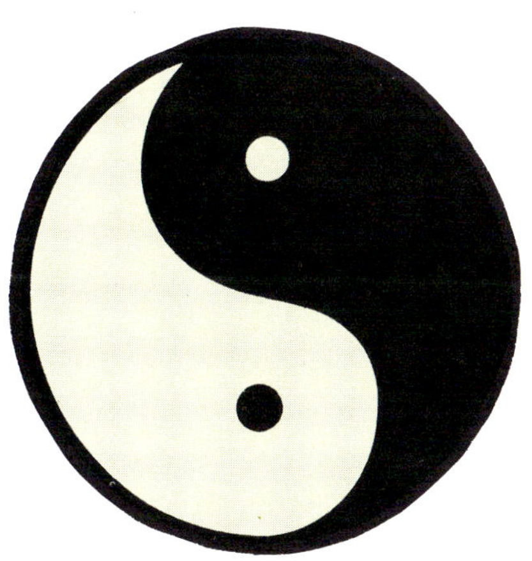

Yin and Yang, the basis of macrobiotics

and are generally consumed during their season of growth. They may be cooked, especially in winter, but the act of cooking itself should reflect *yin* and *yang* principles of balance. Moderate heat, quick cooking and minimum salt preserve *yin* aspects while lengthy cooking, higher heat and more salt lead to *yang*.

Because they are regarded as extremely *yin*, potatoes, tomatoes and aubergines are regarded with caution and usually avoided. Other foods that are central to the pattern of diet include soya beans (used in the form of *miso* and *tamari*), aduki beans, lentils and seaweeds. *Umeboshi*, or salted pickled plums, are recommended for most digestive problems and *mu* tea is taken because it contains fifteen roots and herbs, including *ginseng*.

Foods that are avoided include all processed products, milk, cheese, butter, eggs, meat, refined flour and sugar (fruit concentrates are used as sweeteners, if required). Fish falls into an optional category and is sometimes eaten once or twice a week, preferably in winter. Fruits and nuts are similarly optional and are taken usually as snacks rather than as essential foods.

The macrobiotic approach focuses on nutritious, appealing food and requires that the person eating it should consider its value meditatively and thoughtfully. Food should be thoroughly chewed and eaten slowly.

Diet is important and we are coming to realise that to a large extent 'we are what we eat'. The World Health Organisation has stated that diet is the leading factor in the rise of degenerative illness. Consequently we should aim to eat sensibly and balance our diet. By doing this we are helping to prevent diseases – which are symptomatic of imbalance – from arising in our bodies.

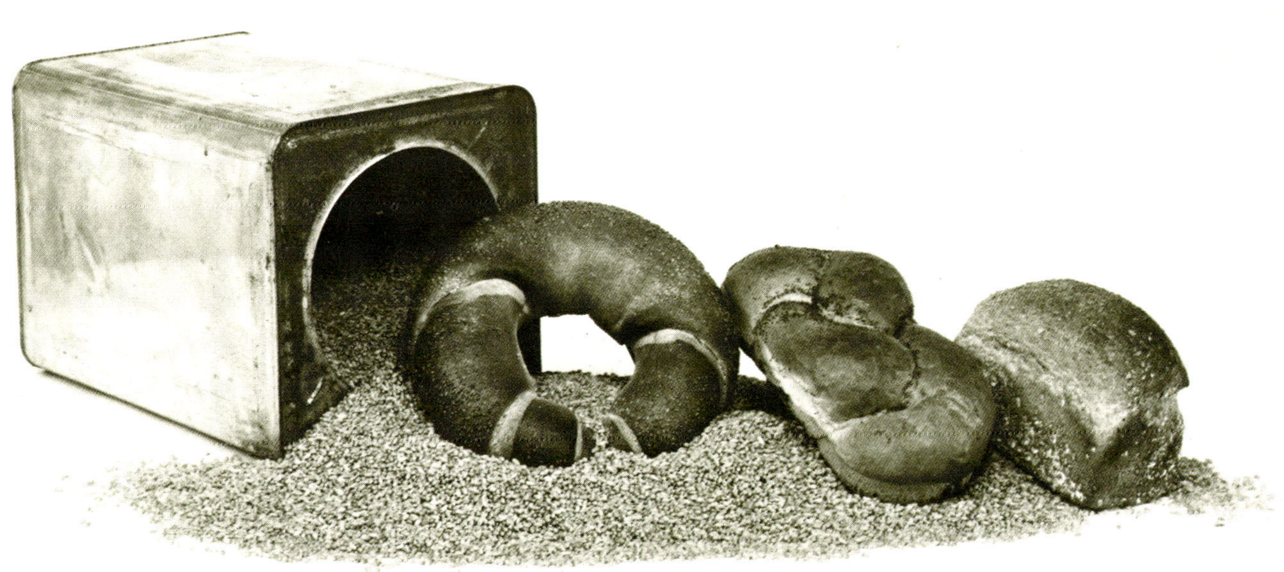

WILLIAM TARA

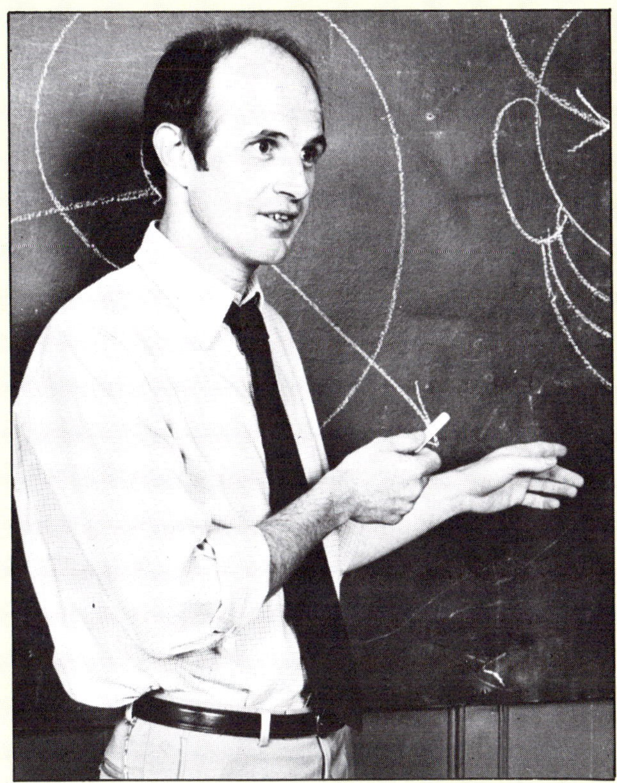

The City of London is renowned for its Stock Exchange, one of the world's most influential banks, and some very materialistic businessmen. To find in nearby Old Street a building devoted to the oriental philosophy of macrobiotics comes as something of a surprise. Nevertheless, at the Community Health Foundation the ancient teachings are alive and thriving.

The Foundation, a registered charity, owes its growth and a following of some 10 000 visitors a year to the drive and enthusiasm of its Director, William Tara, a slim, friendly American. A former theatrical producer from San Francisco, he first used macrobiotics when he was suffering from a large and painful duodenal ulcer and hypertension. Ill health and the drugs he was given by doctors 'made life pretty horrific'. Four months after going on a macrobiotic diet the ulcer that had bothered him for six years had gone, together with the hypertension. When he reported the fact to his doctor he was told that his change of diet had nothing to do with it – just pure coincidence.

Realising that there must be many in the same position as he had been in, he decided to find out more of the macrobiotic philosophy. He took leave of absence from his work and went to Boston, Massachusetts to study with Michio Kushi, a leading teacher of oriental philosophy and medicine, whose lectures and teachings had inspired thousands to take up this way of life.

William Tara found his studies so fascinating that he decided to become more actively involved. At that time in America many new alternative food industries were starting, especially those concerned with promoting organic agriculture. For four years he worked in that field, continued his studies with Kushi and also took courses in shiatsu massage and oriental diagnosis with other teachers. Then in 1972 he came to London, hired church halls and lectured on macrobiotics. A group of fellow enthusiasts joined him to set up a self-help centre. From this came the impetus to set up the Community Health Foundation. Originally a derelict building it required £45 000 to renovate it which came from small donations and voluntary activity.

At the Foundation, he says, we teach people what they can do immediately to improve their health, how they can draw on the teachings of 4000 years of traditional medicine that has been systematically recorded and is available to everyone. 'We are trying to promote macrobiotics as a preventative measure, encouraging people to change their basic nutritional pattern so that they can establish good health.' He explains that macrobiotic nutrition is very close to what most people in the world were eating until about 150 years ago, a diet based on whole grains supplemented by seasonal vegetables, beans, fruits, nuts and 'sea vegetables' (seaweed). If people require animal protein he suggests that they start at the lower end of the food scale, with fish.

All of the activities at the Community Health Foundation are open to the public. They include tuition in the Alexander Technique, shiatsu massage, preventative medicine, oriental diagnosis, yoga, encounter groups, child care and child medicine and nutrition. The educational services of the Foundation have extended to include seminars and workshops at the Imperial College of Science and Technology and many other educational institutions.

In 1978 a Michio Kushi institute was started. This provides an intense study programme for those interested in becoming teachers or health counsellors, or wishing for a deeper understanding of macrobiotics to use in their own lives. Many of those who attend return to their own town or country to start macrobiotic activity and centres on a grass roots level. Groups are being set up in Edinburgh, Brighton, Bristol and Leicester. In Europe there are groups in France, Germany, Portugal and Spain, as well as large macrobiotic centres in Belgium and Holland.

Some of the results that have been achieved through the teachings of the Foundation were published in a series of case histories in 1978 and 1980. These included people who were suffering from both acute and chronic illnesses and who generally showed considerable improvement in their health, and in many cases dramatic cures by changing their diet and lifestyle. William Tara and the Community Health Foundation are part of the developing movement whose ideas and methods are working to transform the lives of people and their environment.

MEDITATION

A popular misconception about meditation is that it is a type of passive introversion, a peaceful but ineffectual form of self-centredness. In fact meditation is quite different from this and as a technique of mind control has very positive benefits for health. Those who practise meditation systematically and regularly believe it leads to increased inner calm, heightened powers of creativity and decision making, increased efficiency in the work situation and decreased mental tension and negative emotions. Accordingly many ailments that are stress-related can be eliminated or reduced by meditation. These include migraine and tension headaches, high blood pressure, heart trouble and menstrual cramps.

The meditative approach to life is not confined to any one spiritual belief system or religion and historically is found co-existing with Buddhism, Hinduism, Sufism and Christianity in different forms. It has been proposed by the researcher R.K. Wallace, who studied Transcendental Meditation, that meditation in itself may actually be an identifiable state of human consciousness similar to, but distinct from, sleeping, dreaming and waking. Essentially meditation produces heightened powers of awareness and deep tranquillity and represents a journey to the inner self.

Meditation has become increasingly popular in the West, partly as a result of the widespread interest in the teachings of Maharishi Mahesh Yogi and the Transcendental Meditation (TM) movement. It is estimated that at present over 6 million in the United States have learned some form of meditation and the practice is also very popular in Britain, Europe, Australia and other Western countries.

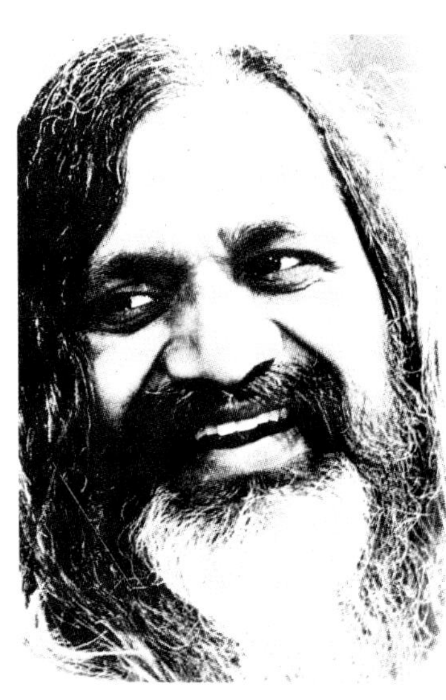

The Maharishi Mahesh Yogi – bringing Transcendental Meditation to the West

The appeal of meditation is that it broadens one's sense of being. Personal anxieties, fears and tensions – which often underly disease – acquire a diminished status and are less all-consuming than they seemed. As Baba Ram Dass says, 'meditation frees your awareness' and opens new horizons of perception.

There are basically two approaches to meditation. The first focuses on powers of concentration, the second emphasises detached awareness.

Concentration

This approach requires that the attention be focused on a meditative symbol, a sound or chant, or a body process like breathing. Sometimes sacred mantras like *Hare Krishna* and *Aum* are used. In some forms of concentration-meditation the teacher gives the pupil a mantra on which to meditate, twice a day. The idea is to turn the processes of thought inwardly until the mind transcends though itself.

Detached Awareness

The focus here is on what is happening *now*. The task is not so much to elevate consciousness to a 'higher state' but to become increasingly aware of the present moment. From that position one gains an awareness of the flux of life and the ebb and flow of human experience.

The *Visuddhimagga* – the Path to Purification – by the 5th century monk Buddhaghosa, describes the meditative approach from the Buddhist viewpoint. In some respects it contains both of the above viewpoints.

One of the major disciplines of the Buddhist meditator is to eliminate distractions, with the aim of attaining a 'unification of mind'. As the practitioner learns to meditate for a long period such factors as agitation, scep-

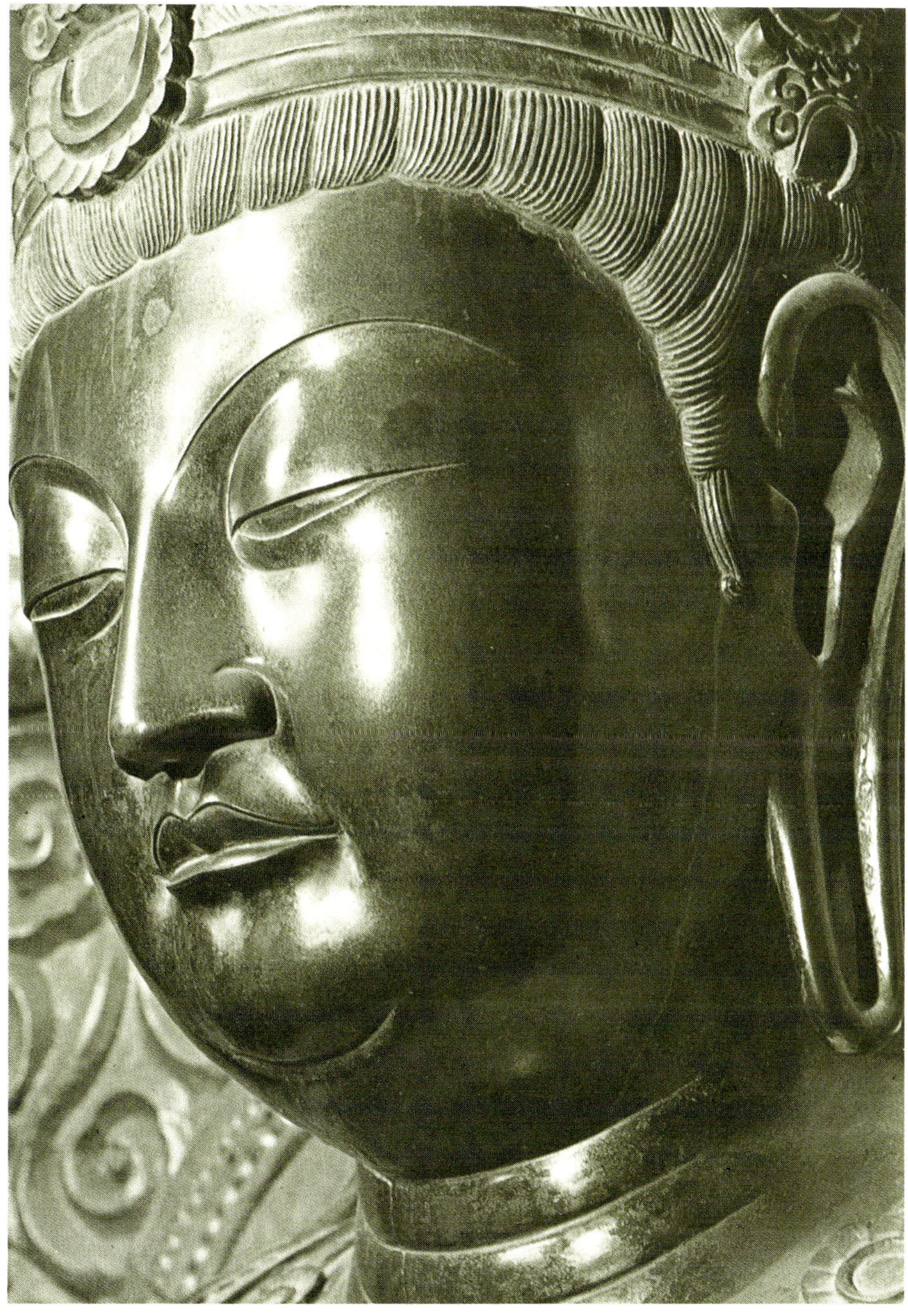

Buddhist meditation: 'unification of mind'

ticism, and doubt disappear and a feeling of one-pointedness (bliss) begins to dominate. The meditator becomes absorbed in thought – a process known as *jhana* – and moves deeper and deeper finally acquiring an awareness of infinite space. Many Buddhists however regard the pursuit of various jhana levels as secondary to the Path of Mindfulness which leads, finally, to *nirvana*. The meditator learns to break out of stereotypes of thought and perceives every moment of the everyday reality as if it were a new event. The ego becomes comparatively less important and the manifested universe is seen to be in a state of total and ever-changing flux. This leads to the sense of detachment from the world of experience, an abandonment of all desires, self-interest and finally the ego itself.

On a more down to earth level meditation provides a deeply felt sense of relaxation which reduces body tensions and stress. Dr Syed Abdullah, a New York psychiatrist, reports a case of a 53 year old woman whom he treated for asthma by prescribing simple breathing techniques and meditation. Gradually she learned to control her bronchial spasms and eliminate the complaint. However she also suffered from atopic eczema, and discovered to her delight that when she concentrated her attention on her skin condition that she was able to heal it also.

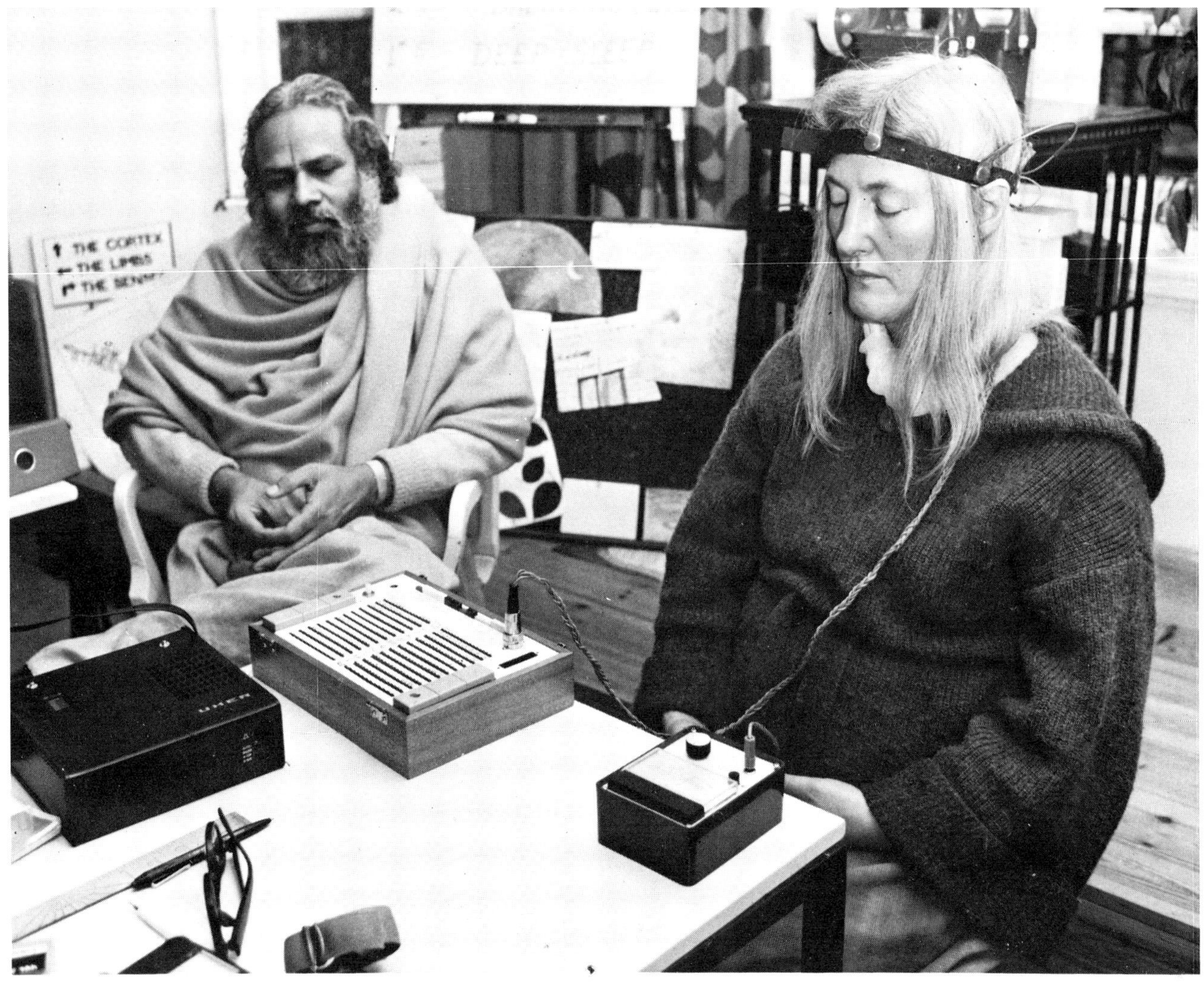

Biofeedback applications in meditation: a session led by Swami Prakashanand Saraswati

Meditation occasionally produces unusual effects although these are by no means the main purpose of the practice. Many thousand advanced practitioners of TM have experienced temporary levitation effects and attempts have been made to monitor the EEG patterns of the brain while the process is occurring.

Dr John Price, a lecturer in mathematics at the University of New South Wales, has practised TM since 1962. In the late 1970s the Maharishi introduced a 'TM-Sidhis' programme and levitation is one of the curious by-products of that approach. Dr Price describes his experiences:

It seemed that in one sense there was a lot of activity taking place in the brain; in another sense this activity was highly structured, highly organised. It was if every neuron in the brain was co-operating with every other neuron . . . Usually a person's nervous system is full of a lot of noise, full of random fluctuations, chemical and electrical fluctuations, but the technique of TM allows the mind to settle down to a very silent, coherent level. The level of rest that TM gives is confirmed electrically in that the EEG shows a very stable coherent picture of the nervous system becoming very clear, very smooth . . . In one sense I knew what to expect on a physical level but there was nothing that could really replace the exhilaration of the experience itself . . .

Meditation does not have to be as spectacular as Dr Price describes it for it to have a positive effect on health. On a day to day practical basis it can be used simply to reduce stress and tension at work or at home and bring about a new level of calm and well being.

NATURAL BIRTH CONTROL

Many women have turned aside from the contraceptive pill, IUDs and spermicides in favour of natural birth control methods. The orthodox familiar methods have their drawbacks: the contraceptive pill suppresses the natural menstrual cycle and may cause blood clotting in women over 35 years of age, especially if they also smoke; IUDs are sometimes uncomfortable and can cause infection, and many women are allergic to spermicides, which are often unreliable anyway.

The Lunar Phase Cycle

Natural Birth Control methods have extended far beyond the 'rhythm method' which is normally only 30-50% effective. Discoveries relating to the so-called Lunar Phase cycle now make Natural Birth Control 98% effective.

The new approach derives from the work of Dr Eugene Jonas, a Czechoslovakian psychiatrist and gynaecologist who studied Roman Catholic women using the rhythm method. He was concerned with the limitations of this technique and discovered that the women in his survey were frequently conceiving on dates which fell outside their expected mid-menstrual ovulation times. When he analysed the timing of these dates he discovered that they fell into a repeating cycle related to the angles between the sun and moon. The women appeared to be fertile when the sun and moon were at the same relative angle as at the precise time of their birth, irrespective of the mid-menstrual ovulation time.

In effect Dr Jonas had discovered a second fertility cycle commencing at birth, repeating in cycles and becoming effective at puberty.

In 1958 Dr Kurt Rechnitz, a Hungarian professor of gynaecology, conducted an experiment in which patients at the Budapest Maternity Clinic combined abstinence during the Lunar Phase cycle with the rhythm method. The success rate of birth control jumped to 98% effectiveness.

In 1968 Dr Jonas established a birth control research centre named Astra in Nitra, Czechoslovakia. In 1970 Astra's scientific council issued a report based on the experiences of 1252 women who had used the Jonas-Rechnitz method of natural birth control for a full year. The official finding, endorsed by the Czechoslovakian medical establishment, was that the method was 97.7% successful.

Research at Nitra ceased after the Russian invasion but further experimentation has been conducted by Dr E. Rolf Schweighart in Vienna, who estimates that 40 000 women have been introduced to the method since 1972.

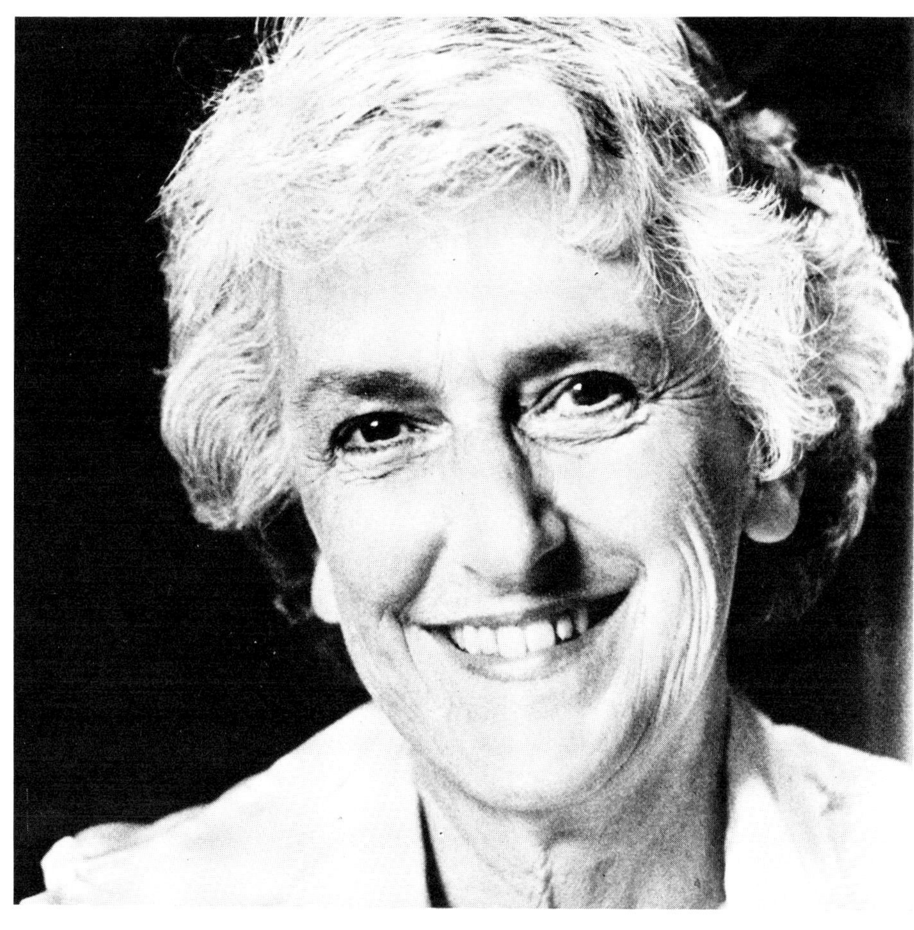

Dr Evelyn Billings, co-author of a new work on fertility control which has earned international recognition. Professor Thomas Hilgers of Creighton University, Nebraska, has described the Billings Method as 'one of the greatest discoveries of this century'

The overall finding is that a woman is most fertile during the 24 hours preceding the exact recurrence of the sun-moon angle present at the moment of her birth, a fact of considerable interest also to astrologers (see article *Astrological Diagnosis*). Since sperms live for three days the fertility period is normally regarded on a broader basis and for contraception purposes is taken as a four-day period repeating every lunar month, that is, twelve or thirteen times a year.

The Ovulation Method

Drs John and Evelyn Billings have developed an internationally recognised ovulation method in Australia to tell accurately when mid-menstrual ovulation occurs. They found that a number of body symptoms changed at different stages of the menstrual cycle. The most important change occurred in the vaginal mucus but there were changes also in body temperature and in the cervix.

During the normal menstrual cycle the mucus secreted by the cervix follows a pattern:

1. Menstrual period
2. A few days with no mucus discharge. The interior of the vagina is moist but there is no exterior wetness.
3. A few days of 'infertile' mucus discharge, which is opaque, thick and white-yellow. It acts as a natural spermicide and forms a plug across the cervix. This mucus is 'tacky' and sticky to touch.

4. For four or five days a 'fertile' mucus is discharged and this period indicates the approach of ovulation. Sexual intercourse during these days could lead to conception since the sperm can swim through the mucus, which is now thin and watery.
5. This is the peak fertility time. The mucus is more profuse and has a quality similar to raw egg-white. It can be stretched between the finger and thumb.
6. After ovulation the mucus becomes cloudy, white yellow and tacky, and then ceases altogether.

By observing these patterns the likelihood of conception or contraception can be systematically monitored. However, other factors are also important.

Body temperature falls lower than usual just before and during ovulation and after ovulation rises by about half a degree. A basal thermometer should be used to record the small changes and temperature should always be taken the same way, whether orally, rectally or vaginally – for purposes of consistency (oral temperature is usually one degree lower).

The cervix is also subject to change. During the infertile phase the cervix remains firm but as ovulation approaches it begins to open. The cervix also gets softer and rises up, making it difficult to reach with the finger. Mucus also makes it feel slippery. After ovulation these changes reverse.

Francesca Naish of the Village Healing and Growth Centre in Paddington, Sydney, has been practising as a Natural Birth Control consultant for five years. Deeply interested in both astrology and natural healing methods, she has been counselling her patients on both Lunar Phase and Ovulation methods and also draws up individual fertility charts.

One of her patients was a woman who was unable to conceive for a number of years although there was no medical reason for this. She did not have blocked tubes and her ovaries were functioning correctly, but her fertility was surprisingly low. She had endeavoured to conceive during the regular ovulation time but without success.

When Francesca calculated her Lunar Phase fertile times she found that they very frequently coincided reasonably closely with her periods. For aesthetic reasons the patient had avoided sexual intercourse during her periods and did not believe she could conceive at that time. However, having overcome her scepticism she tried the new timing and conceived within a few months.

Natural Birth Control techniques, of course, have two major applications. They can be used as a very efficient means of natural contraception with no side-effects whatever, and also as a means of positively anticipating likely conception periods. Above all, such techniques provide women with a deepened understanding of their own fertility cycles and offer new perspectives for responsible family planning.

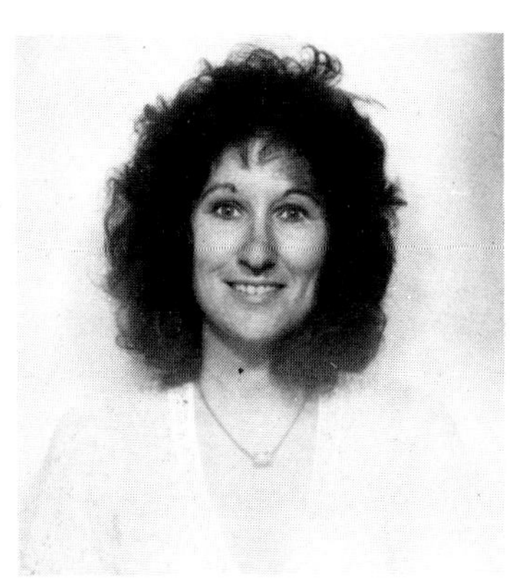

Francesca Naish

Natural Childbirth

There is an increasing tendency for some mothers to prefer their child to be born in the natural setting of the home rather than in the more clinical environment of the hospital. It is relatively rare for circumstances to arise during labour and birth that would demand hospital treatment and over 90% of these factors could be medically predetermined.

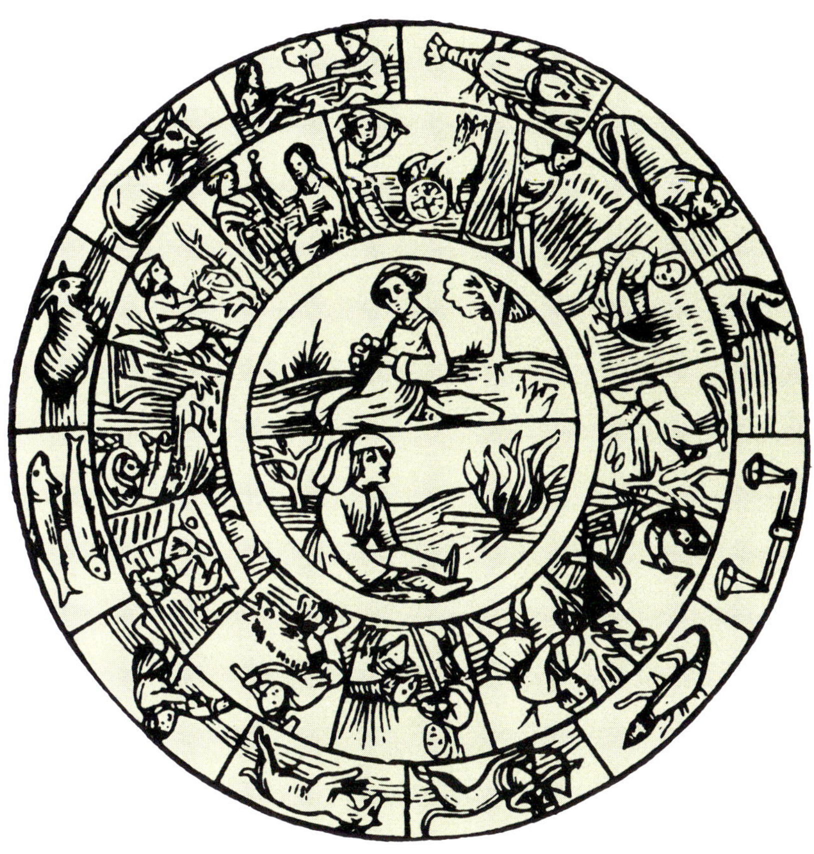

The home has a number of advantages over the hospital in terms of familiar people who can offer friendship and support during labour, birth, and the time immediately afterwards when the baby needs nourishment and protection. In 1976 a survey by the Childbirth Education Association showed that 86% of women who gave birth in a hospital were less than satisfied with the treatment they were given. This is not surprising if we recall that hospitals are primarily places for sick people. In Holland, where 80% of women are instructed in the techniques of childbirth – including correct breathing and relaxation techniques – we also find the lowest mother and infant mortality rate, so clearly there is no evidence to suggest that births at home are more hazardous. In most countries associations exist which provide information on midwifery and childbirth education in order to train both expectant mothers and fathers in parent care and natural birth procedures.

Advocates of natural childbirth often recommend that the mother be surrounded with as many friends as she can feel comfortable with. They in turn provide support for her while she performs her natural breathing (Lamaze) exercises during labour. It has been found that the pain thresholds of women using Lamaze exercises at home in a supportive setting are higher than in hospital, where 50% of women require pain suppressors.

It is vital for the newborn child to be together with its mother during the first days of life. Often in modern hospitals, administrative procedures require the baby to be away from the mother for extended periods and this can have a traumatic and detrimental effect.

Childbirth at home seems to be a very real option for the future.

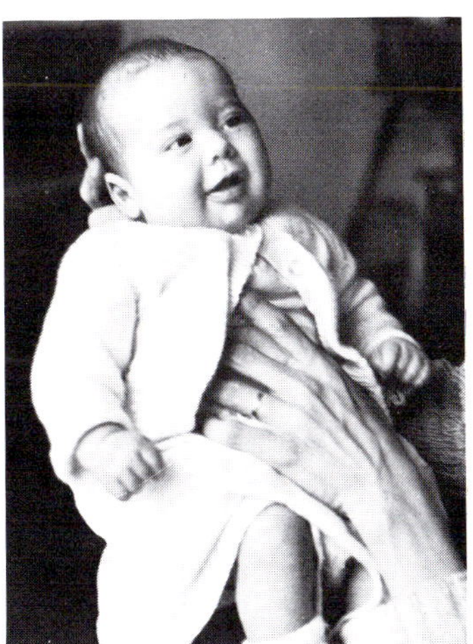

Natural childbirth: back to the home and away from the hospital

NATUROPATHY

Naturopathy is literally a means of treating disease by following the principles and laws of nature. In 400 B.C. Hippocrates referred to 'vis medicatrix naturae' – the healing power of nature – and naturopaths ever since have endeavoured to work with the healing forces present in the body. Naturopaths, as with any practitioners of holistic philosophy, treat people rather than symptoms and do not believe in specific diseases as such. The life force flows through the body in various channels and blockages produce imbalances which manifest as disease through specific organs.

The naturopath focuses however on the complete person and the underlying causes of disease rather than the specific symptoms at hand. Considerable care is taken in compiling a personal medical history, details of lifestyle, diet, exercise and so on. The naturopath recognises that disease can be brought on by a number of factors – poor eating habits, restricted breathing, improper posture, muscular tension or emotional factors – and the aim is to guide the patient back to a state of balance. For this reason a naturopath uses many different modalities in treating a patient. Usually dietary and nutritional counselling and a knowledge of vitamins, minerals and herbs is combined with therapies like osteopathy, chiropractic, acupuncture, homeopathy, iridology or hydrotherapy.

Historically the term 'naturopathy' was first used by the German-born homeopath John Scheel but influential figures in the field also included Henry Lindlahr, who believed that disease derived from 'improper eating, thinking and living', and Father Sebastian Kneipp (1821–1897), the founder of hydrotherapy. Kneipp cured himself of a lung disorder by plunging daily into ice-cold water and then warming himself with exercise. He recommended walking barefoot on wet grass and in cold streams. The idea was that intense cold was followed by resurgence of blood to the limbs, increasing natural warmth.

A number of Kneipp practitioners met in the United States in 1900 and decided to broaden their practice to include all the available methods of natural healing. The American School of Naturopathy was founded in New York and interest in natural modalities of health care increased steadily in the United States until 1960 before falling into a decline. However with the revival of interest in alternative lifestyles and philosophies, interest in naturopathy has again revived.

Naturopathic treatment can be divided under various headings:

Physical: personal hygiene, manipulation of joints and soft tissues, massage, Alexander Technique and other posture therapies.

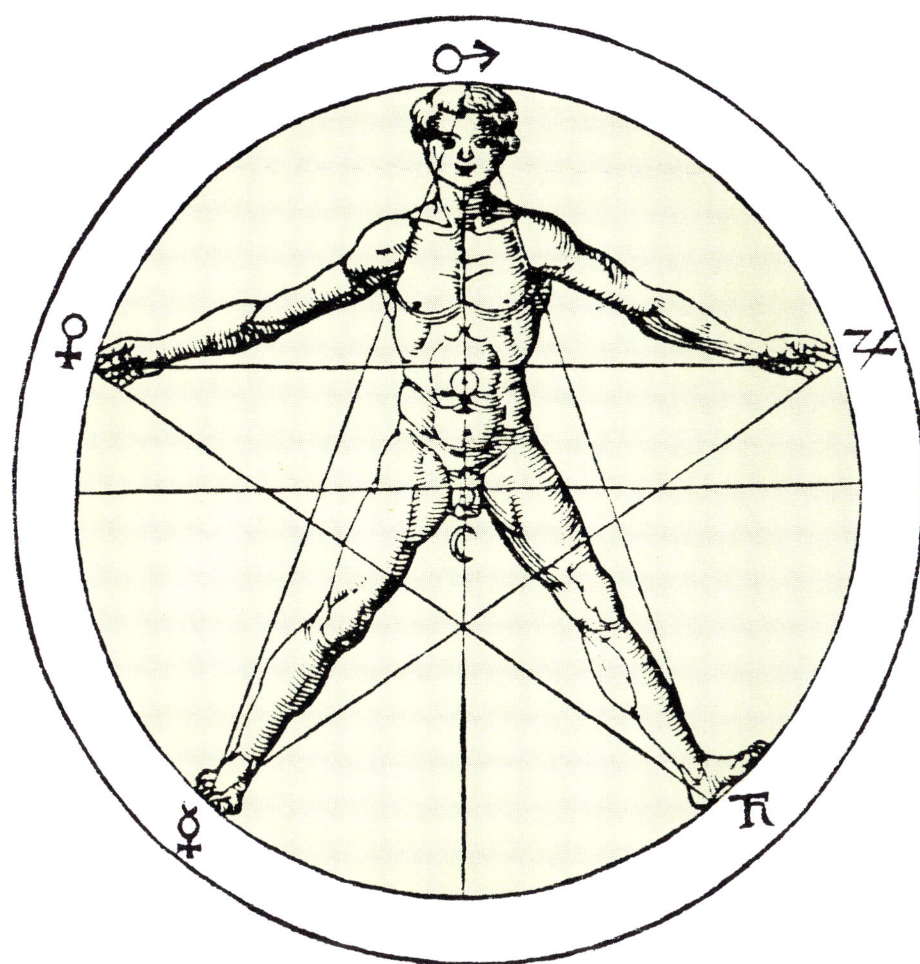

Neurological: spinal manipulation, acupuncture, shiatsu, acupressure, reflexology, pain control techniques

Psychological: counselling, hypnotherapy, biofeedback

Biochemical: diet and nutrition, fasting, vitamin and mineral therapy, herbal medicines, homeopathic remedies.

As naturopath Marti Benedict has succinctly put it, these modalities can be resumed under two fundamental principles. The first is a need to '*nourish* the depleted system with pure food, water, thought, movement and peace of mind'. The second is to '*cleanse* the toxin-ridden body with an internal house cleaning'. However, as she points out, it may be easier for a relatively healthy person to rid himself of toxins than an undernourished person. The latter may require building up first. Accordingly there are no easy short-cuts in naturopathy and each treatment is individually considered and planned.

Toxins can build up in the body as a result of processed and 'devitalised' foods, or chemical preservatives and flavourings. Poor digestion, nervous exhaustion and inability to rest or relax may also compound the problem. Diet and nutrition, though, are the starting point for many naturopathic treatments. Judy Taylor, Director of the Southern School of Naturopathy in Melbourne, has found that 90% of patients attending a natural therapist require vitamin and mineral therapy. Natural vitamins seem to contain more energy than synthetically derived equivalents and she has found that combinations are often useful in assisting absorption. Iron with Vitamin C is a case in point.

Overall, the naturopath seeks to restore vitality and energy to the body, building up the natural capacity for health. Disease symptoms are simply a sign that the bodily condition is less than perfect and the naturopath may turn to any of the holistic healing therapies to return the organism to a state of balance. As one naturopath has said, the essential task is not to treat illness but to induce health.

RUSSELL ATKINSON

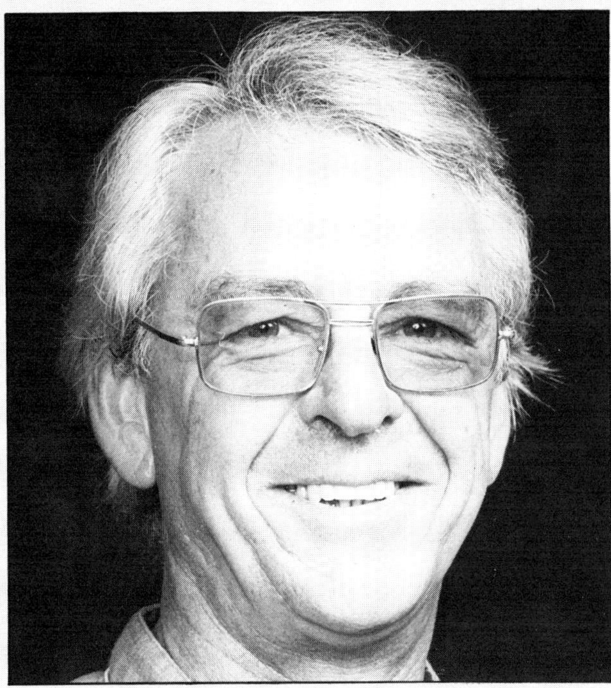

Although he is best known as a naturopath and managing editor of the influential journal *Nature & Health*, Russell Atkinson has also been a pioneering figure in the study and practice of yoga, herbalism and acupuncture in Australia.

Born in the New South Wales country town of Portland in 1930, he moved to Sydney when he was eight, but grew up with a strong inclination to leave the city environment for a more adventurous life elsewhere. Following a brief involvement in advertising, he literally packed his swag and headed north to Queensland where he worked on the fishing boats and later on the cane farms. While there, he chanced upon a book by Yogi Ramacharka titled *14 Lessons in Yoga Philosophy* and decided to take up Hatha Yoga. As his interest grew he decided he would have to abandon the rural life and return to Sydney to study. However in the years after World War II – Russell was nineteen at the time – there was very little available by way of sound instructional material. The revival of Eastern mysticism which took place in many western countries in the 1960s was yet to come and the Bohemian and 'Beat' connections with Zen and other exotic philosophies were still in their infancy and had not yet been reported from the United States. Russell taught himself the rudiments of Hatha Yoga and found a group of friends in the circles of the Young Theosophists. Around this time he also met John Cooper and Jonn Mumford, who would also become influential local figures in the world of yoga.

As Russell recalls, the first public lectures on Hatha Yoga were started in Rowe Street, near the Sydney GPO, by Russian born Michael Volin. These aroused considerable interest through the media and Russell taught there with Volin. Following on from these lectures Russell produced his first book, *Yoga Pocket Teacher*, published in paperback in England. Later he also worked with Dr Alfred Kaufmann – a pioneering osteopath and homeopath who had established a school of chiropractic at Eastwood in the mid 1950s – the first of its kind.

Having explored a variety of philosophies embracing mind/body techniques, Russell Atkinson departed for India on a personal spiritual pilgrimage. The gurus were less in evidence than they are today: Sri Aurobindo and Bhagwan Maharshi had just died and Krishnamurti, whom he met and admired greatly, had no permanent ashram for training purposes. Russell attended his talks and was impressed by his ability to transcend cultural differences; he was humble yet intellectually impressive; lucid yet totally spiritual – and with a very special magnetic presence.

When he returned to Australia Russell felt he should continue to blend the various holistic approaches he had been pursuing and he began to teach yoga, counsel on dietary matters and provide instruction on health and naturopathy. At this time he held weekly classes in Hatha and Raja Yoga with private groups. However soon a change of scale was called for, as public awareness and interest grew. After 'formalising' some of his own studies in advanced massage, herbal medicine and acupuncture, he took a diploma through the Australian Acupuncture College which had established links with Chinese medical practitioners in Hong Kong, and subsequently founded an acupuncture clinic in Gosford in 1972. He also ran courses on herbalism on behalf of the National Herbalists Association and the same clinic has now become the Southern Cross Herbal College, headed by Russell's friend and colleague Dennis Stewart.

Russell joined the Blackmore organisation as their spokesperson on health and diet and related matters and in his editorial capacity on their journal now researches and investigates a wide variety of themes in the area of holistic health and preventative medicine. He finds that his personal direction has changed and he is now much more interested, for example, in naturopathy and diet than in Hatha Yoga. He finds the field of clinical nutrition – the use of food elements to cure and prevent disease – and the related domain of orthomolecular psychiatry (treating mental disease in a similar way) to be among the most exciting frontiers at present. He cites as examples the use of magnesium phosphate and Vitamin B6 for treating chronic kidney stones; the amino acid Tryptophan for acute depression and insomnia and the use of Vitamin B3 and zinc sulphate for treating schizophrenia, as examples of this new research. Another area of interest is the new work being done on cranial adjustment as an alternative or adjunct to spinal manipulation.

At 50 Russell Atkinson remains as active and vigorous as ever. The work and never-ending research meanwhile continue.

DAVID DUGGAN

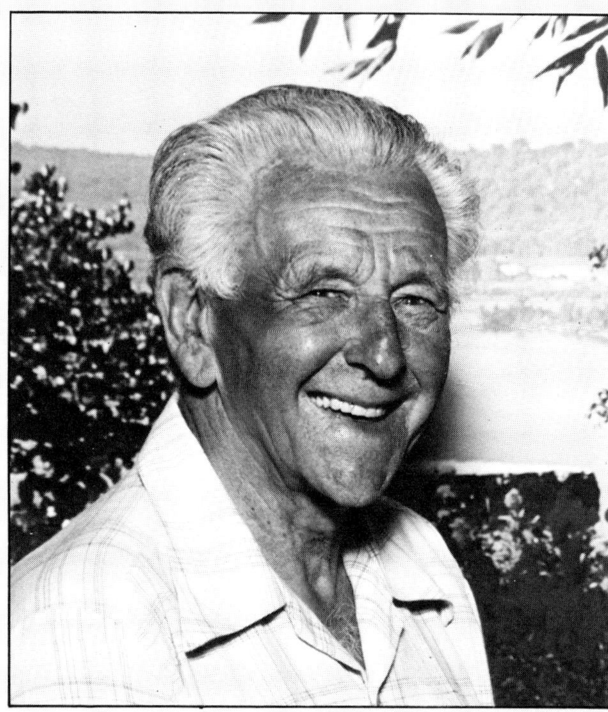

David Duggan looks about 45, says he feels about 40 but, incredibly, was born in 1897. It is more than 70 years since he had a day's illness, and then it was only the usual minor childhood ailments such as mumps and measles. He came unscathed and unvaccinated through the smallpox scare of 1902, and stayed healthy during the great 'flu epidemic of 1918'. He says he has never taken a drug or any other foreign substance into his body. He does not smoke or drink.

His mother was a healer, and she taught him a great deal. He speaks of her with deep respect, remembering, for instance, the great 'flu epidemic when she opened her home to the sick who could not be accommodated in the overflowing hospitals. The house was big and thirty patients went through her home. None of those who came to Mrs Duggan's died, an amazing achievement at the time.

The Duggans (His wife works with him part of the time. She is 79.) do not take holidays. Four days a week are spent seeing patients, beginning at 6 a.m. 'Sometimes we don't get finished until quite late. It has been as late as midnight.' And the people come in their hundreds. The small waiting room often overflows into the corridor of the central Auckland office building.

The people come to avail themselves of the 30 years experience of a man who has dedicated his life totally to helping people.

His skills encompass all facets of natural healing: diet, colour therapy, acupuncture, chromotherapy, radiesthesia, osteopathy, chiropractic, physiotherapy, biochemics, homeopathy, herbalism, acupressure, magnetism.

'We are studying and I'm learning something new all the time. Wonderful things are happening all over the world. Russia has been doing a lot of research on magnetism. They know that a magnet has two different energies. Michael Faraday who discovered magnetism about 100 years ago, thought there was just one current running from north to south and from south to north. But now scientists are finding that that isn't so, that Faraday was in error, and that each of the poles has a separate energy. In the centre was the "Bloch wall", discovered by Professor Bloch, and the lines of force from the south pole would come up into the Bloch wall and would travel from there into the north pole. The north pole energies are sedative and healing. The south pole energies are stimulating. With the north pole, they have been successfully treating many diseases, especially in animals.' Last year, David Duggan broke a small bone in his foot. Within a week after treating it with magnetism, the foot was normal and the pain did not recur. Toothache pain, he says, will disappear within half an hour. He believes the magnet will be one of the greatest tools of natural healing. There are no side effects at all from its use, and he has used it for a number of different complaints. 'We don't treat disease here. We treat the body as a whole. We also have a particular type of massage. We don't use the hands to massage. We only use the fingers, because in the fingers the energy and the power are concentrated, and we can get better results that way.

David Duggan also uses both colour and chromotherapy. All healing, he says, as all else, is colour. Light itself is colour. 'God is colour; every vibration is colour. When we feel sick, what do we say? We feel off-colour, and that's exactly what we are. Intuitively, we know.'

'Life is so full of inspiration and joy and happiness.' He never gets tired because he knows that the strength he needs will be available to him. He does not fear germs. In fact, he sees them as good, since they are part of life, and all life is good. He does not, however, suggest that disease is a good thing, but germs, he says, only attack a body that is not healthy. Germs cannot enter a completely healthy body. So we should not blame the germs. Rather, we should all be trying as hard as we can to make sure we are so healthy that there will be no weak spots for germs or other forms of disease to gain entry. David Duggan is President of the New Zealand Federation of Natural Therapeutics and of the Naturopathic and Osteopathic Association. He is also a member of the Radiesthesia Association, to whom he gives lectures. He lectures at the South Pacific College of Natural Healing and is a minister of the Church of the Kaballah, where he teaches and preaches. And he is a 32nd degree Mason, learning, studying and teaching in that organisation.

The future? 'Well, I won't retire for another 20 years.' And looking at and listening to this vital man, another 20 years seems a conservative estimate.

NEGATIVE IONS

We have all heard the expression 'There is electricity in the air'. The concept is an old one and was noted by Father Gian Baccaria in Turin in 1775; he was interested in the way Nature used atmospheric electricity to promote plant growth. In the 1920s scientists established that the charged molecules in the air – ions – affect both man and nature, and that air with a low ion count or a strongly positive charge exerts an adverse influence on plants, animals and human beings.

A negative ion can be defined as a negatively charged molecule formed by an intense electrical discharge which frees electrons from atoms of gas. The discharge removes the electron – in fact it discharges rather like a bullet – and then loosely attaches itself to other molecules of gas in the atmosphere. The result is a 'negative ion'. Meanwhile the other part of the fractured atom becomes positively charged: a 'positive ion'.

Scientists have established that in cities, where most people live, the balance of ions in the air weighs 5:4 in favour of positive ions and that in this sense the air we breathe is often flat, lifeless and out of Nature's balance. An overloading of negative ions is generally beneficial.

The issue of ion balance was brought to the public notice in 1977 by Fred Soyka, an American executive who worked in Geneva for several years. Soyka found that he began to suffer from 'inexplicable fits of anxiety, depression, physical illness and (a) kind a bottomless despair'. He also had recurrent stomach aches, tension states and malfunctions of the gall bladder which did not seem to derive from any obvious cause. Soyka went so far as to book himself in for an operation to remove his gall bladder but before it could be performed he was called back to the United States suddenly on business. He found that many of his symptoms disappeared. On returning to Geneva, however, the old pattern returned intermittently and he often felt sluggish and lethargic. Finally a German general practitioner, Dr Bernard Wissmer, told him that many visitors to Geneva who were not accustomed to its climate, suffered from fatigues, colds and troubled stomachs and he put it down to 'something electrical in the air . . .' Soyka began to read a large amount of scientific literature on atmospheric conditions and found that certain geographic locations, including Geneva, parts of Central Europe and Southern California, suffered from imbalances in the natural electrical charge . . . because of wind patterns. In such environments people who are 'ion-sensitive' become dull and lethargic and often develop other sicknesses. On the other hand, locations near the sea shore, where waves break upon rocks, and near waterfalls, there is an excess of negative ions and the air is literally pure and invigorating for this reason. After a storm has passed there is also a restoration of the electrical balance and a resultant freshening of the air. Not surprisingly, the Russian researcher A.L. Tchijewsky found that all Russian health spas had an excess of negative ions in the air.

The sorts of 'ion hazards' that occur in the cities include artificial air conditioning, central heating, synthetic fibres, automobile discharge, cigarette smoke and general pollution. Office buildings require vast networks of vents, many of them with sharp angles, to push the air-flow through a large complex of floors and rooms. The rush of air in a constricted space produces friction and an increase in positive ions, and the same occurs when we wear synthetic fibres: friction between the body and the garment produces an adverse positive electrical charge.

Some of the most interesting research into ionisation has been conducted by Dr Felix Sulman in Jerusalem and Dr Albert Krueger in Berkeley, California.

Dr Sulman, who heads the Department of Applied Pharmacology at the Hebrew University in Jerusalem, has made a special study of the effects of ion-imbalance on human emotions and health.

In 1969 he conducted an experiment in which two groups of men and women between the ages of 20 and 65 were confined in rooms containing firstly a positive ion excess and then a negative ion excess. In the first instance the subjects became irritable and fatigued after an hour's confinement. During the second experiment, however, they all exhibited stronger alpha brain waves (inner peace and well-being) and slow, firm pulse (health and mental tranquillity). Psychological tests showed increased alertness and work capacity.

Dr Krueger's work goes back to 1956 when he was approached by senior electronics executive Wesley Hicks to see if positive ions were harmful to health. Hicks headed a company that manufactured electrical heaters which in turn produced positive ions, and he offered Dr Krueger a grant to cover his research. Quite soon afterwards Dr Krueger discovered that a small quantity of negative ions could kill the bacteria that helped colds and influenza

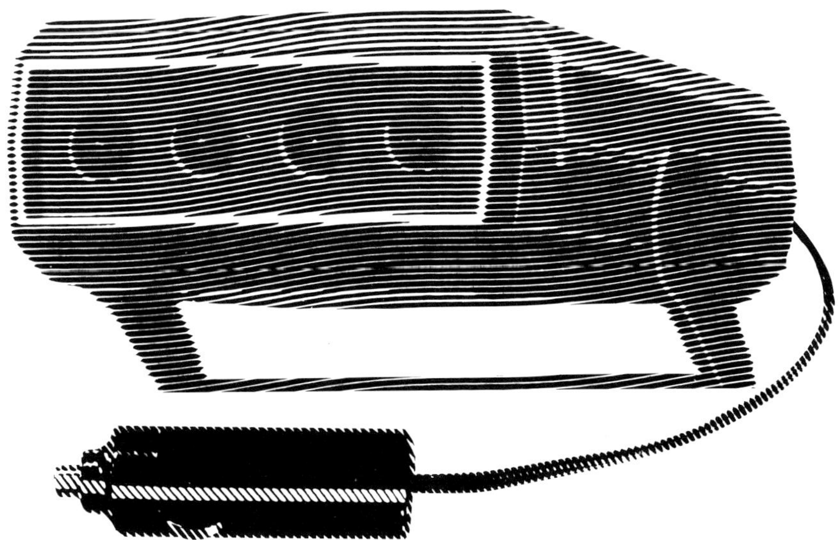

Negative ion producers

to spread. At this stage there was little supporting evidence of such specific correlations. He then experimented with groups of mice that were subjected to different situations : positive ions, negative ions, and a neutral balance. The mice were examined alive and dead and were finally dissected. In 1960 Dr Krueger announced that in his view positive ions caused overproduction of serotonin in mammals, leading to exhaustion and anxiety. On the other hand, Dr Krueger found that negative ions had a calming effect and could counteract a positive ion excess.

If we are agreed that an atmosphere containing excess negative ions is more beneficial to health, what can we do about it, short of camping beside a waterfall?

It is now possible to obtain commercially produced negative ion generators. They are compact units working from a 240 volts A.C., 50Hz power source and generate in excess of 300 billion small air ions per second. Smaller versions, suitable for installing inside a car measure approximately 4 in. × 4 in. × 2¼ in. (11.5 × 10 × 5.5 cm) and work from a 12 volts D.C. power source.

Aside from their general therapeutic value, healers interested in the beneficial aspects of negative ion generators often recommend them to people who suffer particularly from such complaints as asthma and related bronchial problems; influenza; catarrh; hay fever; migraines and sleeplessness. There is now increasing recognition of the effect 'electricity in the air' has on general health and well-being.

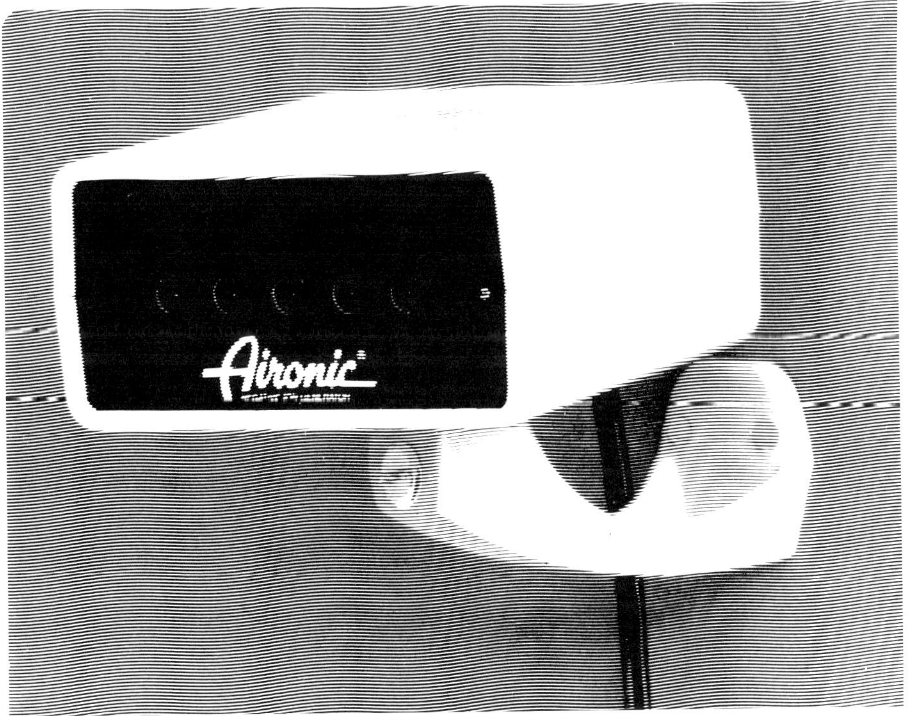

OSTEOPATHY

Osteopathy is often confused with chiropractic since both are manipulative therapies. The essential difference is that historically osteopathy emphasises the relationship of blood circulation to healthy tissue whereas chiropractic pays more attention to the nervous system. Very often practitioners of these two healing arts treat similar complaints: lower back pain and 'slipped discs'; restricted joints; neck manipulation and muscle spasm; and certainly the techniques overlap.

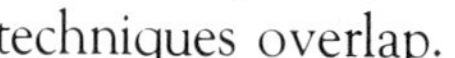

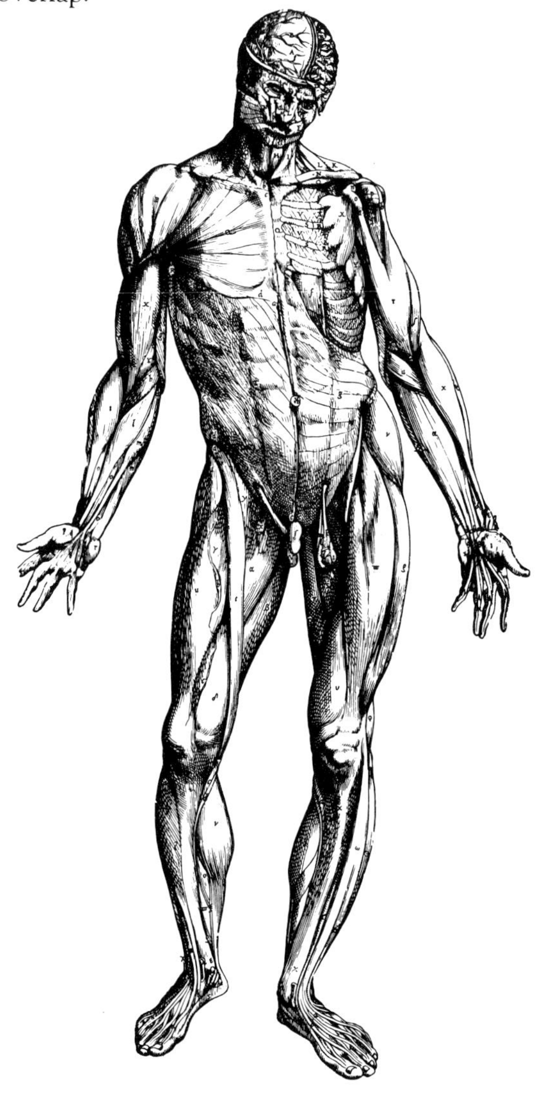

Osteopathy derives its name from two Greek words: *osteo* (bone) and *pathos* (disease), although as a holistic therapy its scope is much wider than this suggests. The system was founded by Dr Andrew Taylor Still (1828-1917), a physician from Missouri. Still grew up in a devoutly religious family. His father was a Methodist minister and passed on to his son a profound respect for man as God's creation. Consequently when Andrew Still's three sons died of meningitis despite all the orthodox medical care provided for them, he turned away from his profession and found consolation in his religious beliefs. He came to believe that illness derived from deviations from the plan God had provided and that man had within him the powers to heal. Still began to study the anatomy of man and animals with rigorous care and attention to detail, and he discovered that he could diagnose medical ailments by touching the body and assessing the speed, heat and quality of the blood flowing in the area. Still called this *palpation*. In some respects Still's approach mirrors the concept of energy flow and blockages found, for example, in Reichian therapy and bioenergetics.

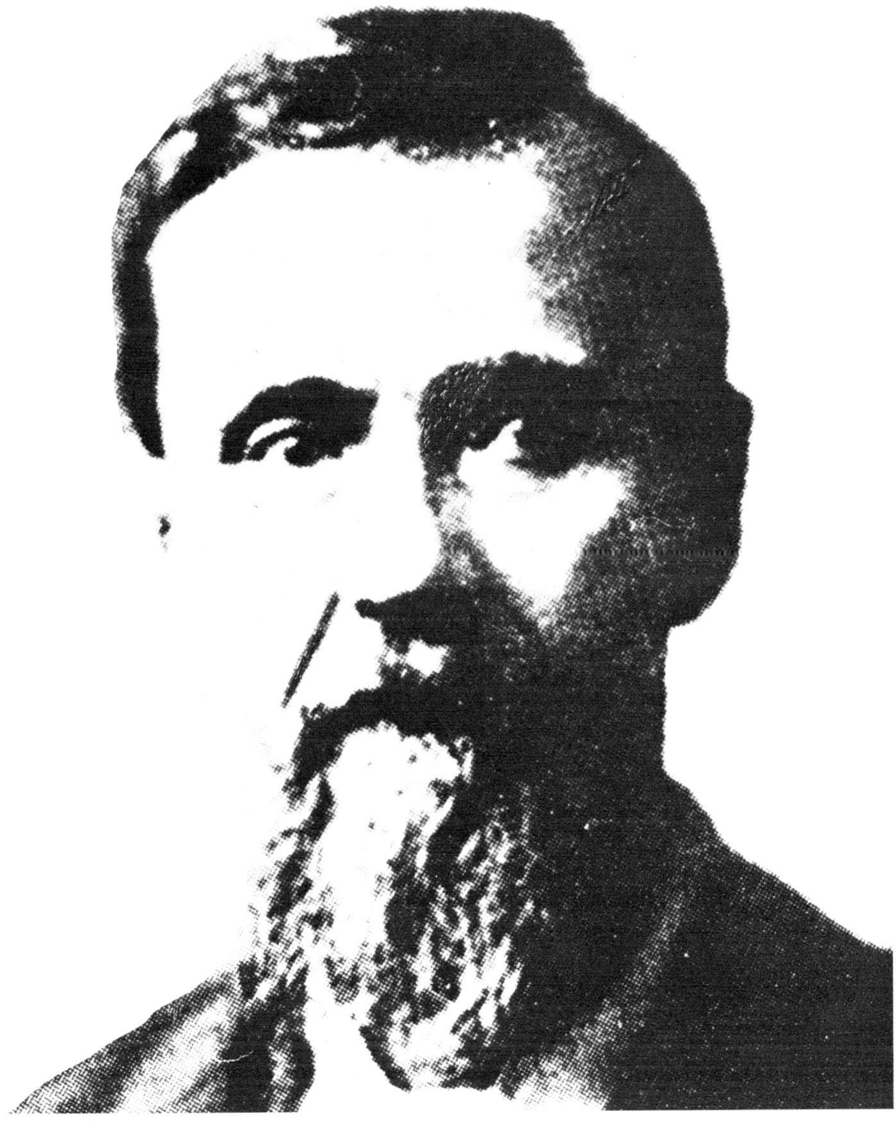

Dr Andrew Still, founder of Osteopathy

In the same way that Daniel David Palmer developed systems of manipulation, Andrew Still found that several illnesses were related to spinal disorders and that these could be treated by manipulating joints back into their correct position. However, whereas chiropractors have been inclined to do this because of pressure on nerves, osteopaths have stressed the factor of blood circulation. Still believed that an abnormal body structure would impede the blood flow and derived the axiom 'The rule of the artery is supreme' to reinforce this point. Still also believed in analysing and treating the whole body, placing emphasis on the movements of the rib cage and the thoracic and pelvic diaphragms and the general alignment of bones. However he recognised that manipulation by itself was not enough. A bone could be repositioned but then fall back into misalignment if the supporting muscle was not developed. Osteopaths therefore often recommend courses of mineral and vitamin therapy to reinforce muscle tone and strengthen the bones.

Dr Still established the first College of Osteopathy in Kirksville, Missouri in 1897, and by the time of his death – at the age of 89 – osteopathy had been recognised in every State of America. The techniques were brought to England by J. Martin Littlejohn and the British School of Osteopathy was founded in 1917. Today it ranks with chiropractic as one of the leading alternative therapies, and one condoned by most allopathic doctors. Like orthodox medical practitioners, osteopaths often take X-rays of the troubled areas of the body and then apply manipulations and massage to correct abnormalities in posture and bone function. Osteopaths are perhaps more inclined to observe the limbs in movement, correcting the action and sensitively feeling the body for clues to malfunction. Chiropractic techniques are usually applied to the patient as he lies quiescent on a bed. Chiropractors like to demonstrate the 'clicking' of limbs back into place (a sound caused by the lubricating fluid in the joints, not the bones themselves) whereas osteopaths insist that manipulations are only useful if the right joint is opened and body movement is restored. The sense of touch is often crucial for this process and a skilled osteopath can identify changes in joints, muscles and connective tissues that a doctor would possibly not notice. Typically osteopathic sessions last around half an hour and require the patient to ease back into correct patterns of body movement and posture. To this extent there is some overlap also between osteopathy and the Alexander Technique.

In recent times osteopaths have been careful to maintain rigorous standards and have worked alongside orthodox medical practitioners rather than compete against them.

Osteopathy is particularly effective in treating lower back pain, some asthmatic and bronchial problems due to lesions of the spine behind the shoulder blades, dislocations, aching joints and some digestive troubles. As such osteopathy is one of the least controversial and most publicly accepted alternative medical treatments and has provided lasting relief to generations of people suffering from back problems – an ailment symptomatic of modern industrial society and 'sedentary' occupations. As such osteopathy is very much a current therapy and in several countries is recognised by health insurance companies.

FRED WESTON

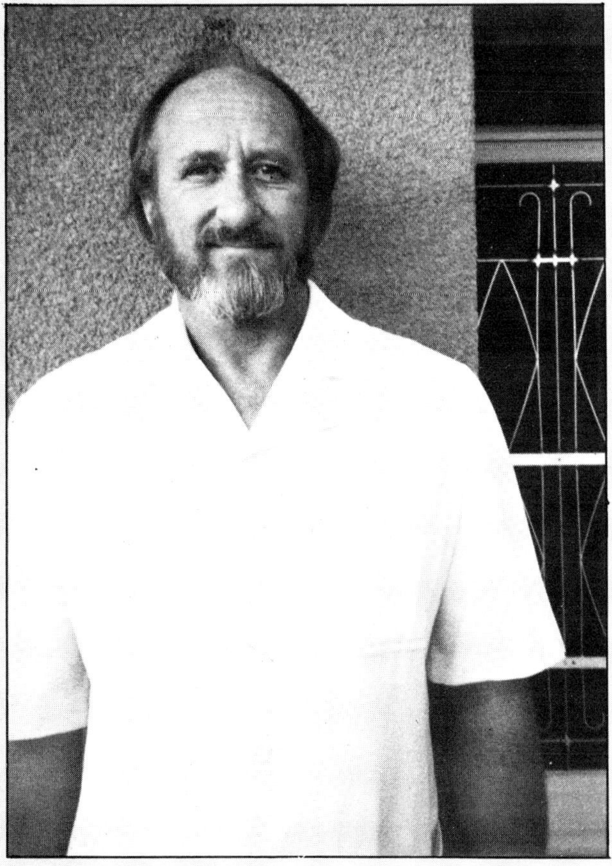

Fred Weston was born in the fruit growing town of Renmark on the River Murray in South Australia on 23 August 1933. According to astrology the Leo Virgo cusp, with 5 houses in Virgo, is the sign of a potential healer. However it would not be for some time that this talent would develop.

After a standard primary and secondary education in Adelaide, Fred entered the sales field selling business equipment, then moved into office clerical work. Soon tiring of this life-style he felt the need to travel. Hitchhiking from Adelaide to Mildura he worked on the grape harvest, then moved down to Melbourne, working a few months as a milko. After a stint as a kitchen hand in the old Monterey Cafe in Sydney's Victoria Building in George Street, he hitchhiked to Cairns in Queensland where he worked in the cane fields, the sugar mills, as a lab technician, and on the M.V. *Marinda* as deck boy running between Cairns and Cooktown.

After a couple of years moving about he returned to Adelaide and shortly after, feeling unwell, he found he had contracted tuberculosis affecting both lungs. Fred spent two years in hospitals and Sanitoriums in Adelaide and soon found a natural interest in things medical. Although he needed medical treatment, he was well enough to help nursing and medical staff with general hospital duties, such as charts, urine tests, blood tests and other simple functions. He also found that he possessed a natural feeling for helping and counselling his fellow patients.

At this time he started reading psychology and anatomy and so understood more about mental and physical aspects of disease. This was a milestone in his future direction. Fred felt he would like to pursue a formal medical training but at this stage couldn't afford the long course of training. Ever-eclectic, he developed an interest in the martial arts of Asia, which led to Yoga, and in turn to Buddhism and esoteric philosophies.

After discharging himself from the T.B. Sanitorium he was told by the doctors that he would not live 12 months on the 'outside'. He re-joined the workforce as a salesman. To show the medicos were wrong he got into ju-jitsu, racing cars, flying and skin-diving with a vengeance. While skin-diving he met three fellow adherents who were training to be chiropractors, and was stimulated by their approach to health care. He was shown some of their techniques and found he had a natural ability. A special lady in his life at this time had a long history of migraine and a 'frozen shoulder' which had been damaged in a car accident. Fred treated her and effected a complete cure. Realising he had natural abilities, he decided to pursue a full understanding and study of holistic medicine.

Moving to Sydney he began studying all fields available: naturopathy, herbalism, iridology, osteopathy, chiropractic. He attended the Academy of Natural Healing, the NSW College of Osteopathy and the Sydney College of Chiropractic. After graduating, Fred taught at NSW College of Osteopathy and practised in Double Bay. He also trained with a Chinese doctor, Dr Casey Wong, who taught him acupuncture. Later Fred practised in a Chinese Clinic in Sydney's Chinatown.

Since his days in Double Bay, Fred Weston has practised as a full-time holistic health practitioner and he continues to be amazed by the way in which the alternative modalities complement each other.

In 1971 Fred moved to the Australian Capital Territory where he established a practice in Narrabundah, and the Canberra College of Natural Therapies. He has taught well over 1000 Canberra residents some aspects of alternative medicine, massage, herbalism, nutrition, zone therapy, shiatsu, Bach flower remedies and other aspects of alternative health care. Fred treats the body-mind as a whole, using the techniques of Wilhelm Reich, Rudolph Steiner, David Boadella, Gerda Boyesen, Stanislav Grof, and others to help people get in touch with the stress aspect of their lives, and enable them physically and mentally to become 'whole again'.

Fred defends the fact that he is not a specialist by recalling that such a person is one who 'learns more and more about less and less until he knows everything about nothing'. And there is a danger, Fred feels, that even the well-meaning natural therapist can be too specialised. True holistic healing must necessarily embrace many fields and approaches. Fred Weston has gone about putting this philosophy and knowledge into practice.

PAST LIVES THERAPY

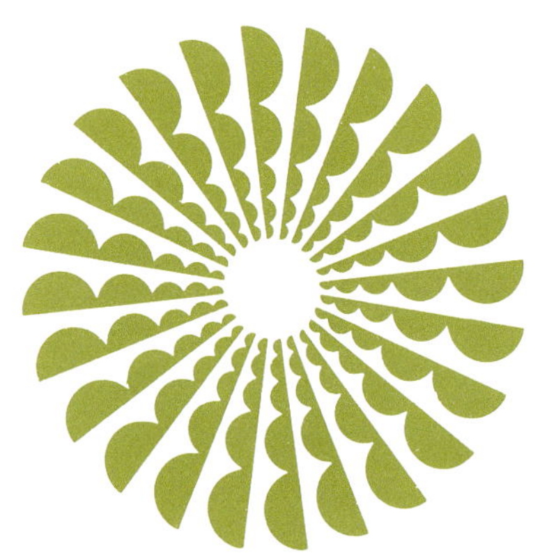

Have we lived in this world before? The idea of rebirth through many lives continues to raise tantalising and intriguing questions about the very nature of our existence. Reincarnation is an ancient and widely held religious belief. It was central to ancient Egyptian religion, occurs in many primitive cultures and is also a major doctrine among many Hindus and Buddhists. Several prominent Western philosophers have also supported a belief in rebirth, including Socrates, Plato, Plotinus, Pythagoras, Spinoza, Leibniz and Schopenhauer.

Reincarnation is, in a sense, closer to the scientific principle of the conservation of energy than the 'special-creation' concept of the soul which contradicts it. The concept of reincarnation could also throw light on cases of remarkable human prodigies where the learning situation does not appear to square with the achievement. One example, from 18th century France, concerned Jean Cardiac, who knew the alphabet at three months, could converse in French when a year old, and in Latin, Greek, English and Hebrew by the time he was six . . .

Claimed cases of reincarnation have been investigated in recent times by Dr Ian Stevenson of the School of Medicine at the University of Virginia. Stevenson's studies, presented in a definitive work titled *Twenty Cases Suggestive of Reincarnation* and also in a shorter essay in honour of William James, have paid considerable attention to cases involving young children where details of the present life can be verified and where conscious or unconscious fraud is unlikely. One of his most interesting cases was that of Shanti Devi, a girl from Delhi who from the age of three began to recall details of a former life in the town of Muttra, eighty miles away. Relatives of the specified person were called in to verify the account, and Shanti Devi was able to recognise other 'relatives' in a crowd, succeeded in identifying the Muttra homestead despite the fact it had been repainted a different colour, and indicated correctly a place where money had been buried and later removed. Shanti Devi made a total of twenty-four statements from her 'memories' which matched verified facts, and there were no instances of incorrect statements. Similar cases investigated by Dr Stevenson included Eduardo Esplugus-Cabrera in Havana, Prabhu Khairti in Bharatpur, India, and Alexandrina Samona in Palermo, Sicily.

While reincarnation as a religious belief remains controversial despite evidence in its favour, a new therapy has developed involving regression into 'past lives'. Practitioners of this approach, which often involves hypnosis, claim that a personal belief in reincarnation is not necessary for the cure to be effective. However, it obviously helps. Some critics have suggested that a past-life regression is nothing other than an exploration of subconscious fantasies but even in such an instance a therapist could still work within the self concepts – real or imaginary – of the patient.

Two of the pioneering researchers in the area of past life therapy are Dr Morris Netherton and Dr Helen Wambach, both of whom practise in California.

Dr Netherton is a psychologist who specialises in counselling. He has been involved in past-life regressions for ten years, but unlike others in the same field, does not make use of hypnotism. His technique is to listen to the speech patterns of his patients in a search for clues presenting themselves from the unconscious. A person might repeatedly use a phrase like 'I'm burning up inside' or 'It makes me see red . . .' and in Netherton's view such expressions may reveal more than might first be apparent. The patient is asked to lie down with the eyes closed and concentrate on recurrent phrases, later repeating them until a mental image presents itself. Netherton has found that such sensory impressions will often flow with a 'rush' once the initial inroad has been made. Through a technique of specific questioning Dr Netherton is able to focus attention on the significance of these images and their relevance to the present lifetime. He writes:

Almost invariably my patients have found that their mental anguish in this life could be pinpointed to a physical situation in a past life. To put it in the simplest terms, a patient who suffers from an acute fear of heights, for example, will discover recurring past-life situations where he died by falling long distances. The past-life falls could easily be called 'creative daydreams' and if a patient wishes to regard them that way I make no objection; the therapy will still work for him. As he detaches himself from the commands of past incarnations he loses the fear he has been suffering in the here and now . . . it is essential for the patient to relive the trauma of each past-life incident moment by moment, fully and completely, in order to detach himself from it.

One of Dr Netherton's subjects was a 34 year old divorced woman named 'Ann' who suffered from ongoing sexual problems with male partners and experienced extreme guilt in each relationship. Over a number of sessions she uncovered a variety of past-life traumas including rape by a priest, the sensation of being crushed by a rope and buried alive during witchcraft persecutions in the Black Forest region of Germany, and also the 'memory' of being betrayed by a lover at a crucial moment. In one of the final sessions Ann also seemed to tune in to the unhappy emotions her mother had felt during her own birth and subsequently went on to relive her mother's feelings that 'no-one would ever love this child'. Ann had frequently used such expressions about her own sexual relationships and felt a sense of overriding futility in her life. Recognition of what seemed to be past-life patterns helped her to distance such emotions and start life anew. Shortly after therapy Dr Netherton was pleased to see that Ann had bought new cheerful clothes, had rekindled her self-esteem and had a more positive attitude towards life in general.

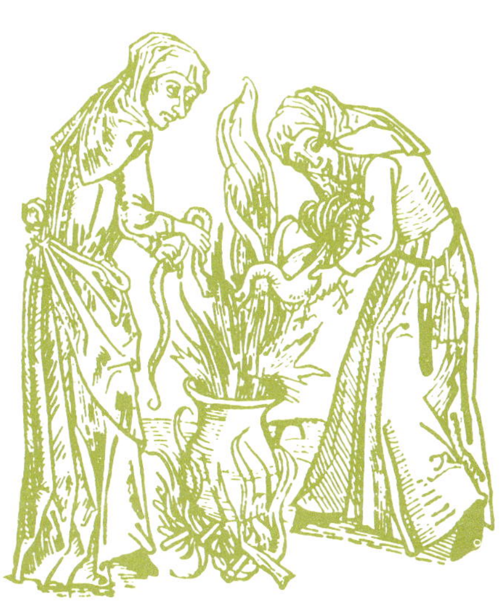

Dr Netherton believes reincarnation to be a fact and notes that past-life therapy works most effectively with patients who are open minded about it. He explains that while psychotherapy recognises repressed anxieties, fears and pain in the unconscious mind, all his therapy is doing that is unusual is to admit the possibility that events from a previous lifetime could still exert an influence on present patterns of behaviour. The unconscious, he feels, is like a tape-recorder and when appropriate techniques are used a memory 'play-back' comes into operation which reveals traumas stretching back beyond the present lifetime.

Dr Helen Wambach's approach is somewhat different. Her past-life regressions make use of hypnosis and she conducts regular workshops in which she seeks recall-information that can be verified against historical data.

One of her students, 'Anna' could regress easily under hypnosis and could also describe her experiences while in that state. When taken back to 1780 she seemed to be a young child living in a country town. Dr Wambach brought her to 1785 and she identified herself as Rachel and her town as Webster, Massachusetts — a real location. Later she regressed into a more recent incarnation in Westfield, New Jersey. She described her life in 1917: the house she lived in, the names of familiar people and a plot to sell government supplies on the black market. Her husband was away in the war at the time and would not have condoned this activity. Dr Wambach visited the town and was able to verify such specific details as the name of the corner store druggist and the town constable. 'Anna' had identified correctly a lane which had been subsequently renamed after it was paved in 1924 and the family burial plot was also located.

Dr Wambach regresses each subject at least three times, to different 'lifetimes'. She believes that if past-life recall were producing fantasy elements that the same personality traits would recur in each recall. There have also

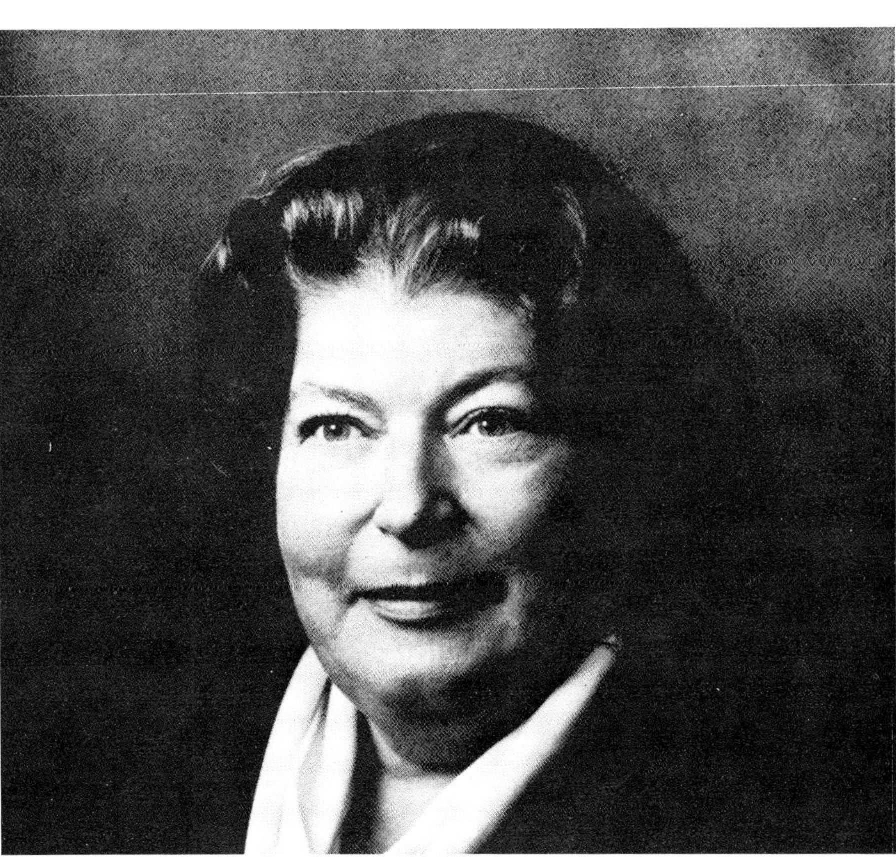

Dr Helen Wambach

been experiments in which subjects were asked to regress to a pleasant incarnation at one of the following times: 1850, 1700, 25 A.D. and 500 B.C.

Dr Wambach was interested to discover that, on the whole, subjects reported comparatively ordinary lives. Around 70% of a 1088 test sample lived 'lower class' lives earlier on and the 7% 'upper class' ones were not especially pleasant. She found that subjects could move from one sex to another but that the recalls produced statistics which reflected the sex split in population. In one test sample in which 78% of the 804 subjects were women, the recalls split into 50.3% male and 49.7% rather than follow the sex-based fantasies the subjects might have had about themselves. A second group that included 55% women returned a very similar split of 50.9% male and 49.1% female. Dr Wambach also found only 11 historical discrepancies in 1088 cases, where she could positively disprove recall data on a factual basis.

Overall, the evidence for the reincarnation viewpoint seems to be quite extensive and researchers like Drs Ian Stevenson, Morris Netherton and Helen Wambach are inclined to believe its validity. Alternative hypotheses regarding subliminal data recall, telepathy and fraud do not fit the total pattern of available evidence. With this in mind the concept of past-life therapy is not as way out as it might first appear. It seems that human consciousness registers sensory impressions and memory patterns that extend back further than the present life span.

MALCOM AND ZOË HAGON

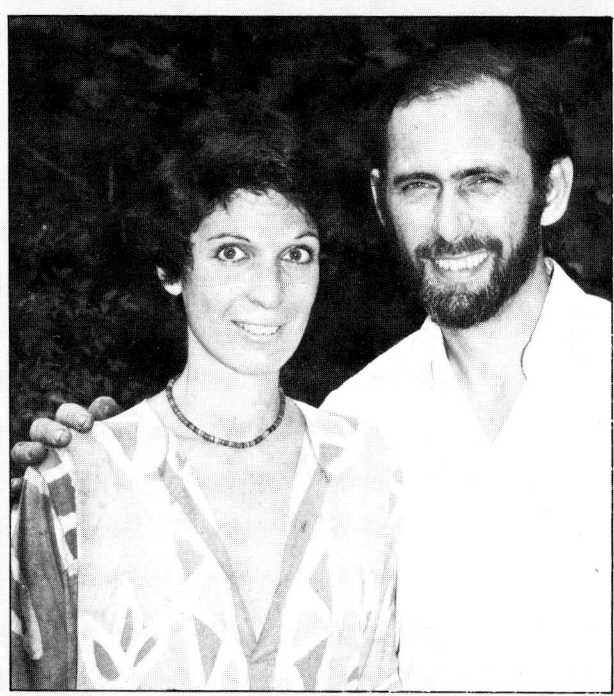

Zoë Hagon grew up in a comparatively private and sheltered environment that could hardly provide an indication of the far-reaching past-life therapy and psychic healing work she is now practising with her hypnotherapist husband Malcom. Raised in England where she trained and graduated as a physiotherapist, she was not content to settle into a conventional medical career. Instead she travelled widely: to Germany, where she lived for a time, to India with a Commonwealth Expedition, to the United States, and finally, Australia. Always nursing a secret desire to act, she forsook her medical background, joined an agency and landed a job in the musical *Hair*. Later she joined the Pageant Theatre Company and then the Queensland Theatre Company. It was during her time with QTC that her future husband hired her for promotions work with News Limited where he worked in public relations.

Malcom grew up in Sydney and similarly developed an adventurous and creative career. He worked in radio, television, public relations and journalism, and was also a keen photographer. After he and Zoë were married in 1974 they travelled as a writer/photographer team through Central and South America collecting material for travel magazines. It was during this time that they developed more than just a curious interest in the psychic field and some of the unusual spiritual gifts they both share in common.

Malcom's sense of the continuity of life is something that has been with him for as long as he can remember and was perhaps heightened by his father's death when he was only ten. He accepted the personal loss but felt nevertheless that his father was still very much with him; he always believed there was far more to life than the superficial reality he found surrounding him. Several years later, at the Sydney Society for Psychical Research, he met a fascinating woman who was to be his mentor and spiritual guide for over a decade. Known by all her pupils as 'Mrs D', she was a clairvoyant, medium and healer who ran courses in self-development. He joined her group, which met weekly, to learn techniques of meditation, psychometry and healing.

Later when Zoë met 'Mrs D' for the first time she felt that she had regained something that she had always known but which she had neglected until that time. It soon became apparent that she had a deep and natural intuition about people which outstripped Malcom's awareness, and he reluctantly found he now had to play second fiddle to her psychic perception. However, he also had something worthwhile to offer: his emergent abilities as a hypnotherapist. As Zoë and Malcom began to find the potential for spiritual healing increasingly important in their lives, they decided to turn their efforts from the comparatively secure work of travel writing and photography and focus their abilities on new approaches to healing.

Today, on a picturesque 1700 acre property south of Oberon, New South Wales, where the Hagons are currently developing the Iona Foundation for Appropriate Industry, Technology and Healing, they run courses in Psychic Development and Healing, and practise a form of past life regression which has startling and effective results. In essence the aim of their past life regression work is to identify the source of any ailments, phobias or compulsions which appear to have a past life origin. Obviously they seek to discover more immediate reasons for disease and sickness, and therefore each patient is thoroughly interviewed to ascertain if regression is in fact actually necessary. Zoë always performs a 'psychic reading' for each patient who comes for treatment, and often finds the impressions gained predictably unpleasant. She believes, for example, that many present day traumas derive from previous lives that ended in violent death, or featured torture or a major crisis of some sort. Often she perceives these details as a series of sensory impressions, and during a session will often pass hand-written notes to Malcom while he is engaged in dialogue with the hypnotically regressed subject.

Malcom uses a technique of progressive relaxation which produces an altered state of conscious comparable to an out-of-the-body projection. Bringing his subjects through their foreheads, 'as if they were glass' he guides them into a cloud of light which then floats back through inner space 'to a life that is relevant to the problem you are facing today'. It may not be the immediately preceding incarnation: many factors can apply, though the Hagons find that accumulations occur and that very often crises have been compounded in more than one lifetime.

Having identified and brought into focus a life sequence pertinent to the problem, Malcom asks the subject to become aware of the surroundings, the other people present, and details of the lifestyle. He then regresses the person to age five or six within that life before subsequently progressing them to the period immediately preceding the crisis. This journeying through the life helps the subject focus on the course of events that led up to the crisis point. Then a decision must be taken: should the subject first stand outside the trauma and view its consequences before experiencing it, or relive it 'blind' and, by passing through it, defuse it of its inherent terror? Ultimately this must be done if the problem is to be laid to rest.

Very often a transition through death to a 'between-lives' existence is experienced and the therapist has to be able to provide steady and convincing understanding and support while his patient is experiencing the crisis period. For this reason Malcom stresses that such work must be done only by an experienced therapist and not by those who are merely idle or curious.

In early 1980 a film entitled *Past Indefinite* was made of two such regressions by the Australian Film and Television School. The male subject, Frank, suffered from constriction in the throat which in turn produced a type of stammer somewhat like loss of breath. When regressed, he began to relive a life as a knight engaged in leading a pillaging expedition with a band of soldiers. During the foray, the soldiers suffered heavy losses and Frank experienced the pain of being hit by an arrow in the leg. He was then captured, imprisoned and then – obviously traumatically – beheaded by his captors. Frank was guided through these terrifying moments by Malcom Hagon, and although he winced with pain during the session, he was finally able to relax peacefully and re-establish his ability to breathe in an unimpeded manner. Frank stated on film that he found the session invaluable in gaining insight into his speech and breathing defect and, as a result of that and previous sessions with the Hagons, dramatic improvement has been made in rectifying the problem.

Past-life therapy is startling and, conceptually, almost unbelievable, and yet its effects are unquestionably profound for those who experience them. Under hypnosis the subject is advised to leave the emotional impact of past-life experiences behind and not let them intrude any longer on the patterns of present life. Malcom believes that the key to the therapy is knowing the right questions to ask and focusing accurately on the cause of the trauma, stored as it is in the computer-like memory of the psyche. Zoë and Malcom have come to believe that their most valuable work lies in 'laying to rest the ghosts of our past that dwell on the fringe of consciousness', and that many people suffer unnecessarily from past-life experiences that cause ongoing suffering and imbalance.

In an overall sense the Hagons believe that we are what we are as a result of what we have experienced, and that past life therapy is a remarkable way of unifying factors of consciousness from both the past and the present – a healing process transcending time itself.

PHRENOLOGY

Traditionally phrenology has been defined as the art of reading the 'bumps' on a person's skull in order to show that conformations of the skull correspond with characteristics of the mind and body. Despite the fact that phrenology for most people has been dismissed as a superstition or pseudo-science modern day phrenologists claim that their art has been misrepresented. In the same way that a tennis player might develop strengthened wrists and forearms and an athlete specific muscles in the legs and torso, phrenologists claim that a similar relationship exists between aspects of the mind that a person chooses to develop and external areas of the skull above specific regions of the brain. Contemporary practitioners spend many years studying charts of these correlations taking into account different skull structures, hair growth and other variables. Phrenologists believe strongly that balanced development of the mind is essential and to this extent their views parallel

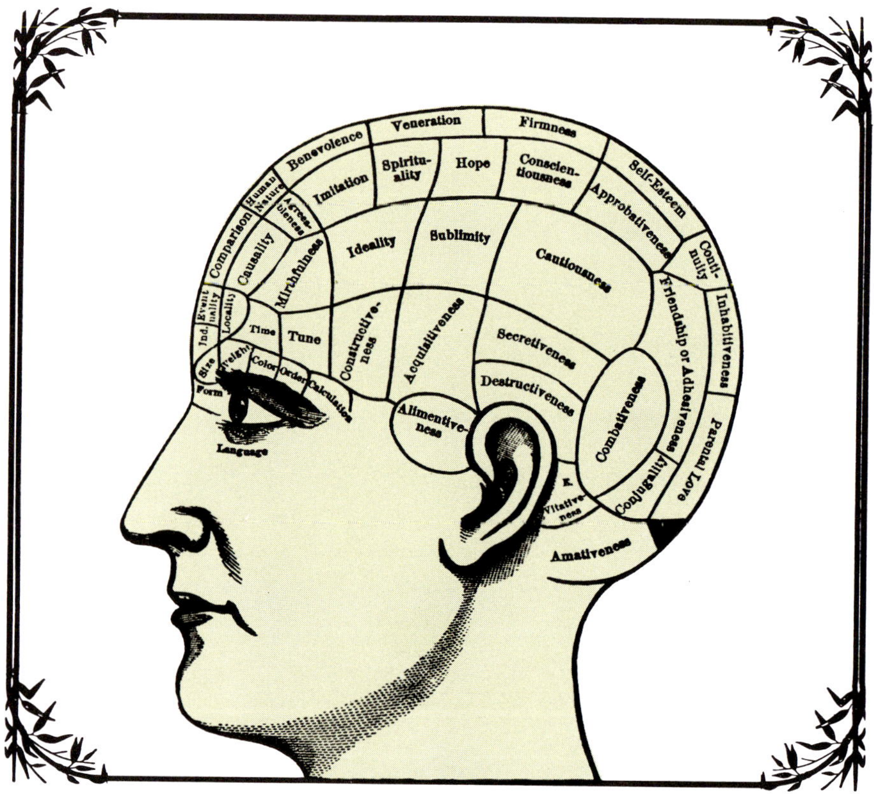

those made by some contemporary psychologists that our technological society has been drawing too heavily on left-hemisphere activities of the brain (associated with analytical thought, logic, sequence and order) and undervaluing right-hemisphere functions of consciousness (artistic endeavour, holistic thought, orientation in space).

Among the notable pioneers in the field of phrenology were Dr F.J. Gall (1756–1828) a successful physician in Vienna and Paris, and his colleague Dr J.G. Spurzheim. Together they wrote a major work titled *The Physiognomical System* and Gall spent many years producing impressive volumes on the brain complete with extraordinarily detailed illustrations.

Later, phrenology was adopted by certain of the English mesmerists who claimed that a somnambulent subject would respond to being touched on specific 'bumps' by exhibiting characteristics of that area of the brain. Several practitioners claimed to have discovered this new application, including a Dr Collyer and the Reverend Laroy Sunderland, although Collyer later repudiated phreno-mesmerism as a delusion.

Traditional phrenological associations are shown in the accompanying diagram.

POLARITY BALANCING

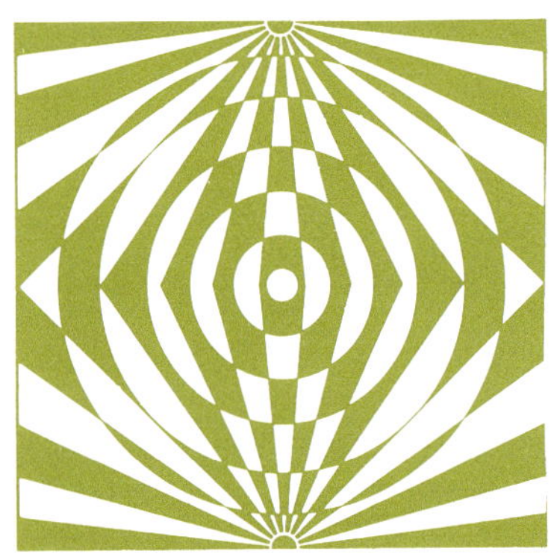

The system known as Polarity Balancing is linked closely to the concept of energy flow and as such bears some resemblance to Wilhelm Reich's 'orgone energy', Yogic 'prana', the Chinese 'chi' force and the parapsychological idea of 'bioplasma'.

The philosophy and principles of polarity therapy were developed by Austrian-born Dr Randolph Stone who had emigrated to the United States when he was 13 years old. A gifted man of far-ranging talents and interests, Stone studied orthodox Western science and also a range of natural healing techniques, finally earning himself doctorates in naturopathy, osteopathy and chiropractic. He also plunged himself into studying the esoteric systems of both East and West, especially where insights into the nature of health and illness could be gained. He read works on occultism and explored the theories underlying acupuncture, herbal medicine, shiatsu and the Indian system of Ayurveda. Polarity therapy is really a blend of these influences coupled with his own insights and personal knowledge. For many years Dr Stone taught and practised, mostly in the American Midwest, before retiring to live in India in 1973, at the age of 84.

Polarity therapists, in recognising the natural flow of energy through the body, attempt to locate areas where it has become blocked or impeded causing emotional tension and physical pain. Pain is defined as deriving from an area 'where the energy has become blocked and crystallised'. As the therapist begins to increase the speed of the energy flow in the body, the blockages break down and toxins are eliminated naturally by one of five means: through the breath, sweat, faeces, urine or emotions.

Dr Stone found that all natural healing techniques had a stimulating effect on the energy system operative in the physical organism. Such energy had a three-fold nature of positive : negative and neutral, known in India as the three *gunas*: Rajasic, Tamasic, and Satvic. Stone noted that the middle of the body was its neutral pole – from the crown of the head down through the spinal cord. The right side of the body was positive, giving off positive energy currents and the left side was correspondingly negative. He recognised the value inherent in the Eastern concept of the *chakras*:

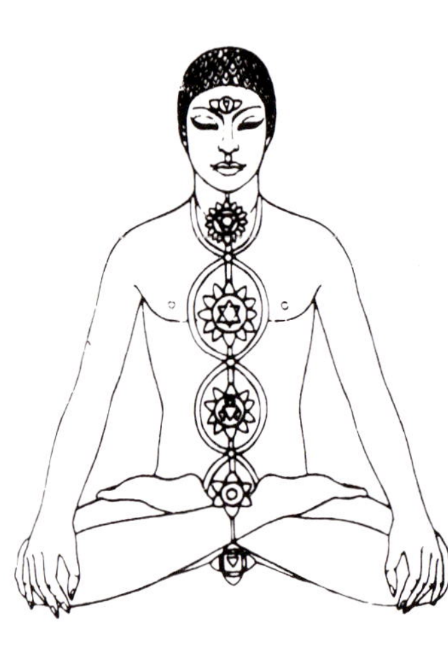

1. The energy centres of throat, forehead and crown associated with spirituality and *ether*,
2. The chakra governing the heart and lungs: *air*
3. The chakra of the solar plexus, stomach and intestines: *fire*
4. The pelvic/genital chakra linked with sexual reproduction and the emotional drive: *water*

5. The chakra of physical activity, associated with the base of the spine and the rectum: *earth*

In his small book *Health-Building* Stone notes the application of polarity balancing:

An excess amount of the positive current produces irritation, pain, swelling and heat in the tissues, organs and areas of the body, due to excess amount of blood in that area, and the opposite or negative pole energy is required to balance it. The positive current is the sun energy of fire and radiant warmth in normal amounts. The right hand *is the conductor of this energy. For negative tension, congestion, spasm and stasis, the right hand contains the antidote, the positive polarity current . . .*

The left hand *is the conductor of the negative or moon current, which is cooling, soothing, refreshing and toning. Place it over the seat of pain, where the positive currents are in excess, giving the above-mentioned symptoms. Wherever the pain is, that excess calls for release of irritation, heat, swelling . . . which the negative current can provide.*

Energy blockages occur as a result of tensions, perhaps brought on by emotional stress, but also from dietary imbalance. To avoid toxin-blockages, the result of improper digestive patterns, Dr Stone recommended a two-part dietary cycle which included a short period for *cleansing* followed by a longer period of *building*.

The cleansing diet, or 'liver flush' includes a drinking mixture containing olive or almond oil, lemon and orange juice, garlic and pepper followed by a herbal tea and fruit or vegetable salads for lunch and dinner. Meat, milk, eggs, coffee, alcohol and carbohydrate foods are excluded.

Following this diet, we come to the time for building vitality in the body. Stone called this the 'maintenance diet'.

In the morning hot water with lemon juice is taken, followed half an hour (or more) later with a non-citrus fruit salad or whole-grain porridge. The main meal of the day is lunch and it should include fresh fruits and vegetables, sprouting grains, beans and seeds. Stone warns that typically the Western diet contains too much rich food and substances which are almost indigestible; quite aside from the fact that most of us eat too much anyway!

Blockages and tensions can also be reduced by a series of exercises:

The Squat

Dr Stone called this 'the youth posture', a way for regaining and retaining vitality. Healthy children often adopt it and in the East generally it is the position for sitting, talking, eating, bearing children and defecating. According to polarity therapists the squat is excellent because it provides a gentle stretch for areas that are often tight: the pelvis, the lower back and the spine. It is recommended as a basic exercise – springing up and down on the balls of the feet – for a few minutes each day.

The Cliff Hanger

This exercise is a powerful stretch and releases tension in the shoulders and neck. Initially one has to find a 'cliff' to hang on to. The edge of a table is excellent:

With your back facing the cliff, rest the heels of your hands on the cliff, letting your fingers hang over the edge, and lower your fairly erect spine until you feel the stretch. As much as possible, use the arms to raise yourself back up, repeating several times with co-ordinated breath: exhale going down, inhale coming up. Then stand free of the cliff and breathe!

The Woodchopper

So-called because the action imitates the chopping of wood with an axe. Polarity therapists stress that it is excellent for the circulation and also relaxes the diaphragm:

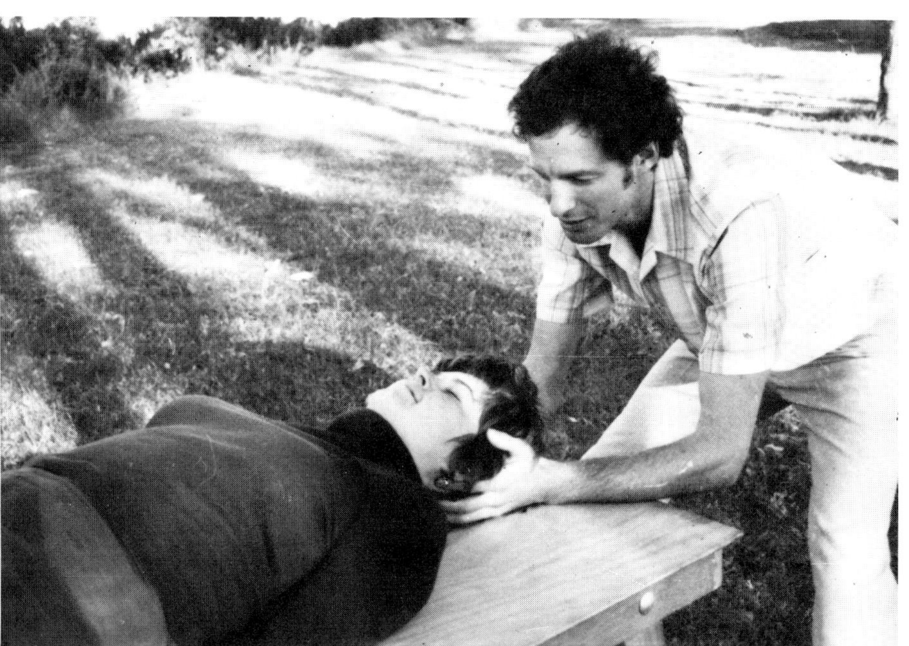

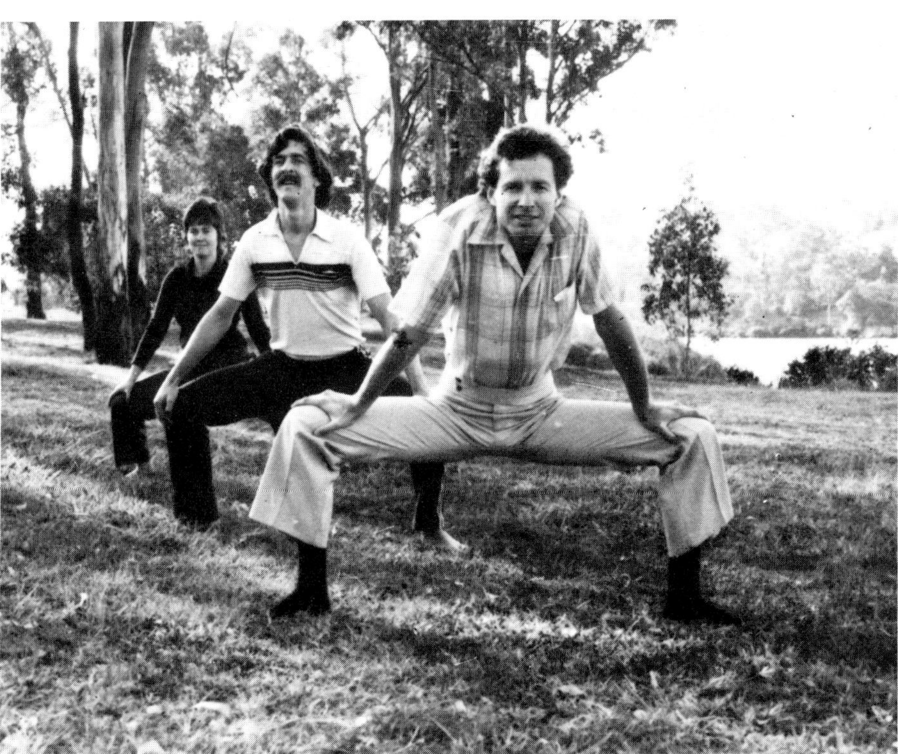

Polarity therapist Gerald Rosenove demonstrating different aspects of his approach. above: *assessing energy flow;* below: *leading friends in 'the squat'*

With the legs comfortably apart for balance, clasp your hands together and swing them up over your head with an inhalation, reaching toward the sky. Then swing forward with a "Ha!" sound (deep, rich and powerful) letting the stroke complete itself between the legs.

Polarity therapy is admittedly eclectic and draws on many sources of ideas and applications for integrating mind and body. In an interview at the Polarity Health Institute, Fall River Mills, California, Directors Sharon and Jefferson Campbell were asked how their therapy techniques compared with massage, acupressure, acupuncture and reflexology. The answer is an interesting one:

Acupuncture and acupressure are based on some of the Polarity principles but their emphasis is different. Some massage people and Rolfers are integrating Polarity with their work and are finding out that by making longer contacts, by working with the energy currents with both *hands constantly on the body, their work is easier and more effective.*

Reflexology generally deals with the feet . . . Dr Stone shows us how the body maps itself many times over — in the hands, the tongue, the limbs, the face, the eyes and in the feet, from several different angles not generally found in foot reflexology charts . . .

Dr Stone incorporated the best of all the natural health practices while adding an energy understanding of how they worked, how they fit together.

Although he has retired to India, Dr Stone is still active, providing clinics for those wishing to experience Polarity balancing as far afield as Calcutta and Bombay. In the United States and in other western countries his work is being continued by such therapists as Pierre Pannetier in Orange, California and other practitioners who have trained at the Polarity Health Institute.

Dr Stone sums up his philosophy this way:

The awareness of life as energy currents, and their regulation as the normal flow, is the key to the natural art of Health-building by regulating the food, drink, the emotions and the mind: all to the pattern of nature and its rational rhythm and keynote.

GERALD ROSENOVE

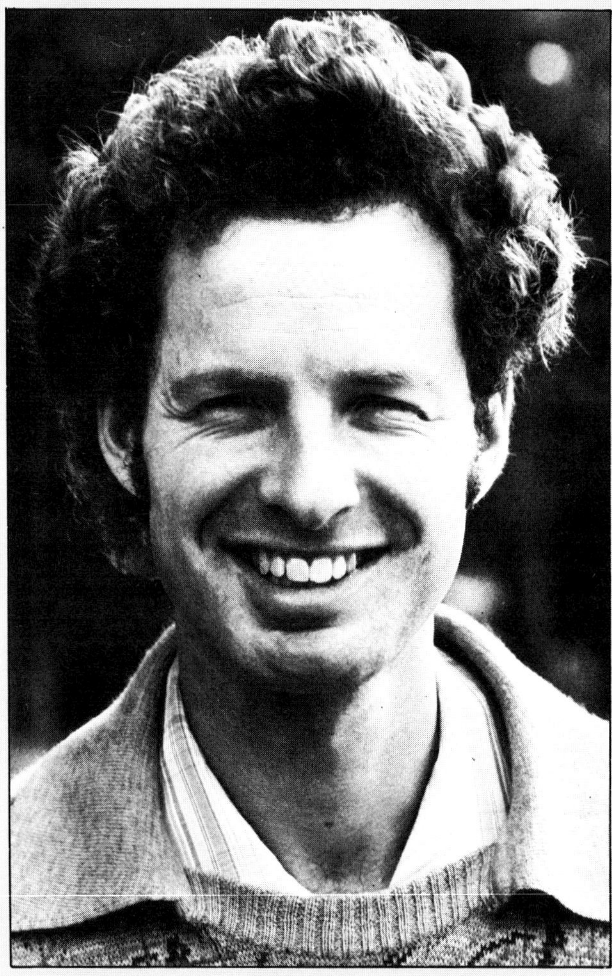

Like many alternative health therapists, Gerald Rosenove adopted his approach initially as a result of family circumstances. His father was a chronic asthmatic and his mother was bed-ridden with acute scoliosis: their solution was to take up Hatha Yoga.

As a result Gerald, who was then 13, became deeply interested in the potential of the human body to cure itself and he still holds to the basic philosophy that one must take responsibility for one's personal disease and imbalance.

Born in Melbourne, Gerald studied fine art and then trained to become a teacher, but became alienated by the over-emphasis on intellectual development in traditional educational methods. Somewhat jaded, he departed for India, staying for a year and visiting several ashrams. He spent six months with Swami Muktananda at Bombay studying Siddha Yoga and it was there that a chance meeting with a member of the American Polarity Health Institute changed his entire future direction. Gerald was given his first personal demonstration of natural healing, experiencing the pulse balancing and energy flow testing that he now practises in his therapy.

After returning to Australia in August 1978, Gerald contacted the Polarity Institute on Orcas Island near Seattle, Washington. Its founder, Dr Randolph Stone, had retired in 1972 but the polarity work pioneered by him was continuing and attracting increasing international recognition. Gerald undertook training at the Polarity Health Institute and believes he is still the only Australian to have studied there although others have participated in workshops run by Stone's protege Pierre Pannetier who is based in Orange, California.

Gerald Rosenove now lives in Queensland but does not confine his activities to that State. While he works alongside Reichian therapist Peter Eedy at the Taringa Health Centre he is also active touring, conducting workshops, counselling and participating in New Age groups in Melbourne, Sydney and Canberra. He was involved in the important conference at Brisbane's Griffith University: *Visions For The Future: an exhibition of change* in October 1980 and believes that there is increasing acceptance of new therapies for health. While his attention has been on polarity energy, he recognises that the balancing of positive, negative and neutral in the body has equivalents in acupuncture, Buddhism, yoga, Taoism and other mind/body philosophies. Within his own frameworks of analysis, for example, he uses the Yang/Yin distinction to refer to the flow of energy through the body with the right hand of the healer acting to stimulate (positive, Yang) and the left hand (negative, Yin) to soothe energy imbalances in the patient.

Gerald Rosenove is a strong advocate of the work of Dr Randolph Stone and at present is the leading exponent of his polarity energy balancing techniques in Australia.

PRIMAL THERAPY

Arthur Janov has worked for thirty years in psychotherapy specialising in child psychology and psychiatric work. He has become world-famous for his work on Primal Therapy and now directs two institutes, in Los Angeles and New York.

Primal Therapy, in essence, is an attack on neurosis. Mental illness, he believes, has its origins in Primal Pain which has been carried around since childhood. Perhaps this 'Pain' (differentiated from more superficial pain, of a physical nature) derived from a serious humiliation, rejection by a parent or by some sense of terrifying isolation. Such events might have built up to an overload situation but at that stage they became unconscious : a child understandably finds it difficult to comprehend and resolve such traumas and the Pain is blocked.

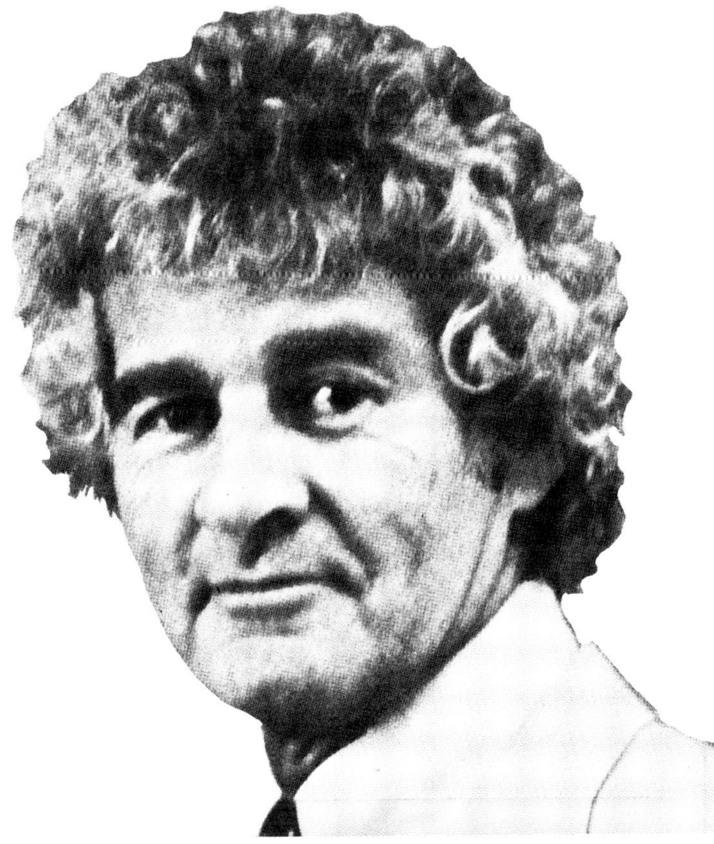

Arthur Janov – acknowledging Primal Pain

In his writings Janov emphasises that as Pain and repression establish themselves a new self emerges: *the unreal self*. This persona engages in a smothering process, increasingly shielding out the Pain and refusing to acknowledge its very existence. In his most recent work *Prisoners of Pain,* Janov writes: 'The real self is simply the part of us which contains all our buried feelings and needs. The unreal self is the part of us that carries out the burial . . .'

In his earlier, famous book *The Primal Scream* Janov had noted that the split between these two selves could derive from a single major event in childhood around the ages of 6–8. He now believes that the germs of neurosis can arise much earlier but it is around the age of 6 that the unreal self begins to 'crystallise'. By the teen years the character has become fairly fixed and neuroses express themselves through emotional and intellectual patterns. Religious fanaticism in the late teen years, for example, may result from the need for a protective, loving father, or there may be emotional outbursts, idiosyncratic speech patterns and various obsessive habits.

Neurotics develop these 'secondary defences' to shield their real feelings and they may indeed be concocted to help the person adjust to the outside world. Nevertheless, from this point onwards the only way for a person to become 'real' again is to reverse the process of neurosis. This is exactly what Primal Therapy sets out to do. A neurotic is caught in the bind of either feeling Pain or struggling against it, so Primal Therapy gradually dismantles the pattern of defences which shields the person from the experience of Pain. Janov notes: 'Until we feel the Pain, we suffer'. Pain heals, while suffering is the chronic state of not having healed . . . Primal Therapy seeks to uncover the deep emotions, which Janov believes to be truly rational. Neurotic behaviour derives from blocked feelings and it is the therapist's task to reach beneath these defences. In Primal sessions the suffering has to be converted into Pain for the healing to occur.

As the therapist dismantles the layers of defence he defers the acting out of tensions and guides them towards a climax. This is a very sensitive process and the therapist has to be careful not to plunge the patient in too quickly. Janov believes that healing takes place in the 'Primal Zone' . . . an area of consciousness where feelings are *accepted and integrated*. This is approached by guiding the patient towards a peak . . . the suffering builds up but then the patient begins to directly experience the underlying Pain, which floods the consciousness during the moment of self-recognition accompanying the Primal Scream. This is followed by a profound sense of relief, because conflicting facets of the self have been integrated.

The process has to be conducted with the utmost care because if the therapist were to push the patient too quickly the sense of 'overload' could occur again, producing further repressions and neuroses. For this reason Janov and his colleagues emphasise that Primal Therapy must only be conducted by specially trained and skilled practitioners.

Primal Therapy treatment may extend over one or two years. Initially therapy is individually based and the therapist seeks to get behind behaviour and speech barriers thrown up as defences. There may also be a need for the therapist to redirect the patient away from *external* authority figures (parents, the therapist etc.) and towards *inner* reference points. After two or three weeks of individual sessions the patient then joins a group which may include as many as sixty people. However, as Janov indicates, this is not an encounter session. The people present are there to learn from within themselves and not from others. The therapists guide the patients towards such self-recognition. It is necessary for the opening-up process to be complete, since anything less would still result in buried elements of neurosis. And the process of *feeling* is ongoing : many patients experience Primals after therapy has theoretically concluded.

Janov emphasises that is possible for a person to indulge, knowingly or unknowingly, in 'fake' Primals. These episodes, known as abreactions, are in themselves defences which are easier to experience than real Pain. The clue is that abreactions do not involve the experience of true and profound feelings but only shallow emotions. The patient may scream, cry and thrash around but in the final analysis such a performance is only a hysterical display. Abreactions may involve suffering, but not the experience of Primal Pain. True Primals strike to the cause of repressions and move through all levels of consciousness from the intellectual and emotional through to the *visceral* level of experience where the earliest traumas occur.

Primal Therapy is thus a process of 'neurosis in reverse', a means of directing consciousness back to the very origins of repression in early childhood and towards the integration of all layers of the self.

DR GLYN SEABORN JONES

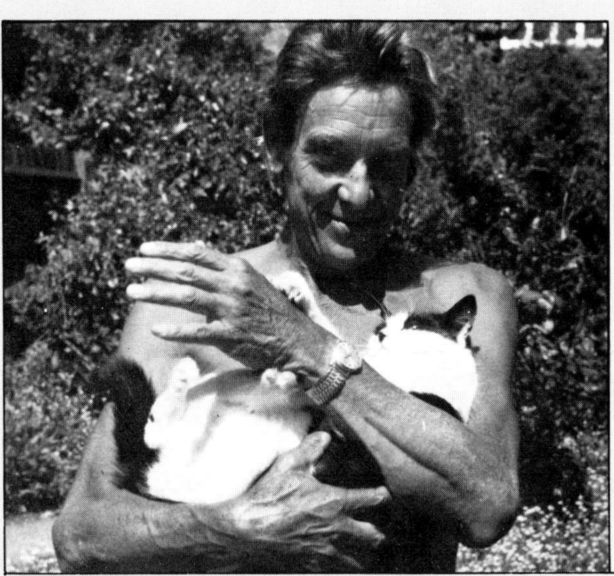

When Dr Glyn Seaborn Jones talks about primal therapy the subject of cats tends to crop up. He likes them and not simply because they are soothing company. They also provide an apt analogy with the results he works to achieve with his clients. Cats, he says, are perfectly content to curl up and just *be*, simply to exist. They don't demand a constant bombardment of stimulation and distraction as most people do – tea, coffee, whisky, radio, television, newspapers and chatter. It is by the temporary withdrawal of these things, while at the same time giving appropriate therapeutic support to his clients, that he helps to bring about an integration of their whole personality and organism. He calls his approach to primal therapy, *Intensive Rhythm Therapy*. *Intensive*, because, while undergoing it, temporarily it becomes the most important thing in the client's life. *Rhythm*, because the aim is for the client to find his own natural rhythm according to his own energy, capacity, needs and upbringing.

To his work Dr Seaborn Jones brings a background of theoretical and practical experience in philosophy, psychology and psychotherapy. A former classical scholar, he studied Latin, Greek and ancient history at Jesus College, Oxford, and, after serving in the RAF during the war, returned to study philosophy, politics and economics, following this with a Ph.D at London University in philosophy and psychology. He worked in psychoanalysis with an analytic group and for eleven and a half years was with a research group at the Tavistock Clinic. In his work he employed a combination of the theories of Freud and Melanie Klein with Gestalt. Becoming dissatisifed with purely verbal techniques and increasingly interested in bodily aspects of behaviour he studied bioenergetics with John Pierrakos, psychomotor therapy with Albert Pesso and, when group leaders from Esalen came to London, attended their seminars in Encounter methods.

It was in the 1960s that he developed his Intensive Rhythm Therapy. He uses a three-week isolation period during which the patient is cut off from his family, his friends and all distractions. He asks him to sign an undertaking that during the three weeks he will abstain from alcohol, nicotine, sedatives, pain-killers, tranquillisers, anti-depressants and all other drugs. The patient also agrees to refrain from reading books, newspapers or magazines. He is provided with paper and drawing material for doodling and painting and is encouraged to express primal feelings and any creativity that comes from within. Swimming and walking is also permitted. He finds that when his clients' minds are freed in this way from external stimulus and input, their whole organism tends to integrate and the natural healing process begins to take place. Prior to this three-week period, for which there is normally a wating list, the client has individual therapy sessions with him and afterwards there is a follow-up of similar sessions, which last about a year. There is then a phasing out, when clients join *Reciport* sessions, a system of reciprocal support, carried out in groups, where the principles of primal therapy form the basic approach.

He finds that the effects of primal therapy are most dramatic in younger people between the ages of eighteen and thirty. The degree of change in their character, personality and mode of life is so considerable that you could call it a transformation. 'People who have known the person before and afterwards can hardly believe he is the same individual'. Although older people, he finds, do not display such a marked change, they do feel very much better; there is a steady reduction of their anxiety level and life becomes enjoyable.

During the fifteen years of his work in primal therapy no client has ever left without completing the three-week isolation period. He tells of one young man undergoing it who appeared to be obeying all the rules but was then discovered to be taking a night coach to the provinces in order to provide himself with a distraction. 'He was', says Dr Seaborn Jones, 'using the coach window as a "television screen". I had to explain to him that travel by night coach was not allowed, but it hadn't occurred to me to put it on the list of prohibitions!'

In addition to his work in primal therapy, he runs training groups for professional therapists who are disenchanted with using only verbal techniques, and their instruction includes primal therapy method. He also takes part in a television series called *Predicaments*. People are invited to write into the programme if they feel they would benefit by discussing their own predicament in the studio. One such issue concerned 'feeling worthless'. What has impressed him about the series is that people seem to benefit simply by revealing quite openly what they have been keeping as a 'guilty secret' for a long time. When they reveal it in the studio, often to family and friends watching, they experience enormous relief, sometimes with a profound effect on their lives.

PSIONIC MEDICINE

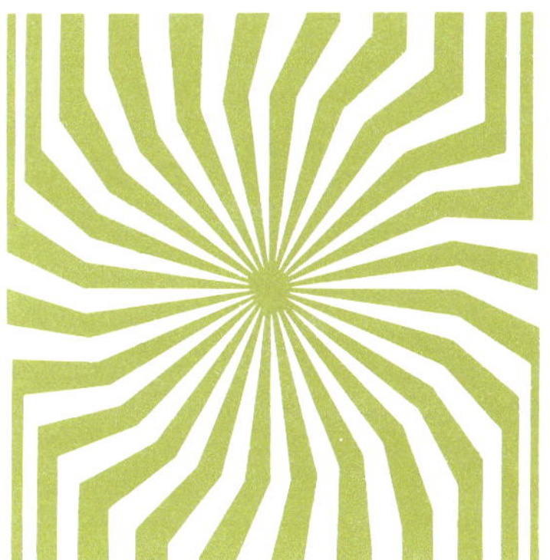

Psionics grew out of medical radiesthesia and the work of such pioneers as Dr Albert Abrams and Dr Guyon Richards. It was developed by Dr George Laurence, who was a member of the Medical Society for the Study of Radiesthesia and a physician of many years standing. Dr Laurence was particularly interested in the nature of chronic disease. He preferred to avoid the use of drugs and surgery and considered that medical radiesthesia and related techniques offered more fruitful possibilities.

Psionics makes use of the dowsing faculty but also includes aspects of homeopathy and various 'vitalist' theories of energy flow. Laurence applied a holistic philosophy to the nature of disease and held the view that disease was related to protein balance. Toxic substances would tend to cause various organs to fall out of balance with the intrinsic vitality of the body as a whole. Laurence borrowed Samuel Hahnemann's idea of 'miasms' in introducing homeopathic concepts to his work. Hahnemann had posited the idea of disruptive factors affecting the body's natural curative capacity and reasoned that such 'miasms' interfered with the vital energy flow in the organism. Miasms prevented the body from satisfactorily recovering from chronic diseases. Inherited miasms linked one generation to another: imbalances underlying chronic diseases arising in one generation could be passed on, manifesting as symptoms in successive generations. Such factors as diet, stress and environmental factors could trigger the flow of hereditary miasms or toxic residues and bring on new attacks of disease.

Psionic medicine aims to diagnose body imbalance taking such factors into consideration and focuses on the *original and basic cause* of disease, not necessarily the more obvious factors. It is an effective treatment which avoids the use of synthetic chemicals.

According to Dr Laurence a high proportion of mental illness derives from inherited miasms in conjunction with acquired toxins, and miasms relate very specifically to familiar complaints. Laurence emphasises syphilis and TB as the main hereditary miasms, and measles, chicken pox and whooping cough as the dominant acquired ones. Dr Aubrey Westlake, a founding member of the Psionic Medical Society (established in 1968), believes that the hereditary TB miasm underlies such diseases as asthma, hay fever, sinus complaints, and several types of mental illness and may also be connected to leukaemia and diabetes.

Although the idea of toxic residues and inherited miasms seems very unorthodox, a report in *Scientific American* in 1974 drew attention to the fact that viruses often remained in the body without revealing themselves in the form of infection, and could subsequently 'cause or trigger degenerative disease in man'.

Psionic Technique

Dr Laurence's system depends on the idea that everything in Nature radiates a vibration which can be perceived as being either in or out of balance. Health is a state of balance – 'a balanced harmonious behaviour of energy patterns'. Chronic imbalance on the other hand gives rise to disease.

Psionic medical practitioners use the so-called W.O. Wood chart to register pendulum readings which reflect degrees of balance or imbalance. Health is represented as zero on the chart *(illustrated)* and deviations are marked as 'plus' or 'minus' readings. There is a three-way variable because different factors are brought to bear at each point of the triangle. A sample of blood from the patient is placed on the right hand corner; this is the 'patient's witness'. The so-called 'diagnostic witness' – consisting of samples of tissues, organs and diseases in homeopathic potency – is placed in the left hand corner, and proposed homeopathic remedies are located at the apex. When the forces from the three corners are in a state of balance, indicating an appropriate cure has been ascertained, the radiesthetist's pendulum swings up and down the zero line and does not deviate. Since there are potentially a large number of diseases that a patient could be suffering from, Dr Laurence and his colleagues draw also on detailed medical histories to provide clues and also use a classificatory system correlating diseases with colour. Laurence found that infections reacted differently to different colours and if he exposed the patient's 'witness' to a certain colour the reaction could point towards a specific group of possible diseases, and provide a short-cut to diagnosis.

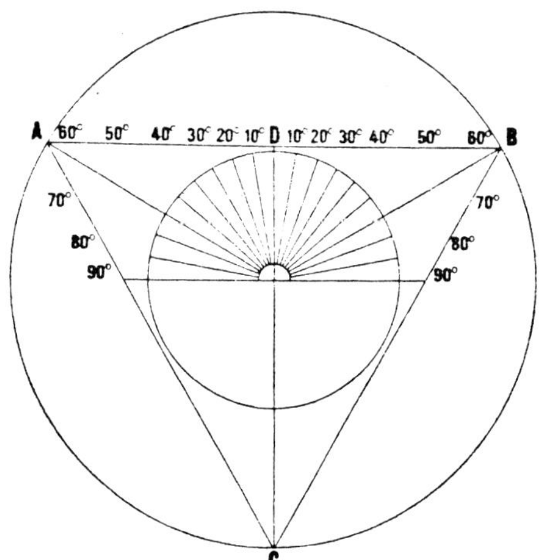

A diagnostic chart of the type used by practitioners of medical radiesthesia and psionic medicine

Psionic medicine's great claim is its use in treating chronic diseases by determining the underlying causal factors. It draws attention to the fact that holistic medical treatments can only be effective if they recognise the presence of miasms and acquired toxins and seek to remove them. Psionic medicine is also preventative since its techniques enable hereditary miasms to be detected and eliminated in children – breaking the otherwise ongoing patterns of potential disease transmitted from one generation to another.

PSYCHIC SURGERY

While spiritual healing is acknowledged by some doctors as a possible psychosomatic treatment for illness, psychic surgery is much more controversial. In recent years the popular press has abounded with tales of miraculous cures and equally vehement claims of fraudulence and deception. Do the healers of the Philippines, for example, really penetrate the skin of their patients, withdraw diseased body tissue and tumours from the body and then heal the parted skin without trace?

According to leading American surgeon William Nolen, who spent two years researching the subject, the Filipino healers use concealed mica flecks to make incisions, substitute betel-nut juice for blood and employ advanced techniques of sleight of hand to simulate 'psychic surgery'. He also believes that the material 'extracted' from the bodies of patients is non-human, and notes that when he subjected himself to an operation he recognised a 'tumour' removed from his body as animal fat – probably from a chicken.

It is commonly claimed by sceptics that the psychic surgeons conceal the objects they will later withdraw (animal tissue, blood substitutes) and pinch the skin in folds to give the impression of an incision by the fingers. Any cures that are effected are thus purely psychosomatic and have no basis in actual surgery. While this is certainly the case with a wide range of psychic healers, the available evidence is contradictory and it is necessary to keep an open mind about the nature of the healing experience. It is possible that in both the Philippines and Brazil authentic healers are being imitated by sleight-of-hand charlatans anxious to exploit a huge captive audience of willing subjects.

There are currently around 30 Filipino healers, including Juan Blanche, Benji Belacano and Alex Orbito in Manila; Jun Labo, Tony Agpaoa, Philip

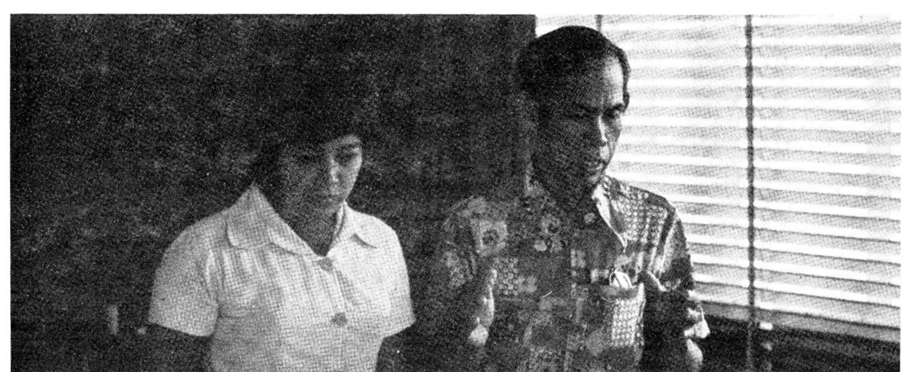

Benji Belacano and his assistant

Malicdon and Placido Palitayan in Baguio City, and Josephina Sison in Pangasinan. The degrees of commerciality surrounding these healers, and their claims to authenticity, vary enormously. Several of the healers appear to be working in conjunction with international travel agents and making considerable incomes from their healing performances. Graham Gambie, an Australian investigative journalist, writes for example that Tony Agpaoa has contracts for 20 tour groups and uses four assistants to treat 200 patients simultaneously. Jun Labo '. . . sports a permanent wave, a diamond ear-stud and heavy gold jewellery. He works out of a lavish hotel disco catering mainly for wealthy Japanese businessmen . . .' It is also evident that while payments for psychic surgery used to be voluntary, the tour groups are now fixing donations in a large number of cases – at between $175 and $2000 per operation. Belacano, Blanche, Sison and Placido are among the few who have not succumbed to commercialisation of their services.

In September 1974 a number of court hearings were held in the United States before Judge Daniel H. Hanscom. Their purpose was to resolve complaints against a number of travel agencies that arranged package tours to the Philippines for psychic surgery. The hearings involved 48 witnesses, 134 exhibits and culminated in a report 2388 pages long. Judge Hanscom finally described psychic surgery as 'pure and unmitigated fakery' and ordered the travel agencies to stop promoting the controversial healing tours. Two of the witnesses, Carol and Donald Wright, were initially favourably disposed towards the psychic surgeons. However Carol Wright changed her mind after analysing a 'tumour' which she found to be 'a flat piece of membrane that had been stuffed with cotton and blood clots to look like a round tumour'. Donald Wright meanwhile claimed that a Filipino healer had confided in him and explained how animal tissue and organs could be used in sleight of hand techniques. After watching a number of psychic healers in action the Wrights claimed that several well known figures – including Terte, Alex Orbito, Tony Santiago, Jose Mercado and Placido Palitayan – used sleight of hand.

Another witness, Phyllis Douglass, received treatment from Tony Agpaoa for breast cancer. Her husband subsequently had a part of the removed tissue analysed by a pathologist who stated that it came from the bowel of a small animal.

Dr Thomas Hausen from West Germany and two Filipino physicians, Augustus Damian and Leopoldo Lazatin, visited Josephina Sison at her chapel and watched her 'opening up' her patients using only her hands. She wore a sleeveless blouse and apparently had no facility for concealing substitute animal tissue. After watching Sison perform, the three doctors were convinced she was genuine. However when Dr Hausen had a Sison 'tumour' analysed in West Germany it proved to be part of a plant. Dr Hausen said later : 'I still can't believe that I was tricked . . . I'm a medical man, trained to observe surgical procedures. I'm not easily impressed or fooled . . . I just don't know how they did it'.

Alex Orbito no longer allows specimens to be taken away and claims that foreigners have substituted animal liver and tissues in scientific analysis – giving him a bad name. Juan Blanche believes that most of the healers are fraudulent, and visited several of them himself, in the role of a patient, to discover their methods. However a conjuror assisting in a research project organised by Ateneo University noticed a small razor blade dropping from Blanche's finger-nail during a 'psychic operation'. No-one else present observed this deception.

A similar tradition of psychic surgery also operates in Brazil where the Spiritist movement influenced by 19th century Frenchman Allan Kardec continues to flourish. According to Kardec, who authored such works as *The Spirits' Book*, *The Medium's Book* and *Spiritualist Initiation*, . . . everyone is a spiritualist who believes that there is in him something more than matter . . .' Several Brazilian healers claim to perform psychic surgery under the guidance of spirit physicians while others use techniques closely resembling those of the Filipino healers. In his book *The Unknown Power* (1975), Guy Lyon Playfair described the work of such healers as Antonio Sales who used no anaesthetic and relied on the guidance of spirit physicians in eye operations, and Lourival de Freitas who claimed the assistance of the spirit of Emperor Nero. Other healers like 'Maria' and 'Zeca' used various instruments in surgery. Maria employed scissors and pincers and Zeca orthodox surgical instruments, withdrawing diseased material from the bodies of his patients with apparently no possibility of sleight of hand. However in his later book *The Indefinite Boundary* Playfair writes that Zeca had later been caught in a 'deliberate and premeditated fraud' on at least one occasion.

If so many psychic surgeons are fraudulent are there any who are genuine? One has to remember that such judgments depend very much on whether a healing practitioner has actually been caught deceiving his patients, and the track record of the Filipino and Brazilian psychic surgeons is not very impressive. Possibly there may be exceptions.

Jose Pedro de Freitas – known to the world as Arigo – began to acquire an international reputation as a healer in 1956 after operating on a Brazilian politician, Lucio Bittencourt, for a tumour of the lung. X-rays taken after an operation on Bittencourt showed that the tumour had disappeared.

Dr Andrija Puharich was one of several American doctors who investigated Arigo's healing operations in the village of Congonhas de Campo. Arigo claimed to be guided by the spirit of a German physician named 'Dr Fritz' who spoke to him through his right ear. Consequently instead of diagnosing 'eye trouble', for example, Arigo might announce that a subject was suffering from 'retinoblastoma'. He was often able to make extremely specific medical diagnoses merely by looking at patients, despite the fact that he had had minimal education, read no books and had spent most of his life in menial clerical or labouring jobs. Unlike some of his Filipino counterparts, Arigo did not charge a fee for his services. Dr Puharich and his medical colleagues were extremely impressed, and puzzled, by his diagnostic abilities:

A good healer, and I don't limit this strictly to Arigo, has the ability to somehow match, in his head, a knowledge of what is wrong with the chemical nature of an individual and fill that missing link in the chemical puzzle with the right type of chemical. In the case of Arigo, he had this ability to an extraordinary and even a superlative degree. He would prescribe every known pharmacological agent to patients, and he would do this in a way totally unknown to modern medicine.

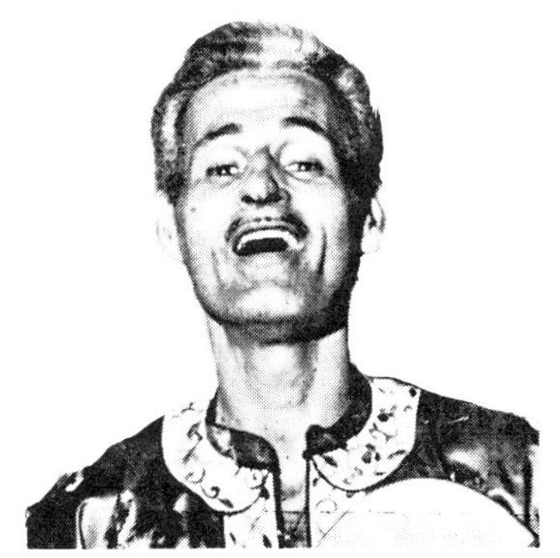

Brazilian healer Lourival de Freitas

Arigo also performed hundreds of 'psychic'operations in Dr Puharich's presence, during which he used an ordinary knife or scissors in surgery without anaesthetising his subject or sterilising his instruments. On no occasion did the operation cause pain. Sometimes the surgery was extremely delicate. Puharich watched Arigo remove cataracts from an eye without producing any ill-effects whatever.

Australian writer and editor, Clare Downs, has also reported a personal experience of psychic surgery in the Philippines which clearly did not involve sleight of hand and was accompanied by extraordinary photographs.

Clare visited the psychic surgeon Benji Belacano in Manila and told him about her rare liver complaint. Benji performed several operations on her which she was able to observe closely and a series of close-up photographs were also taken. They have since been published in the Australian journal *Simply Living*. Clare watched incredulously as Benji held his hands four inches above her skin and parted it – without touching it – between her breast and stomach. Photographs of her operation show the yawning incision quite clearly without any possibility of body-fold deception. Clare writes : 'It is hard to convey how it feels to have your skin part and curve inwards to expose a pool of blood which sits there, quietly'.

In view of the conflicting evidence available it is extremely difficult to pronounce one way or the other on the authenticity of psychic surgeons. Thousands of visitors to the Philippines have claimed astonishing cures while an equally large number of patients have returned to their homes still suffer-

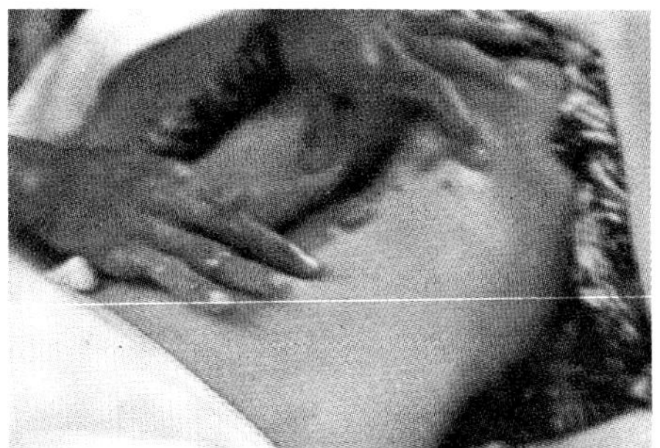

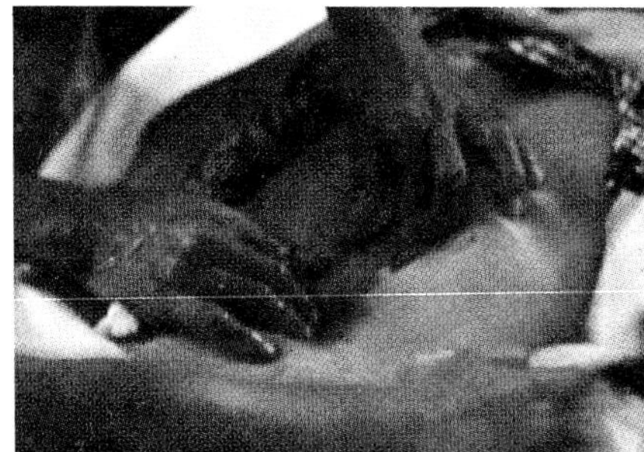

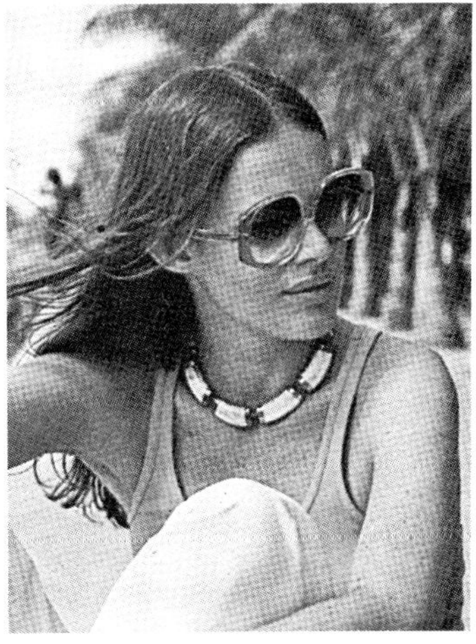

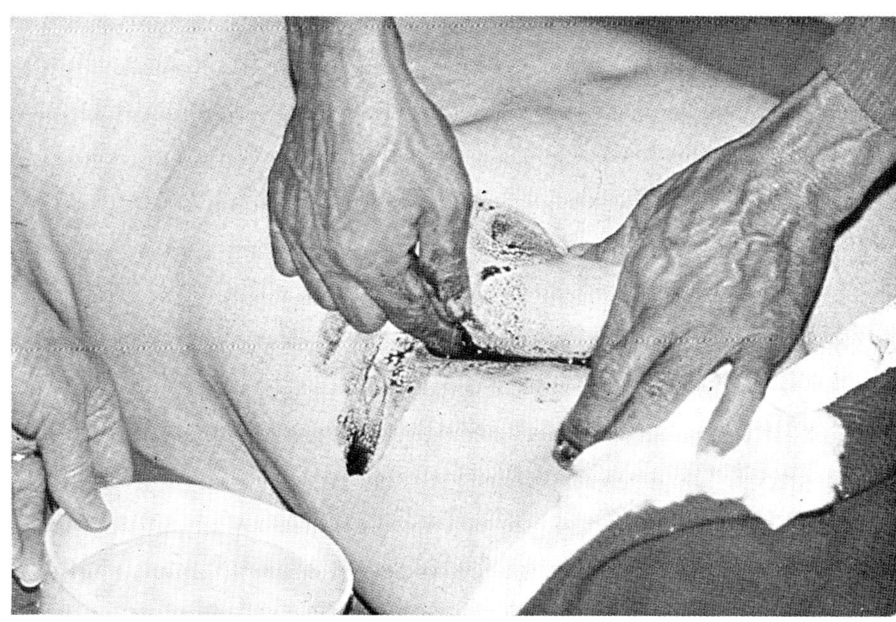

Australian journalist Clare Downs visited psychic surgeon Benji Belacano in the Philippines. These photographs show the dramatic effects of his 'psychic surgery'

ing from their original illnesses. Some psychic surgeons – like David and Helen Elizalde who normally reside in Australia – are now travelling to other countries to demonstrate their powers, and recently gave a healing performance at Stansted Hall in Essex. Among those who received treatment included the editor of *Psychic News*, Maurice Barbanell, his wife Sylvia and American acupuncturist Alan Papier. The results were impressive and Papier was moved to comment : 'I do not pretend to explain how it works. There is no reason why psychic surgery should not work . . .'

It is perhaps appropriate to sound a note of caution about psychic surgery while admitting that there appear to be genuine cases as well as obvious instances of fraud and deception. There is no doubt that psychic healing can certainly produce psychosomatic cures but Clare Downs' documented experience, in particular, points to a quite different mode of surgical operation from that known to orthodox medicine.

PSYCHOMETRY

Psychometry is a diagnostic technique of determining the characteristics of people who are not present by means of objects that have been in their possession. The theory was conceived and named by the psychic researcher Dr J.R. Buchanan who believed that every object or event that has ever occurred has left its impression in the 'ether' or 'astral light'. Psychometry has played a major role in spiritualism since mediums claim to be able to sensitively perceive events and activities on the astral plane.

The technique of psychometry involves holding in the hand or close to the forehead such objects as a watch, ring or jewellery, that have been the close personal property of the one from whom an 'impression' is required. A medium using psychometry will relax with the eyes closed, hold the object carefully and then begin either to speak or record internal images. Quite often in a spiritualist meeting details of sex, age, physical description, health and personal circumstances can be given in detail.

Australian therapist Malcom Hagon combines psychometry with relaxation. In his recent book *Journey Within* he writes:

A good method here is to breathe in deeply and then slowly exhale, concentrating as you do on each part of your body, and purposefully letting it go loose. Start at your toes and end up at your scalp. Once peaceful, turn your thoughts to the object you are to read.

It is important to be aware that from the very beginning that objects are very much like records or tape recordings, in that, as well as being physical, they have impressions stored within them which, under the right circumstances, can be tapped. This information takes two forms: the inherent memory of the object, and the other impressions which have been transferred to it by its owner or owners. The strength or intensity of these impressions will vary . . .

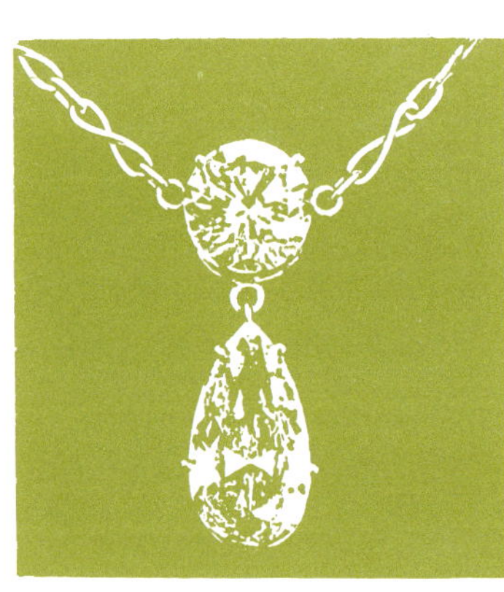

Following various experiments, Dr Buchanan discovered that if medical substances were used in psychometry the students often exhibited the symptoms that would result had the substances been swallowed. Later he found that it was possible for some people to diagnose illness simply by holding the patient's hand.

Psychometry is allied to radiesthesia and radionics as an intuitive art and has been used effectively by some holistic practitioners to diagnose specific causes of pain, ongoing medical ailments, misalignments of bones in the body or traumatic past events that continue to influence the present state of health.

PSYCHOSOMATIC HEALING

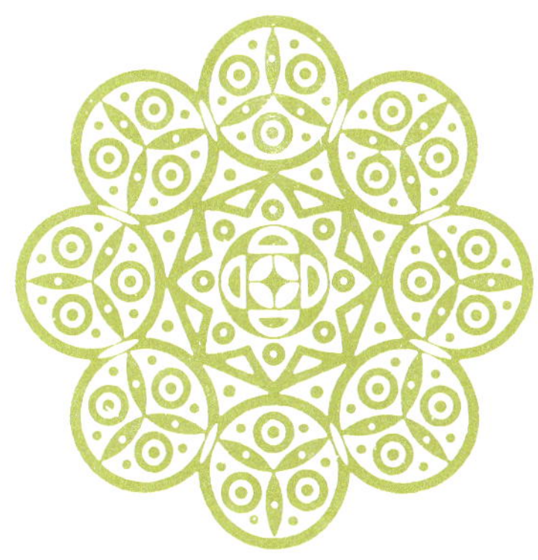

We live in an age where heart attacks and cancer are the two major killers. This situation has led many to ask: Is there any connection between the increasing pressures of our modern lifestyle and the rising incidence of these diseases? Are they related to stress?

The issue of the inter-relatedness of mind and body has only just begun to gain new consideration in medical circles. Until recent times any specific links between mind (psyche) and body (soma) in relation to the cause of disease have been difficult to demonstrate clinically, even though many individual doctors have believed for some time that such connections exist.

Professor Hans Selye of the University of Montreal regards stress as an extremely important factor underlying illness. However, he points out that stress should not necessarily be equated with the *intensity* of lifestyle. Stress is best thought of as deriving from the perception of events in our lives and is a reflection of our ability to deal with the demands of those events. Stress may be measured by such factors as general irritability, depression, high blood pressure, impulsive and aggressive behaviour, inability to concentrate, accident proneness, emotional tension, sexual problems, insomnia, migraine headaches and a variety of other symptoms. Selye notes that people react differently to the demands made upon them. We all learn to adapt to pressures but stress arises when the processes of coping begin to fail. We then have to develop daily priorities for regaining equilibrium – by slowing down or altering the pace of life, and so on. Otherwise we risk a breakdown of health beginning perhaps with relatively minor conditions like skin complaints and intestinal upsets but leading possibly to more serious illnesses.

Studies have been made to determine whether stress is related to the incidence of cancer and heart attacks, and consideration has been given to the question: Are certain personality types more susceptible?

In 1959 the Californian cardiologists Dr Ray Rosenman and Dr Meyer Friedman put forward the hypothesis that a behaviour pattern known as 'Type A' correlated with the likelihood of heart disease. Such a person was typically extremely competitive and aggressive, scheduled more and more activities into less and less time, was in too much of a hurry to derive any sense of beauty from the environment, did not delegate easily, exhibited explosive speech patterns, had trouble sitting and doing nothing, and exhibited lip-clicking, head-nodding, fist-clenching and other related traits. The Type

A person, in a business setting, might appear to be extremely productive and full of confidence but underneath feels inferior and prone to failure.

Recently a panel of 25 noted American cardiologists, epidemiologists and psychologists convened under the auspices of the National Heart, Lung and Blood Institute and concluded that the evidence for the Rosenman/Friedman hypothesis is substantial and that such a personality type *does* have a high risk of coronary disease.

A similar relationship seems to exist between psychological factors, stress, and the outbreak of cancer. According to Dr Charles Garfield of the Cancer Research Institute at the University of California, 'The evidence demonstrating that malignant processes are related to certain psychological conditions is formidable.' This opinion is shared by Dr Lawrence LeShan former head of the psychology department at the Institute of Applied Biology. After studying 250 cancer patients and administering personality tests, LeShan compared them with 150 non-cancer subjects. The following factors emerged:

• 77% of cancer subjects but only 14% of healthy subjects showed extreme tension over the loss of a close relative or friend.
• 64% of cancer subjects as opposed to 32% non-cancer, showed signs of not being able to adequately express anger, resentment and aggression towards other people, but bottled up their feelings.

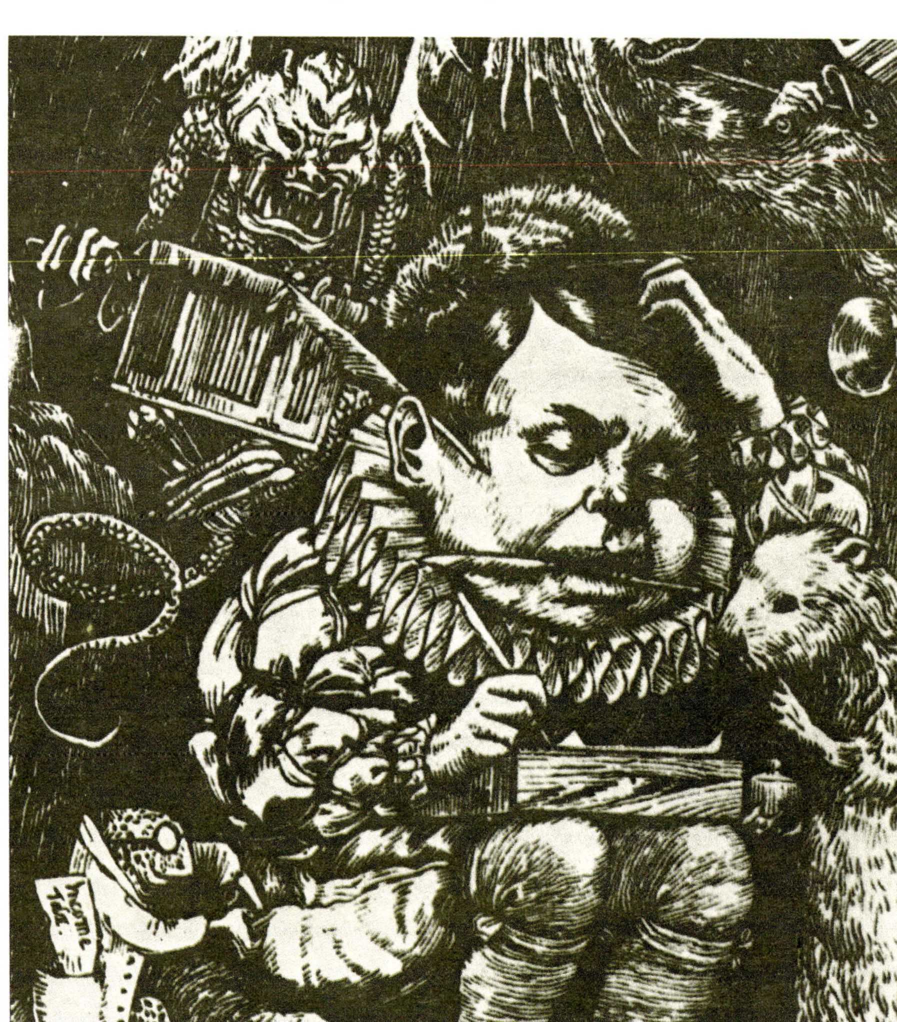

The demons of stress . . . a cause for cancer?

• 69% of cancer patients had low personal esteem and culpability while only 34% of the control group showed this characteristic.

LeShan also found that typically cancer patients had experienced an emotional trauma six to eighteen months prior to the development of the disease.

Dr Carl Simonton, a physician specialising in the treatment of cancer, extends the hypothesis of Drs Friedman and Rosenman beyond heart patients and believes that there is also a 'cancer' personality. The most pronounced characteristics are:

• a tendency to hold resentment and a marked inability to forgive.
• an inclination towards self-pity.
• a poor ability to develop and maintain meaningful, long-term relationships.
• a very poor self-image.

Dr Simonton places great emphasis on Professor Selye's discovery that chronic stress suppresses the immune system since this is the mechanism for destroying or keeping at bay the cancerous cells present in the body. During the 'May Lectures' held in London in 1974 Dr Simonton stated:

All human beings have cancer cells within them. The problem is not the cancer cells but the breakdown of the body's ability to deal with them and rid itself of disease. I see cancer, therefore, as having much in common with diseases like tuberculosis, the common cold and so forth. We are continually exposed to many dangerous agents both from within and without, but it is only when we become susceptible to them that the disease actually develops.

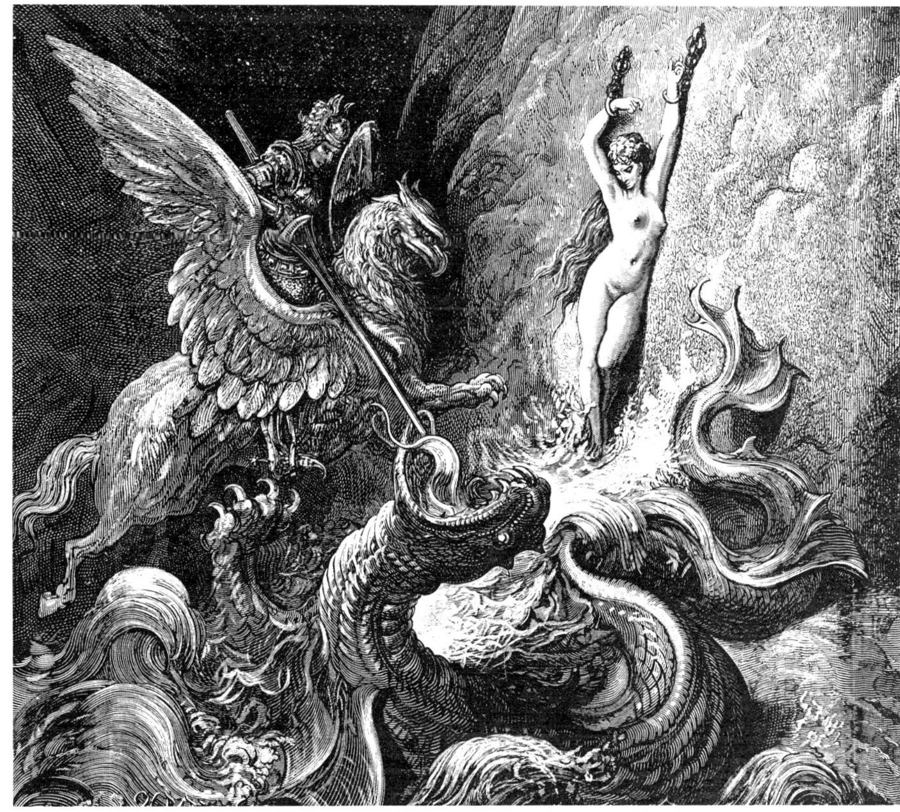

Using visualisation techniques can be a powerful means for treating psychosomatic illness. This illustration by Doré for Ariosto's Orlando Furioso *could be regarded therapeutically as symbolising the conquest of malign disease entities*

Dr Simonton practises at the Cancer Counselling and Research Centre in Fort Worth, Texas. One of his most distinctive techniques, as an adjunct to orthodox radiation therapy, is the use of guided visualisation and relaxation to enable the patient to focus on the cancerous growth. Three times a day, every day, the patient visualises the disease, the treatment and the body's own immune mechanisms (white blood cells) acting positively and victoriously over the disease. Dr Simonton has found that patients with a positive attitude towards their disease have a much more favourable clinical response to treatment than those with a poor attitude.

Dr David Bresler of UCLA has used similar psychosomatic techniques to reduce pain. One of his patients, a cardiologist with rectal cancer, was in excruciating agony. Dr Bresler asked him to visualise his pain and finally it emerged in the form of a large, vicious dog snapping at his spine. The patient was asked to imagine himself making friends with the dog, talking to it and patting it on the head. As the patient succeeded in this he found the pain subsiding, and after a few sessions it became quite manageable.

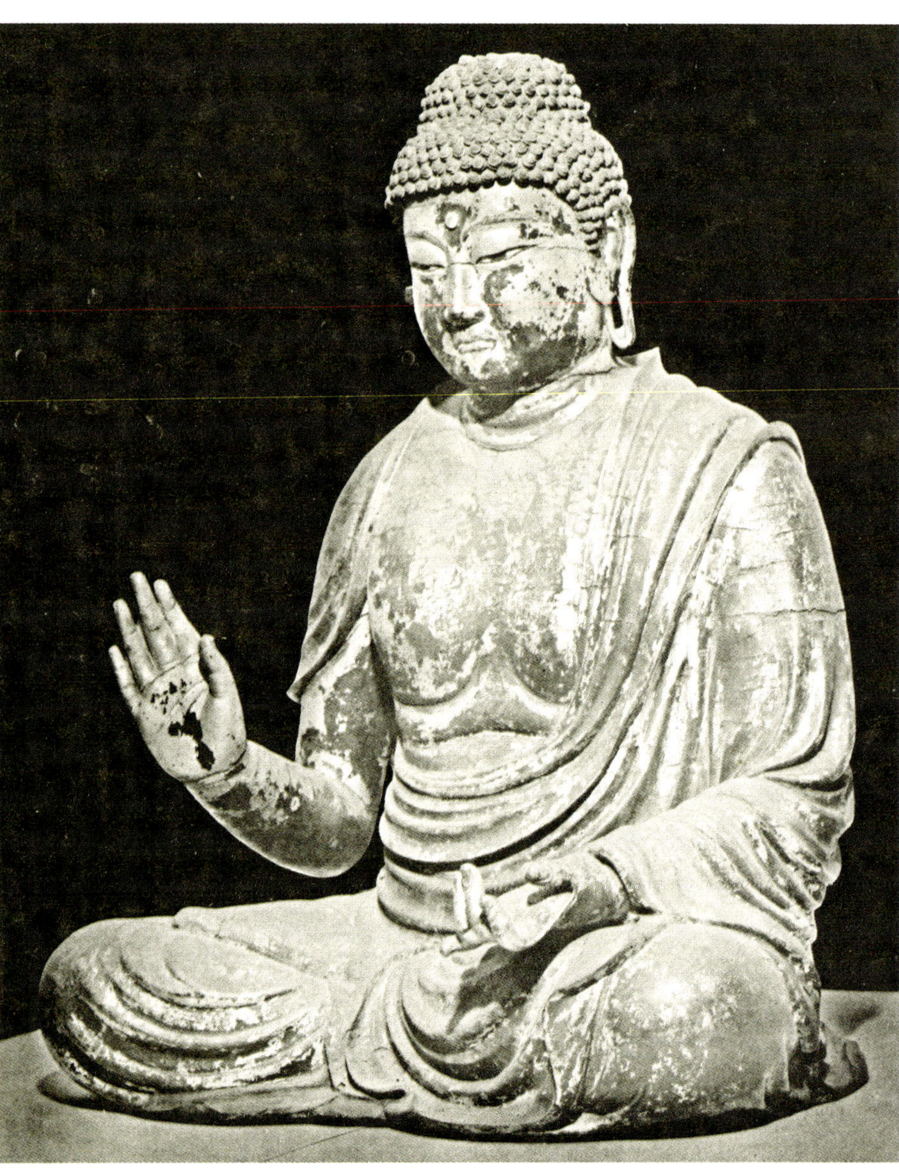

Meditation; new directions in cancer treatment

The Australian psychiatrist Dr Ainslie Meares has similarly been involved in treating cancer by using mind-over-body techniques. Dr Meares lived for a time in a Zen monastery in Japan and has a profound respect for Oriental techniques of meditation which he believes reduce anxiety levels considerably. At present he is treating some cancer patients by asking them to participate in intensive meditation. He has described several examples of cancer regression in *The Medical Journal of Australia* although he emphasises that meditation as a total cure has not yet been proven experimentally.

Nevertheless, the evidence for the inter-relatedness of mind and body as a factor underlying health, and, conversely, disease, seems to be well established. Orthodox doctors are paying more attention to the healing modalities which recognise the psychosomatic origin of many stress-related diseases.

At present in the department of behavioural medicine at Beth Israel Hospital in Boston, patients suffering from high blood pressure, chronic pain and arthritis are being taught to exercise, meditate and change their lifestyles and attitudes towards themselves. Dr Kenneth Pelletier of the Psychosomatic Medicine Clinic in Berkeley, California, asks the same thing of his patients. Stress patterns are eliminated and new regimes of diet and exercise are introduced. Dr Pelletier believes that psychosomatic factors play an important role in holistic medicine and health care and are now receiving the recognition they deserve.

PYRAMID ENERGY

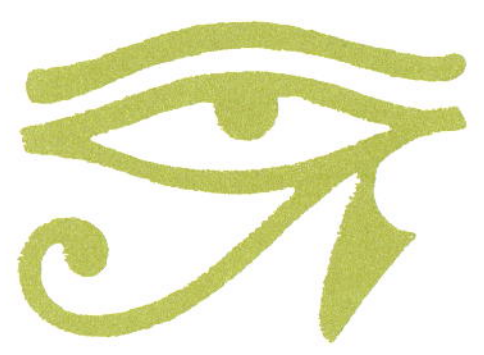

The Great Pyramid at Giza remains as an awesome reminder of the architectural skills of the ancient Egyptians. Although it is no longer the highest building in the world it is still the largest, with a base of 14 acres and containing 90 million cubic feet of stone — more than the quantity in all the churches and cathedrals built in England since the time of Christ. It seems that the Great Pyramid had a polished limestone face that could reflect light like a beacon, and it is noteworthy that the word 'pyramid' itself translates as 'glorious light'.

Several aspects of the Great Pyramid are impressive. It is aligned exactly to magnetic north and its position is at the exact centre of the earth's land mass. The north-south axis (31.9E) is the longest land meridian and the east-west axis (29.58.51N) is the longest land parallel. The Great Pyramid is also so mathematically perfect in its construction that it can be used to calculate the distance of the sun almost as accurately as by the means available to modern scientific technology. In essence there is something special about the Great Pyramid, both in terms of its proportions and its cosmic significance.

The pyramids at Giza: a 19th century photograph

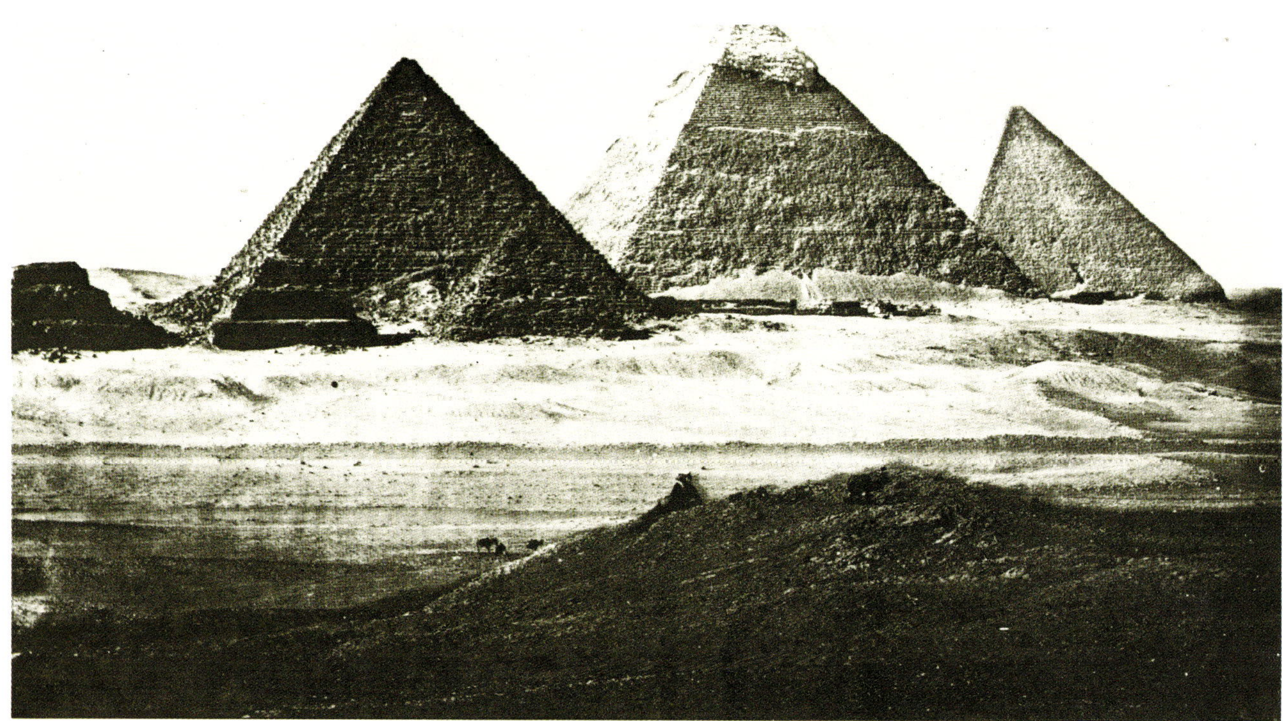

In the 1930s a French explorer named Antoine Bovis took refuge from the sun in the pharaoh's chamber which is located at the centre of the pyramid one-third of the way up from the base. He found it very humid but was surprised to find that the bodies of a dead cat and some other desert animals had not decayed there but had simply dehydrated. Bovis wondered whether the structure of the pyramid itself had something to do with this effect so he later made an exact model of the pyramid, aligned it north-south and east-west and placed a dead cat inside it in a comparable position to the central chamber. He found that once again the body dried out but did not decay.

Later the Czechoslovakian radio technician Karl Drbal began exploring the potential of pyramid models and found to his complete amazement that a blunted razor blade placed beneath the apex of such a pyramid regained its sharp edge. While in the army he had been puzzled by the fact that a razor blade left in full moon light lost its sharpness and the pyramid model proved to reverse the effect! Drbal was granted Czechoslovakian patent 91304 in recognition of his discovery and nearly twenty years later Professor William Tiller of Stanford University vindicated Drbal's experiment. He found that blue Gillette-type razor blades rely on a row of crystals along their edge for their sharpness and that these crystals distort under the effect of polarising moonlight. He similarly found that pyramid models could be used to reinstate the sharp edge. Dr Lyall Watson, author of a number of works on metaphysical themes, notes in *Supernature* that he has been able to keep an ordinary

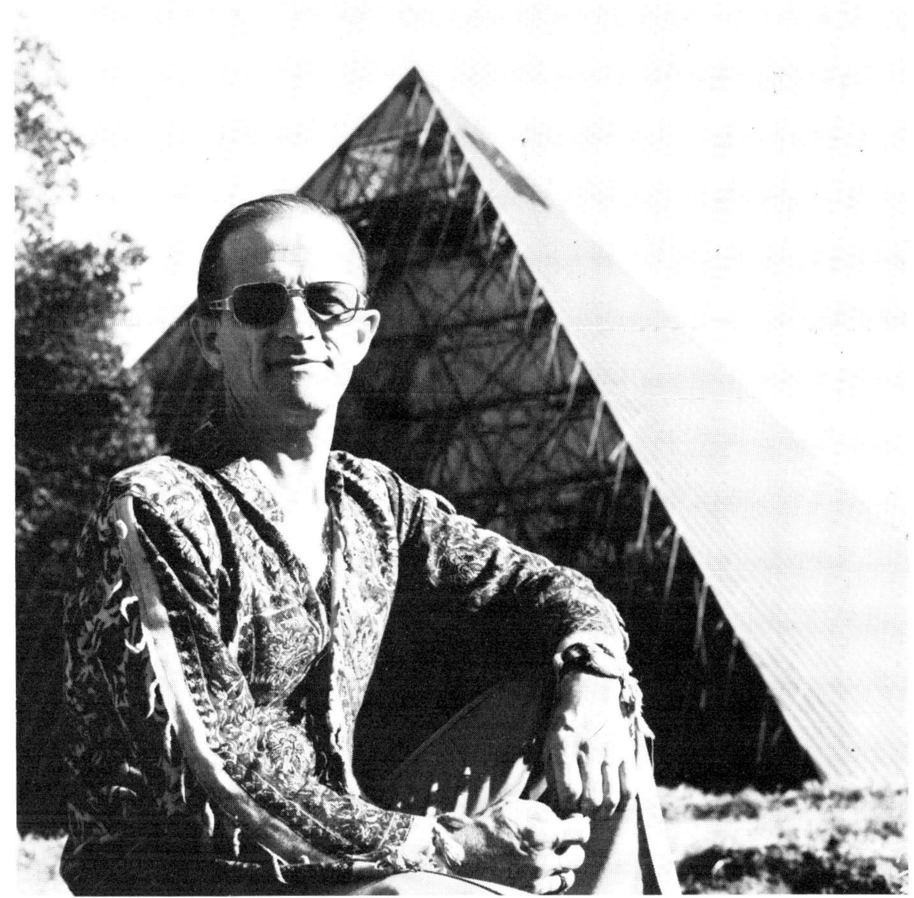

Researcher Graydon Rixon seen here in front of the 'glass pyramid' in Sydney's botanical gardens

Wilkinson Sword razor blade in continual use for four months using a pyramid model and he believes that the shape of the structure has a lot to do with it: 'We can only guess', he writes, 'that the Great Pyramid and its little imitations act as lenses that focus energy or as resonators that collect energy, which encourages crystal growth. The pyramid shape itself is very much like that of a crystal of magnetite, so perhaps it builds up a magnetic field . . .'

In Australia, researcher Graydon Rixon has made a lengthy study of pyramids. In his recent book *Discover Pyramid Energy* he summarises some of his findings:

- Pyramid models arrest the bacterial breakdown in meat and can also be used to dehydrate vegetables and fruit without diminishing their flavour.
- Cheap wines and liquors become milder and more palatable after a night in the pyramid while juices lose their bitterness.
- Plants are stimulated in their growth when placed under a pyramid.
- Vitamins increase their potency.

Quite aside from these factors Graydon Rixon has also experimented with meditation under the pyramid and finds that it substantially stimulates thought activity while also aiding general powers of awareness and sensitivity.

Pyramids come in different shapes. The variety with closed sides may be used for experiments with objects separated from their life source (fruit, wine, tobacco) while an open sided model is more suitable for energising such objects as plants that are still connected to their life source. Large open models are used for personal meditation. According to Graydon Rixon the energy zones in these shapes differ slightly: 'The energy in the closed sided pyramid is centred in a tight ball shape in the area one-third of the way up the pyramid, directly under the apex. With the open frame pyramid, there is a subtle difference. The energy starts in the same area one-third up from the bottom but then rises in a solid core of power to the top of the frame.'

Pyramids seem, therefore, to have definite meditative applications and their shape appears to produce a magnetic effect on the enclosed space which stimulates mental awareness. Pyramids remain something of a mystery nevertheless and no-one is quite sure exactly why they produce this effect. Perhaps in the years to come we will know more about the links between geometric figures and energy patterns – secrets that the builders of the Great Pyramid at Giza have not passed down to us.

ALAN GEFFIN

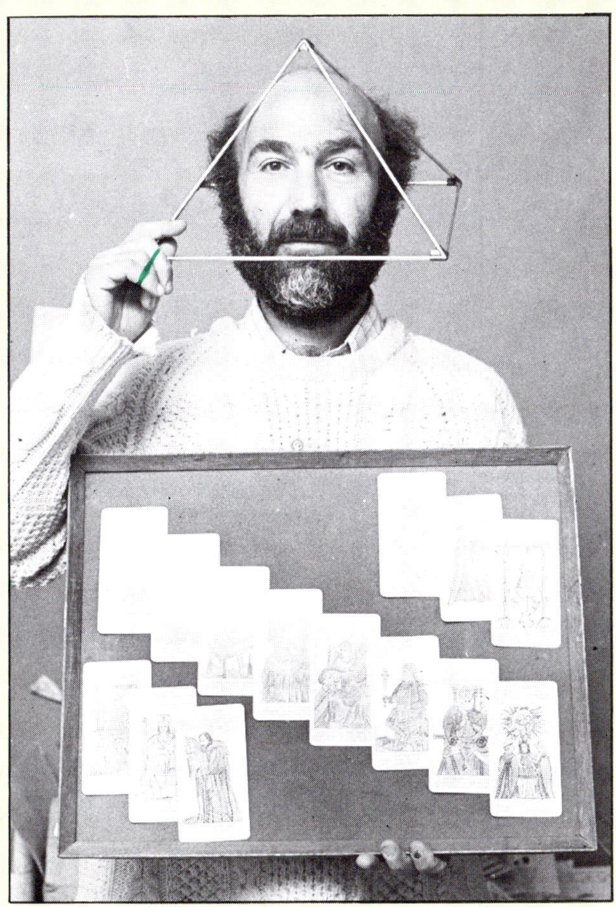

The Great Pyramid at Giza is certainly not the first thing that comes to mind as you approach the peace and calm of Chalvington, near Hailsham, deep in the Sussex countryside. Nor are Alan Geffin and his wife Jessica the sort of people you would normally associate with near-miracles. They are level-headed, have a delightful sense of humour and are completely rational. So when they begin telling you about pyramid energy and what they have seen it do you sit up and pay attention.

Pyramid energy is close to Alan Geffin's heart and has been for a number of years. It all started when he gave up his job as an accountant and went into business for himself. His new ventures included the introduction to the Western world from Japan, of the Biomate, for calculating biorhythms. It was when he was exhibiting these at the Festival of Mind and Body that he met the biggest manufacturer of model pyramids in America and signed a contract to introduce them into Britain.

A firm believer that anything he offered to others must first be seen to live up to its promise, Alan Geffin and his wife began a seriesof experiments with the frame pyramids which are built exactly to the proportions of the Great Pyramid of Giza. The results startled them. In his own words 'one saw what in ordinary terms would be called miracles'.

The first test consisted of placing a 9 inch base pyramid over some alfalfa seeds for just over a week. As a result the covered seeds germinated considerably faster than the others. Jessica then found that when she cut a tomato in two, placed half under a pyramid and left the other outside the latter formed a mould in a few days while the covered half did not decompose. They have also placed an electric light bulb on a lead under a pyramid and watched its brightness increase.

Alan regularly keeps a bottle of water under an 18 inch base pyramid and drinks from it daily. He is convinced that in some fashion energy is absorbed into the water. One of the many correspondents who keep in touch with them reported that after two weeks under one of Alan's pyramids ordinary tap water tasted as if it had come fresh from a natural spring. And not only water is affected. On a radio programme a test with wine was carried out with a professional wine taster. From a bottle of cheap wine two glasses were poured. The wine taster was asked to drink from both. Without his knowledge one glass had previously been placed under a pyramid. This glass of wine he found very acceptable. Of the other he said he would not have it in his house!

Honey, meat and fish react positively, too. A dish of liquid honey placed under a pyramid forms a crust which dissolves when taken out and returns when replaced. Another of their correspondents reported that he had placed small pieces of meat and fish under his small frame pyramid for one month while equal portions were left uncovered. After a month these were putrid. The pyramid portions were given to his cat who ate the month-old scraps with relish.

Jessica Geffin tells that her own cat loves being put under a pyramid and demonstrated the fact. If the pyramid is taken away the cat returns to the spot where it was. However insects are not so appreciative. Flies avoid pyramids.

At one of the Festivals of Mind and Body Alan Geffin tried an experiment relating to alpha brain waves, those which reflect states of relaxation. Over the head of a woman who was wired to apparatus for testing brain waves he slowly lowered an 18 inch base pyramid. As it descended over her eyes the television screen to which she was linked recorded considerable activity and her alpha level was seen to increase. It has been reported that large pyramids under which one can sit have been used with overactive children. Alan says that not only do they love playing under them but were very much calmer while inside. They have received reports, too, that many people are more relaxed and experience relief from migraine.

Alan Geffin says that many people believe that the Great Pyramid at Giza has a message for mankind that will one day be understood. Perhaps pyramid energy is just one manifestation of that message. Meanwhile he has given a great deal of pleasure and no little mystification to thousands of people.

RADIESTHESIA

The practice of radiesthesia, a form of 'medical dowsing', has its origins both in traditional divining and modern spiritualism.

Forked divination rods are mentioned in records from ancient Egypt and also in the writings of Cicero and Tacitus. In the 16th century Sebastian Minister included engravings of mineral diviners at work in his book *Cosmography* and similar illustrations appear in George Agricola's *De Re Metallica*, published in Basle, which made reference to 'forked rods'. In 1663 Robert Boyle, the so-called 'father of chemistry', published an essay in England which describes the typical activity of a dowser:

A forked hazel twig is held by its horns, one in each hand, the holder walking with it over places where mineral lodes may be suspected, and it is said that the fork by dipping down will discover the place where the ore is to be found . . . When visiting the lead mines of Somersetshire I saw its use, and one gentleman who employed it declared that it moved without his will, and I saw it bend so strongly as to break in his hand.

The practice of dowsing has continued to the modern day and practitioners seek a variety of things: water, buried treasure, wires, oil and missing objects.

However, spiritualism has also played its part. In the 19th century some spiritualists used a technique in which a golden or silver ring was attached to a silk thread and suspended above a disc of parchment. The latter bore the words 'yes' and 'no'. The spiritualist would hold the thread between the thumb and forefinger and address questions to a spirit summoned in prayer. The answers were given by the movements of the ring over the disc. Later, French spiritualists replaced the ring with a pendulum which could be suspended over a glass. The pendulum would rattle against the glass – one tap for 'yes', two taps for 'no'.

The French priest Abbe Mermet gained quite a reputation for his techniques of radiesthesia and appeared to be able to pinpoint a source of water several thousand miles away. He included in his analysis details of where to drill, the nature of the water source, temperature and flow. On other occasions he used his powers for such diverse functions as identifying the location of missing persons and diagnosing ailments by using only a photograph of the afflicted person. His book *Principles and Practice of Radiesthesia* was extremely popular with the public and summarised his research over a forty-year period.

Radiesthesia took a more medical turn when Mlle Chantereine claimed to be able to diagnose samples of polluted water by holding a pendulum

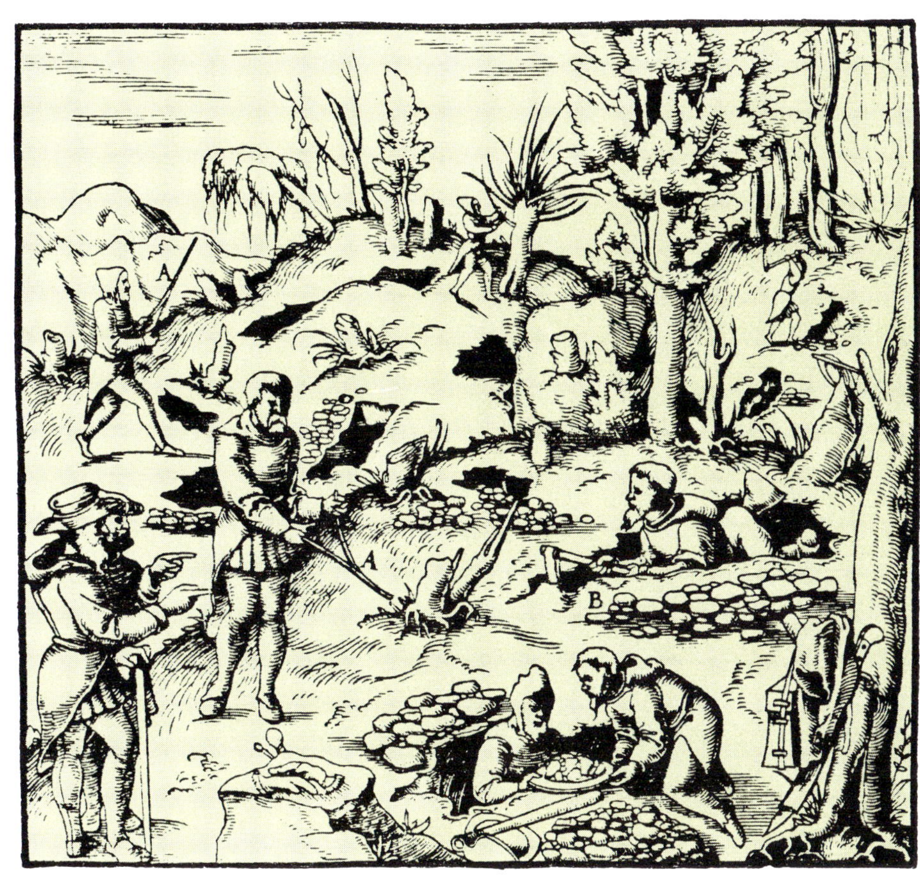

Dowsing more than 400 years ago . . . an illustration from George Agricola's De Re Metallica

in one hand and, one by one, samples of bacterial cultures in the other. Later, when the British Society of Dowsers was founded and followed in 1939 by the Medical Society for the Study of Radiesthesia, several medical men turned their attention towards the new techniques. They included Dudley Wright, Winter Gonin and founder member Guyon Richards.

In medical radiesthesia the practitioner uses a pendulum in association with a geometric rule or pattern. Different diseases are indicated by different positions. David V. Tansley, a leading contemporary practitioner, notes: 'A certain point on the rule will represent optimum vitality and if the pendulum begins to swing into a clockwise or anti-clockwise direction before it reaches this point, then this will indicate the lowered point of vitality . . .' In general, there appear to be four basic movements: clockwise and anti-clockwise; left to right across the body; and away and towards the body at right-angles to it. However the meaning of a pendulum's motion has to be individually determined for personal purposes of interpretation. One could take a silver coin and ask the question: 'Is this a coin?' The answer would have to be 'yes', so that direction would be regarded as affirmative. If one then asked 'Is this made of chalk?' the resultant action would demonstrate the movement for 'no'. Other questions like 'Is this made of silver?' would yield the yes/no category since silver coins are partly alloy.

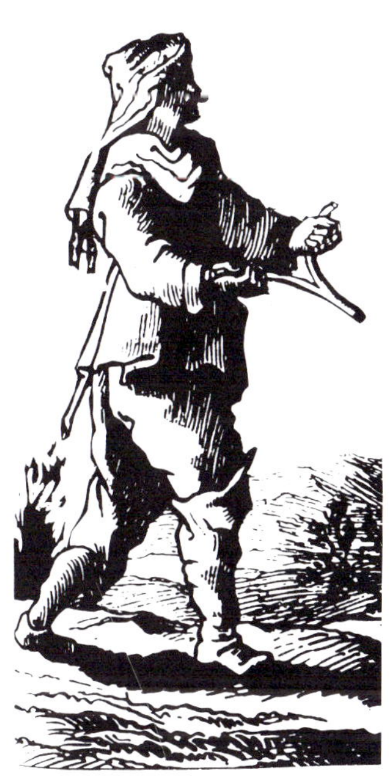

Does radiesthesia work? The answer is yes: for some people. However the reasons why the bob of a pendulum or dowsing rod yields accurate information may not be the same as the reasons given by the practitioner. In 1854 M.Chevreul of the French Museum of Natural History investigated radiesthesia and concluded that although no deliberate fraud was intended the pendulum moved because of involuntary muscular actions. Many sceptics maintain similar arguments today and feel that when dowsers are successful, for example, in locating water:

• they usually recognise features on the earth's surface that indicate underground water.
• they benefit from the fact that if a well is dug deep enough almost anywhere, there is a reasonable chance of bringing up underground water.

Often the dowser may be drawing on years of experience to recognise the terrain where water is likely to be found. He is so sensitively attuned to his hazel or metal rod that an unconscious response triggered by memory can translate into an apparently involuntary and 'mystical' gift for locating water. In 1980 a televised experiment was held in Australia which removed the element of the 'familiar terrain'. The experiment involved several of Aus-

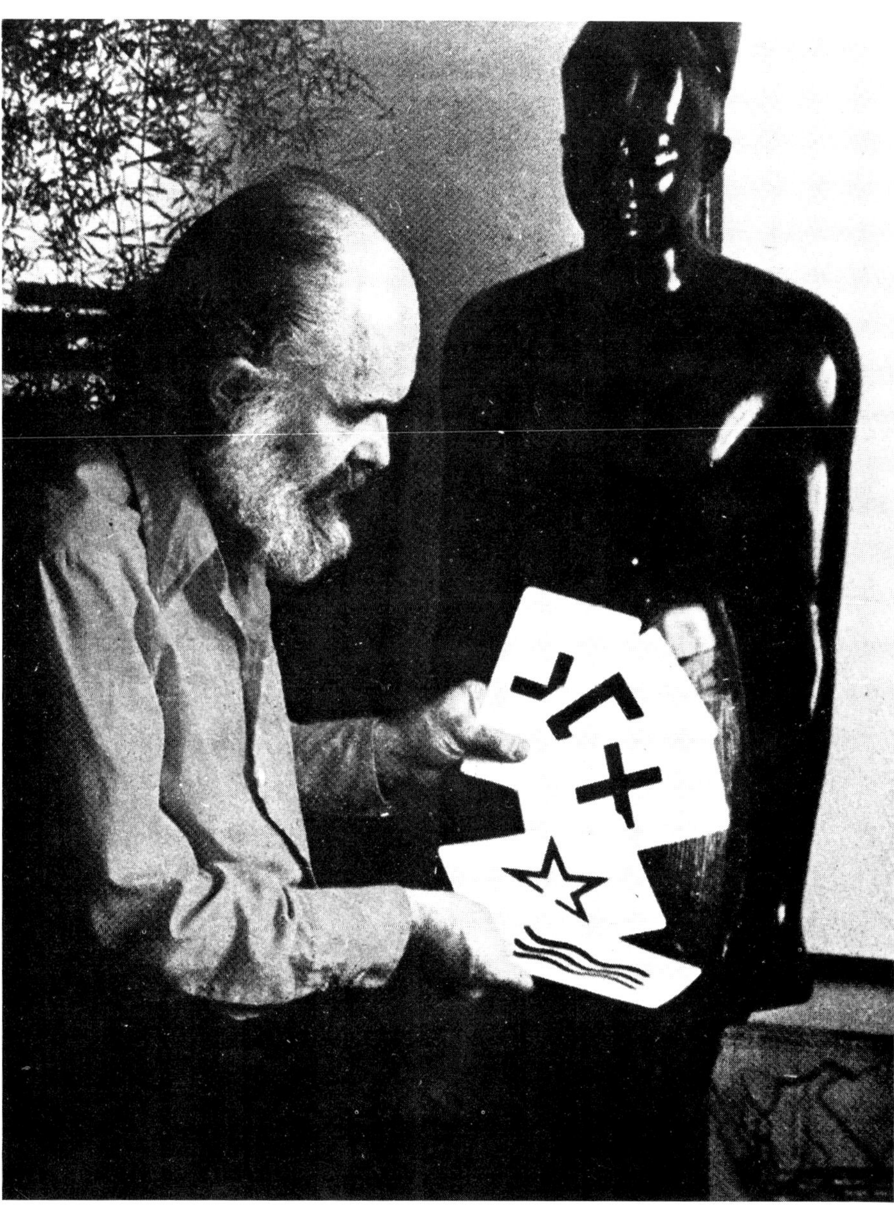

Noted American conjuror Randi, who has also investigated the claims of dowsers, seen here with a set of Zener cards used in psychic research experiments

tralia's leading dowsers and was supervised by the American conjuror Randi, who has been strongly critical of the 'psychic' performances of Uri Geller, which he believes are cleverly staged. Randi's role in the dowsing experiment was to challenge the dowsers to put their abilities to the test. During the experiment water was switched on at different times in various pipes which had been placed in the ground and covered with earth. The dowsers had to walk over the area above the pipes and attempt to identify the one in which water was flowing at a given time. The overall tally of 'hits' versus 'misses' did not exceed those of a chance result and for some dowsers the success rate was actually below what could be expected by random guessing. No evidence of a psychic component emerged.

Nevertheless, despite its controversial history, radiesthesia has played a part in the development of alternative medicine, especially in terms of the development of the allied practices of radionics and psionic medicine. These are described in other chapters of this book.

RADIONICS

With the increasing use of machinery in radiesthesia a new 'science' was born : radionics. The pioneer of this development was Dr Albert Abrams who was born in San Francisco in 1863. Abrams qualified with a medical diploma in California and then graduated with honours from Heidelberg University. His wealthy inheritance enabled him to undertake postgraduate work in Heidelberg, Berlin, Paris, Vienna and London.

In 1910 while Abrams was examining a patient's cancerous ulcer he noticed that a small area of the abdomen produced a dull note when it was 'percussed' (This is a technique in which the doctor taps the middle finger of the left hand with the tip of the middle finger of the right hand while the left hand has contact with the body). Subsequently he discovered that this dull note only occurred when the patient was facing west. Abrams felt that perhaps he was dealing with an 'electronic' phenomenon affected by the Earth's magnetic field. Abrams then wired his patient to a healthy person and discovered that the 'emanations' from the cancer produced a dull note in the same area of the healthy subject's abdomen.

In subsequent tests Abrams found that the same effect was produced by wiring a piece of malignant tumour in a container to the healthy man : still the dullness occurred. The implication was that diseased tissue was affecting his nervous system, altering the percussion note in the abdomen.

Abrams felt that 'radio waves' might be involved and called the new method *radionics*. As it turned out, different diseases produced different areas of dullness in different parts of the body. However cancer and syphilis both appeared to produce dullness in the same part of the abdomen. Abrams now used his electronic skills to introduce a variable resistance box into his circuit. It was found that cancer produced dullness with 50 ohm resistance while syphilis did so with 55 ohm resistance — he had discovered a means of differentiation! Abrams referred to his discovery as 'the electronic reactions of Abrams' (E.R.A.) and he now ordered some specially constructed, highly accurate resistance boxes.

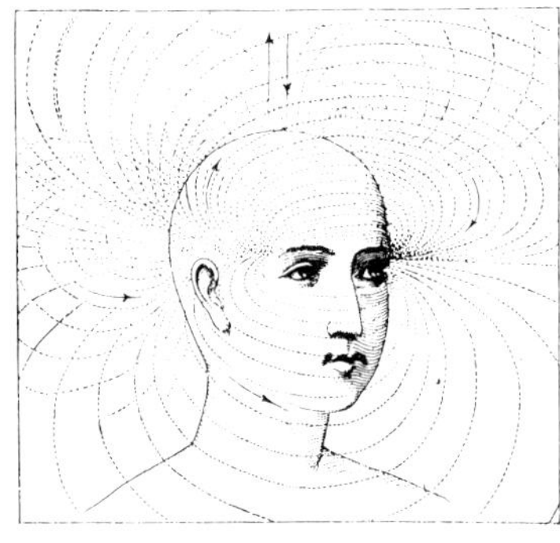

Abrams kept making new discoveries. Over the years he found that he no longer needed diseased tissue to obtain his results — a drop of blood on tissue paper was all that was required. The advanced resistance technology enabled him to differentiate between different diseased tissues. Abrams also found that when quinine was put to the test with a sample of malarial blood, the 'radiation' from the quinine appeared to neutralise that from the contaminated blood, eliminating the dull note in the process.

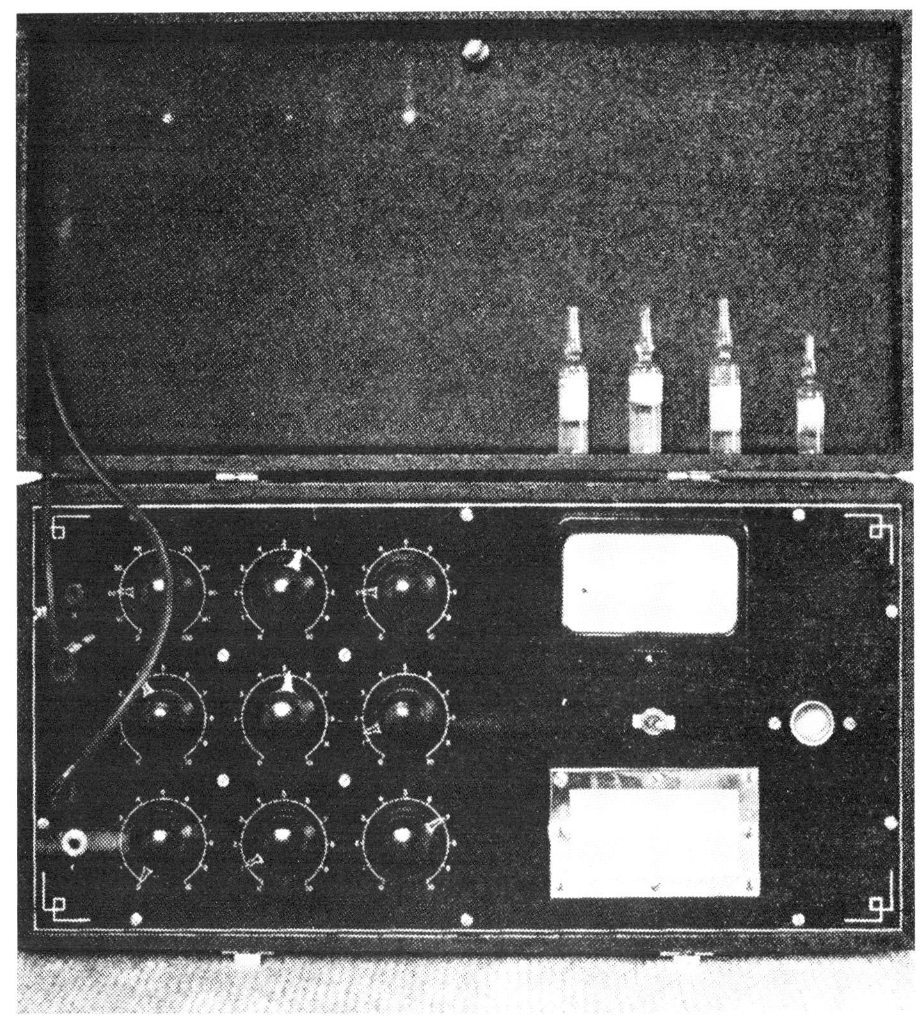

A radionics 'black box'

While many doctors were intrigued by Abrams' discoveries others were critical and a few set out to discredit the new invention. According to Francis King, 'this versatile machine was subjected to abuse by cynical physicians who dispatched the blood of healthy animals for diagnosis. A chicken was diagnosed by Abrams as suffering from syphilis and a sheep as "suffering from acute motor-neurotic tensions with a pre-clinical neoplasm caused by the strains of modern life" '.

The controversy continued until 1924 when a committee was set up by Sir Thomas Horder under the auspices of the Royal Society of Medicine to test the new devices. In the first test, twenty-five successive trials were successful and the committee finally reported that 'no more convincing exposition of the reality of the phenomena could be desired'.

Abrams died the same year, before the pronouncement was made. Meanwhile the prejudice of some cynical doctors remained, despite the endorsement of Sir Thomas Horder's investigation. A revival of interest occurred, however, when Dr Ruth Drown in the United States and George De La Warr in England continued to research using modified forms of the so-called Abrams 'black boxes'.

Dr Drown modified the instruments and used a rubber 'detector plate' instead of the human abdomen. She also replaced the resistances with a rotary pattern of dials. Dr Drown claimed that she could diagnose disease and also treat a patient from a distance, using the blood sample as a 'link'. However she was not able to substantiate her claims scientifically. In 1950 tests on the 'black box' at the University of Chicago were so discouraging that Dr Drown withdrew from the investigation. She was harassed by the American Medical Association and later charged and convicted for medical quackery although charges of fraud had not been adequately substantiated. She finally died, dispirited, in a California prison but maintained to the end that there was 'a resonance between the whole human body and each of its parts' – a viewpoint now widely recognised by holistic health practitioners.

During the 1940s and 50s George and Marjorie De La Warr undertook extensive research into radionics at their Oxford laboratories. They had copied Dr Drown's instruments with her permission but sought to improve them. The De La Warrs replaced the rubber plate detector with small bar magnets and standardised the use of flat strips of spring metal, formed into a near-circle beneath the dial. Now they attempted to correlate various parts of the body with the diseases to which they were prone, and effective remedies. Eventually some 4000 such correlations or 'rates' were assembled. The De La Warr instrument included a series of cards identifying the diseases with parts of the body but also called for the operator to tune in mentally to the disease and its location. The standard instrument, which is still used, has nine dials on a panel, a magnet set at 90° to the dials and a plate for the patient's blood sample.

George De La Warr's innovations also included attempts to interpret 'radionic emanations' in terms of sound, and the use of a colourscope that treated patients with light of different wavelengths. De La Warr argued that waveforms of sound altered as they passed through the body and similarly reflected changes in body tissue caused by disease. De La Warr also produced a controversial radionic 'camera', an object which resembled a washing machine in shape and size, and which could allegedly produce a photograph of a subject's internal condition by tuning in to a drop of blood. The camera, however, only appeared to work if specific people – presumably of an open-minded nature – were present. The experiments with the camera were not able to stand up to objective scrutiny, however, and a judge in a legal case brought against the inventor by an unhappy client commented that 'the totality of the evidence suggested that the camera was completely bogus and the photographs were fakes'.

This is not to say that radionics devices are not sometimes effective in producing accurate diagnostic results. In the same way that a crystal ball may work for a sensitive fortune-teller by enabling that person to focus attention and bring about an altered state of consciousness – in turn leading to heightened perception and accurate intuitions about a client – the radionics device may similarly be used as an aid for the healer. The elaborate system of cross-referencing diseases and parts of the body and the use of sophisticated electronic equipment may similarly act as a 'focus', allowing the radionics practitioner to channel attention psychically towards the patient whose blood sample (= life essence) is used for diagnosis. De La Warr himself often referred to the concept of 'radionic rapport' and in this respect was philosophically aligned with the idea of energy flow and interaction which seems to underlie many of the alternative healing therapies.

REFLEXOLOGY

Reflexology is a therapy which focuses on the reflex points in the feet, although there are other points throughout the body. It is said that there are around 72 000 nerve endings in each foot which connect to other parts of the body. By applying massage to those nerve endings an impulse is conveyed to other organs. When a person is ill, eats the wrong food or fails to exercise sufficiently, circulation in the feet slows down and crystalline deposits – mostly of uric acid and excess calcium – form around the nerve endings in the feet and elsewhere. Reflexology uses massage to crush the crystalline deposits, allowing them to be reabsorbed into the blood, and at the same time stimulates the nerve endings. This has an effect on organs and glands that could be functioning below their normal level, affecting the overall balance of the body.

Although reflexology bears some resemblance to ancient Chinese and Indian medicine, it was introduced to the United States as a system in its own right around 1913. Dr William Fitzgerald called it 'zone therapy' and used it for its anaesthetic effects. Subsequent pioneers of this type of therapy have included Dr George Starr White and Dr Joe Shelby Riley. Riley's pupil, Eunice D. Ingham, was a leading figure in formulating contemporary techniques of reflexology and presented them through seminars to the American public from the 1930s onwards. She focused almost entirely on the zones of the feet and brought to her study a vast amount of anatomical and physiological knowledge. Her special approach came to be known as the Ingham Reflex Method of Compression Massage and her work is the basis of most forms of modern reflexology.

As with acupuncture, acupressure and polarity balancing, considerable attention is paid in reflexology to energy flow : the vitality of the body depends on the circulation of energy through myriad pathways, or meridians, and good health reflects this process.

The 'reflex' part of reflexology is based on the fact that a reflex is an involuntary response to a stimulus and the reflex response of an organ depends upon a clear neural pathway between the point of stimulation and the organ itself. When the reflexologist presses on different points on the feet he produces impulses which are transmitted to the ganglia – the nerve cells outside the spinal cord and brain. The impulses then travel vertically to organs on the same side of the body as the applied stimulus, and are part of the autonomic or involuntary nervous system. The response of the organ is a 'reflex' action.

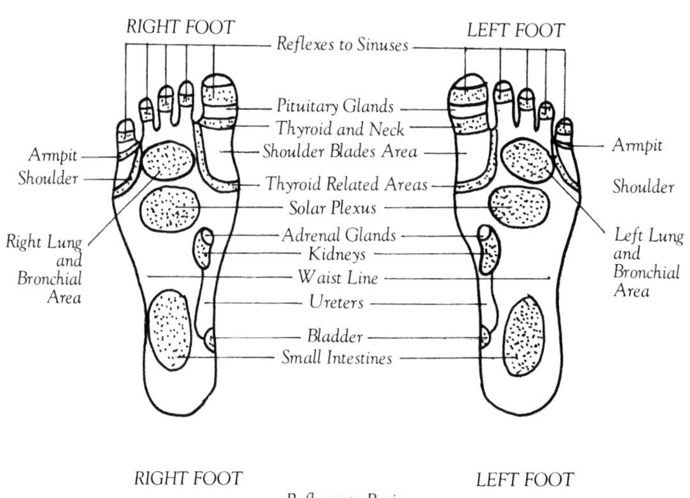

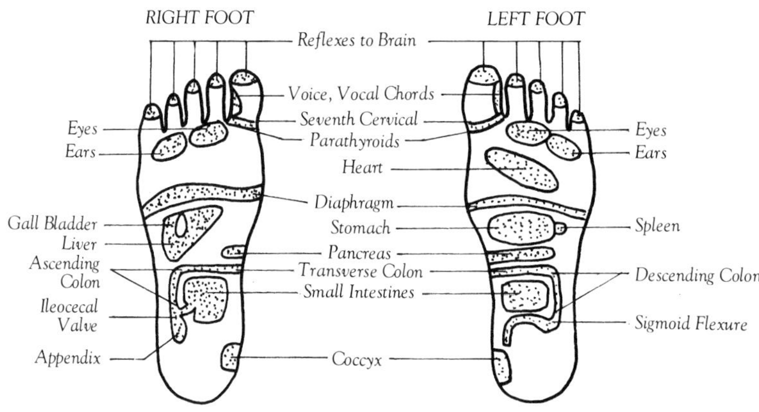

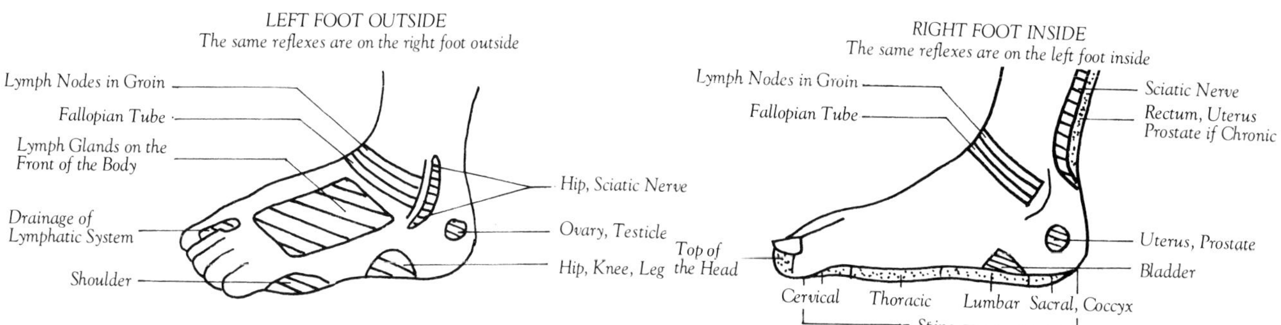

According to reflexologists every organ needs to be able to contract and relax. If crystals or calcium deposits impede energy flow, organs are adversely affected. Conversely a skilled reflexologist can use foot massage to remove blockages and activate the organs, thus restoring good health holistically.

The massage technique depends upon use of the thumb, which maintains steady pressure while the other hand is used to stabilise the foot. The thumb is bent at 90° at the first joint and has to apply pressure at precise points to be effective. In between, it glides across the skin.

Pressure is applied just for an instant and is then released by straightening the thumb. The thumb then remains flat against the skin and is subsequently raised vertically above another pressure point. In this way the thumb makes little 'steps' across the foot. Pressure points in general are about one-sixteenth of an inch apart.

A good reflexologist develops a rhythm in applying pressure. The thumb tip faces in the direction of flow which on the sole of the foot is always from the toes to the heel or from the outer edge of the foot to the inner. The reflexologist begins first with the left foot and then the right. If the upper surface of the foot is being massaged the practitioner usually commences with the outer heel and moves around to the inside, and also works upward from the heel to the ankle and down the upper surface of the foot to the toes. However, not all reflexologists agree on this direction. Polish-American practitioner Anna Kaye, for example, prefers to work in lines of force rising from the base of the foot up to the ankles rather than moving down to the toes, while Lew Connor and Linda McKim of the California Reflexology Institute recommend the downward action to the toes.

The reflexes in the toes are important because they relate to the lymphatic ducts, and stimulating this area helps, in the final analysis, to remove toxic substances from the body. According to Eunice Ingham about three-quarters of the body's toxins accumulate in the lymphatic duct on the left hand side of the body. The area between the big and second toe is pulled to 'drain' the lymphatic system.

During a reflexology session the patient sits comfortably in a chair and rests the legs outstretched so that they are approximately level with the masseur's shoulders. Usually bare legs are covered with a light cloth to retain body heat, aiding blood circulation. Relaxation is important and the patient is encouraged to let tension flow from the body through progressive 'loosening up'. The practitioner should also be relaxed so that the thumb can move evenly and rhythmically over the skin.

Sessions tend to last around 45 minutes and are usually given twice a week, although the degree of systematic massage will depend, for example, on such factors as the amount of crystalline deposits in the feet. Reflexologists resist crushing too many crystals in one session because when they are released into the blood there is a temporary increase in toxicity in the body and the patient can feel ill for several hours, or longer. Reflexologists also avoid pressing on injured limbs or swollen areas since pain increases tension which has a counter-effect to the healing process.

Massage is not recommended for people undergoing drug medication, pregnant or menstruating women, or people who have just eaten a large meal. However in general it is a form of bodywork with a wide range of applications as the accompanying diagrams show. Essentially reflexology has to do with energy flow and removing blockages so the body can be revitalised. The techniques are applied to suit the individual characteristics of each person.

AMOS HOLLIS

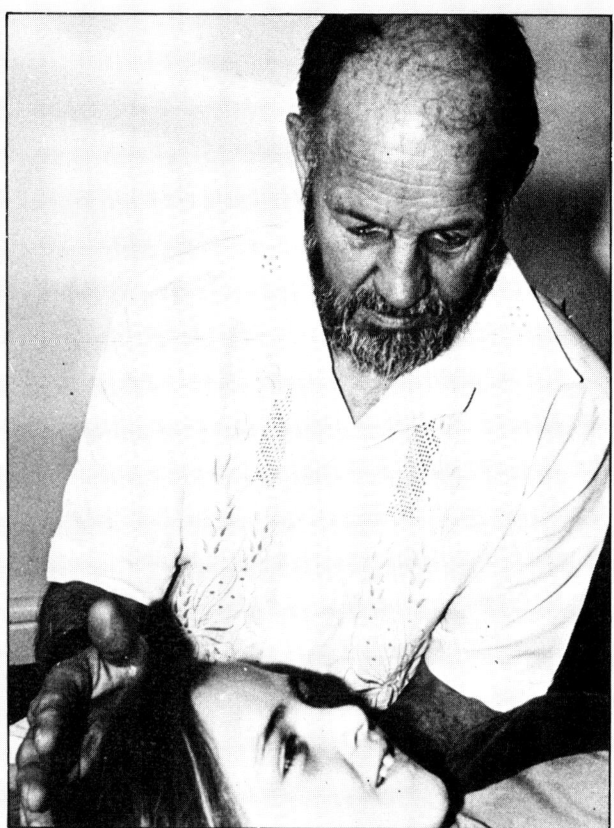

Like many holistic practitioners, Amos Hollis uses more than one therapeutic technique in his healing approach. Although he is best known for using manipulative therapy to bring the 'life force' through to the patient, he also applies the methods of zone therapy, foot reflexology, biofeedback, iridology, ear therapy, acupressure, colour therapy, and 'soulhealing' through regression.

Between the years 1936 and 1938 Amos served with the St John's Ambulance and immediately afterwards with the Royal Army Medical Corps in the British Army. He became interested in alternative healing practices, undertook chiropractic training with a registered practitioner of the Chiropractors Association of Australia, and followed this with a course in Hong Kong through the auspices of the Chinese Finger Pressure and Acupuncture Association located in Kowloon. He is also the Chapter President of the South Australian branch of the Christian Spiritual Regeneration Movement whose headquarters are based in the Philippines, where the Reverend Placedo Palatanyan conducts his Psychic Healing Centre. Amos sometimes uses the techniques of 'laying on of hands' himself, particularly to conclude a healing treatment, and he finds that this assists the healing process and induces complete physical and mental relaxation.

Since February 1980 Amos has practised from the Life Force Healing and Research Centre in Adelaide and he has been involved in both healing and teaching other holistic practitioners. He has tended to focus on patients requiring help for the elimination of headaches, reduction of migraine attacks, painful menstrual periods, back pain, haemorrhoids, asthma, varicose veins, arthritis and other areas where the ailment lies at least partially in the nature of the mind/body relationship.

Initially Amos uses a combination of foot, zone and manipulation therapy to allow toxic waste material to pass from the body through the life-force energy channels. The effect of this is to stimulate both the circulatory and lymphatic systems of the body and to allow its self-regenerating and healing aspects to function effectively. Here a laying on of hands may follow, and also nutritional advice and herbal remedies if required.

Amos uses biofeedback techniques in order to allow patients to reduce tension, alleviate pain from headaches and gain more muscular use of their limbs if they have been semi-paralysed following a stroke, for example. He candidly admits that his techniques are not effective in cases of gross paralysis and if any cases arise where more orthodox medical treatment is required he refers his patients to an appropriate specialist.

Over the years Amos has found that around 30% of patients show a marked improvement after the initial treatment and 60% do not have to return to him at all. The other 10% represents the unresponsive segment that do not show improvement . . . but nevertheless a 90% response rate is impressive, after all.

Often, the day after the healing session the patient will experience adverse reactions which are the result of the body purging itself of the contaminating functions. For example there may be copious urinary or bowel output, unpleasant odours, and the feeling that one is 'off-colour'. Marked improvement invariably occurs immediately afterwards as the building-up process begins.

As a holistic educator, Amos Hollis has been offering courses at his Centre in human body functions, demonstrations of 'life-force' healing therapy, iridology, ear therapy, reflexology, nutrition, diet, herbal remedies and basic physical fitness. His classes are held on a regular basis and are designed, appropriately, to teach people how to look after their own health. Like most holistic practitioners, Amos Hollis is as much interested in prevention as in treatment and feels that the general public should take more interest and care in the area of personal well-being.

REICHIAN THERAPY

Wilhelm Reich was born on 24 March 1897 in Galicia, Austria, the son of middle-class Jewish parents. His father was volatile and autocratic, his mother attractive and warm in temperament. However she committed suicide after Reich revealed to his father that she was having an extra-marital affair. Soon afterwards Reich's father developed pneumonia and tuberculosis and also died.

Reich was obliged to manage his father's farm while he studied. With the advent of World War One he joined the Austrian army but in 1918 was able to enrol at the University of Vienna. His chosen pursuit was medicine and he qualified as an M.D. in 1922. During the same year Sigmund Freud founded a psychoanalytic clinic in Vienna and Reich worked with him. However as with several of Freud's other colleagues, differences soon began to appear. Freud refused to give Reich personal analysis and did not share the latter's strong Marxist leanings.

In 1930 Reich moved to Berlin, became more closely affiliated with the Communist Party, and helped establish 'mental hygiene' centres in Germany. His politics alienated him from most other psychoanalysts and his radical views on sexuality were not acceptable to the German Communist Party who expelled him in 1933. Reich subsequently lived in Denmark, Sweden and Norway before moving to the United States in 1939 to accept a faculty position in medical psychology at the New School for Social Research in New York.

By this stage Reich was already an accomplished author. He had already written *The Function of the Orgasm*, which analysed bioenergetic aspects of sexuality; *Sexual Revolution* on sexual repression and social norms; *The Mass Psychology of Fascism* on the roots of authoritarianism, and *Character Analysis*, a major work on character types. The last of these books has been extremely influential and deals with Reich's concepts of character and body 'armouring'.

Reich believed in the concept of bioenergy flow through the body and considered that repression of the emotions and sexual instincts could lead to blockages resulting in rigid patterns of behaviour (character armour) and the tightening of specific muscle groups (body armour). As such blockages increased, the energy flow in the organism was impeded and in chronic instances would lead to a marked deterioration of health.

For Reich, sexual energy was the essence of human existence. The climax of orgasm was a completely satisfying release from tension that allowed sexual energy to be discharged in an act of physical embrace and love. Reich later

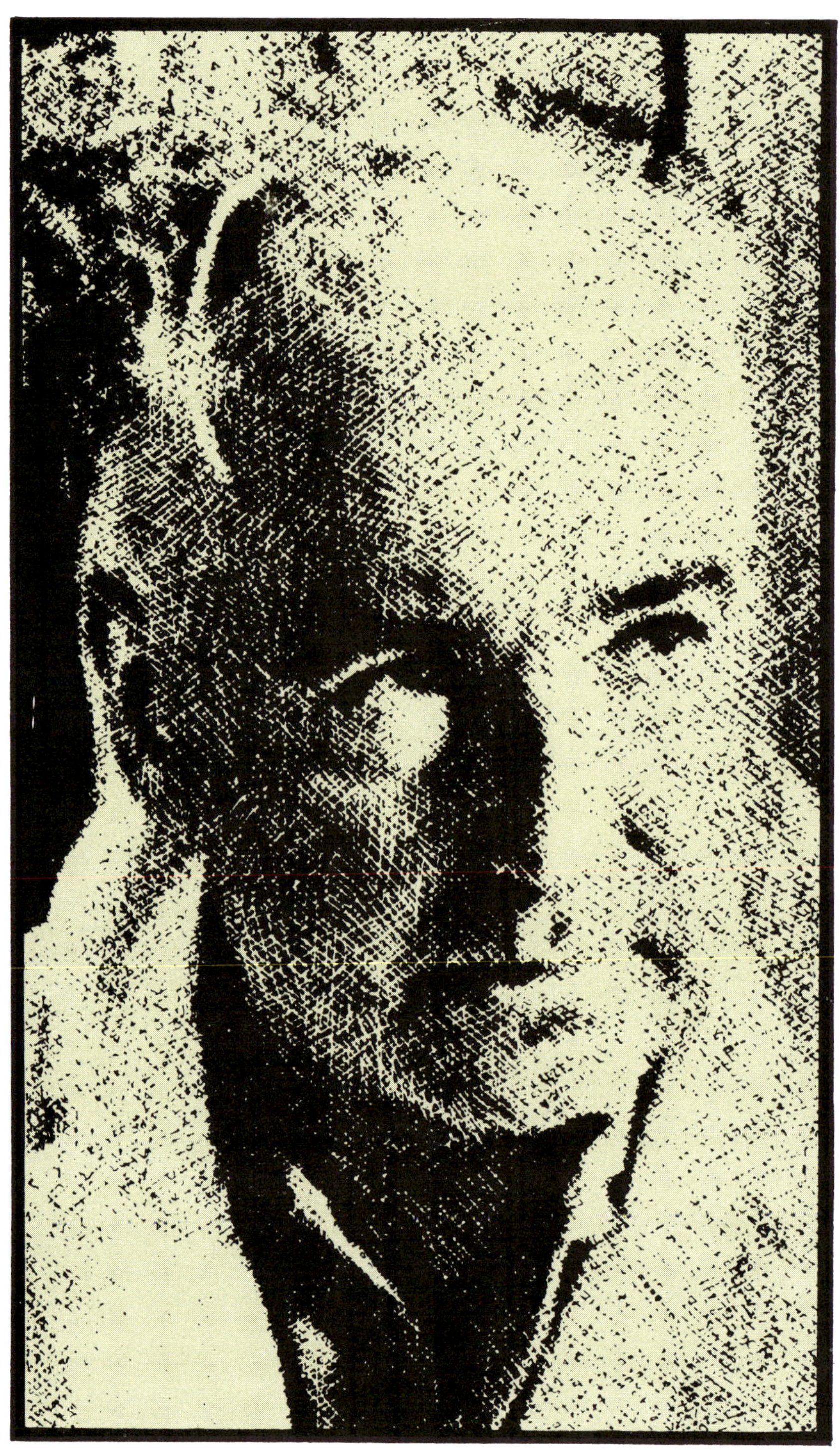

Wilhelm Reich: from Freud to Bioenergy

postulated his formula of 'biological tension and charge' which involved four stages : mechanical tension, bioenergetic charge, bioenergetic discharge and relaxation (see article on *Sexual Therapy*). He noted that the full orgasm had an almost transcendent quality, involving loss of ego and a profound sense of peace. By contrast, people who felt guilty in sexual expression worked against the current of 'orgone energy' and produced frustrations and emotions that were subsequently repressed. This brought with it the neurotic, negative behaviour that Reich termed 'character armouring'. Sexual energy produced an effect on the autonomic nervous system which, in turn via sympathetic and parasympathetic actions, caused a tangible influence on specific organs in the body. While a healthy organism would normally exhibit patterns of contraction and expansion — a type of rhythm of life — in the case of an 'armoured' organism this was a permanent state of contraction.

Reich was appalled by the fact that mass neurosis appeared to be the norm in Western society and believed that such character patterns derived from defences against the free flow of sexual energy.

Reichian Therapy

In essence Reich's therapy is a dismantling of layers of pent-up emotion. Reich divided the body into seven zones at right angles to the spine and centred in : the eyes, mouth, neck, chest, diaphragm, abdomen and pelvis (including the legs). He believed that orgone energy was bound up in chronic muscular spasms and that it was necessary to free this energy progressively. Reichian 'bodywork' therapy entails dissolving the armour, beginning with the eyes and working down the body. Several approaches are used:

Deep breathing Breathing conforms to patterns proposed by the therapist. The patient may feel the stream of bioenergy in the form of prickling or tingling sensations.

Deep massage Pressure is applied to muscle spasms. Sometimes such areas of tension are pinched to loosen them up.

Facial expressions The patient 'makes faces' expressing certain emotions while keeping eye contact with the therapist and maintaining certain patterns of breathing.

Chest-work The therapist pushes down on the chest while the patient exhales or screams. Such bodywork is designed to removed blockages to breathing.

Convulsive reflex-work Convulsions break down the armouring. The therapist may work with the disruptive effects of coughing, yawning etc.

Stress positions Stress positions may be maintained to produce an effect of bodily irritation. This may lead to tremors or 'clonisms' which similarly break down the body armour.

Active movements The therapist may encourage the patient to kick and stamp and move parts of the body vigorously, as a 'loosening up' exercise.

In general a Reichian therapist penetrates from outer, accessible layers of armouring to deeper and deeper levels. It is important that such probing occurs at a pace that the patient can handle. Different effects are noted in each of the body segments:

The eyes The eyes may appear dull and lifeless. The patient is encouraged to roll them from side to side and perhaps open them wide as if in a state of sudden amazement.

The mouth This area also includes the muscles of the chin, throat and back of the head. The patient may be asked to cry, shout or suck, or move the lips in various ways, in order to loosen up the muscles concerned.

The neck Screaming and yelling may be used to free up tensions here also.

The chest Any armouring here will show up when the patient breathes or laughs. Inhibition of breathing is a means of suppressing the emotions and may require the use of special gestures involving the arms and hands.

The diaphragm Armouring tends to reveal itself via body posture in this segment. The spine may curve forward, constricting outward breath. Such armouring is loosened with breathing exercises and the so-called 'gag reflex'.

The abdomen This segment includes the back and abdominal muscles which are often tense if a person is defensive. Armouring is loosened up in these muscle regions.

The pelvis and lower limbs With strong armouring the pelvis is pulled back and may stick out, revealing signs of deep-seated repressed anxiety. There is also a tightening of the pelvis, inhibiting sexual expression and pleasure. The patient may be asked to strike the couch with the pelvic region or kick the feet until a sense of freedom in this region develops.

Reichian therapy is thus a systematic loosening of body tensions aimed at releasing the natural energy flow through the body. The techniques have exerted an extensive influence on the Human Potential Movement, particularly in the area of bodywork therapies like Bioenergetics, Rolfing and the Feldenkrais method of body movement.

PETER EEDY

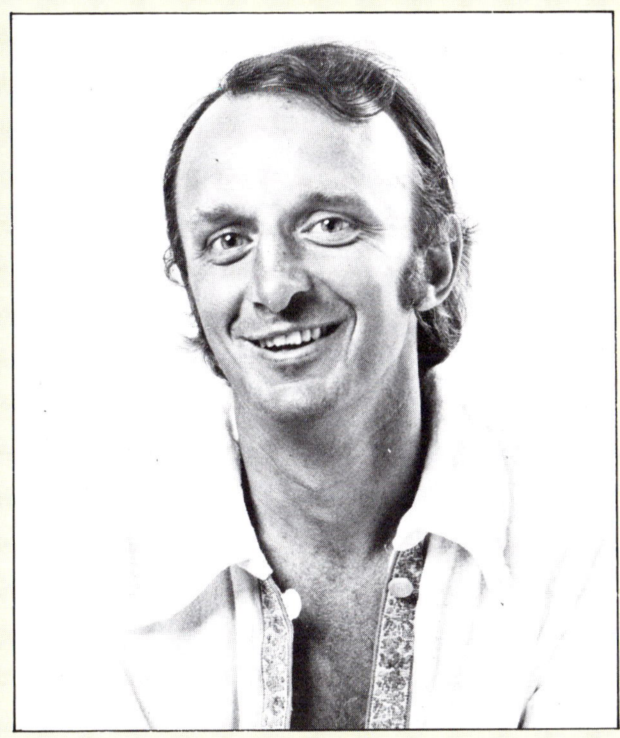

In recent years Peter Eedy has become a well known figure in the Australian counter-culture. He was a mainstream force behind the 1973 Nimbin Aquarius Festival and also organised the first Down to Earth Festival in 1976. In 1978 he established the Taringa Growth Centre in Brisbane which has since become a location for many alternative healing modalities including Reichian therapy, Rolfing, Polarity therapy, Touch For Health, Herbalism, Dream gestalting and Bioenergetics. Often he has worked with his sister Ruth who utilises many forms of massage in her work, including Reflexology, Brazilian toe massage and Energy Distribution massage.

Peter was born in Sydney in 1944 and grew up in Redfern and Waterloo. He left school at the age of 15 to become apprenticed as a chef and in the meantime decided to further his knowledge in areas of special interest. After a period of travel he used the University of Sydney library resources and read the collected works of Freud from cover to cover. This was in the late 1960s and the war in Vietnam was at its height. Peter had been a member of the Communist Party and believed in the concept of forcibly changing society. Since aligning himself with the Human Potential movement he now feels — with most adherents of the 'new consciousness' — that individuals must transform themselves and help raise the general levels of social awareness that way. However in those earlier days there seemed to be fewer options for change available. Freud meanwhile was heightening Peter's awareness of sexual repression in society and other emotions that people bottled up inside themselves.

In 1970 he came across the work of Austrian-born psychoanalyst Wilhelm Reich for the first time and was profoundly impressed. He seemed to share with this author a concern to discover the actual origins of sexual repression. At the Nimbin Festival three years later he spoke on Reich and subsequently conducted a lecture tour of six university campuses on Australia's eastern coast. The reaction among students was generally positive and favourable and with his friend Libby Scott, Peter has been compiling a book which draws on these lectures and also describes his own transformation of consciousness from Marxian influences through to Reich and other holistic philosophies.

In England Peter undertook personal therapy and trained with Nadine Scott and several members of the Boyesen family. Gerda Boyesen remains one of the leading neo-Reichian therapists and has evolved a technique of massage coupled with 'psycho-peristalsis' — sounds from within the organism related to blocked energy flow — that Peter regards as being the most important discovery in psychosomatic medicine this century (see entry : *Bioenergy* in this volume).

In 1974 Peter began conducting neo-Reichian workshops and lectures in Vienna — where Reich himself had trained in the University medical school — and helped re-establish links between local therapists and the neo-Reichians in England. The following year he held similar workshops and training sessions in California.

Later, after returning to Australia and meeting the former Australian deputy Prime Minister Jim Cairns — who similarly admired Reich — he decided to work with Dr Cairns and help the Down To Earth Festival, and invite several prominent overseas figures to attend. Wilhelm Reich's daughter Eva, a noted therapist in her own right; Dr James Prescott, Arthur Lincoln Pauls, and Len Harris — an Esalen masseur — came to Australia under Peter's sponsorship. The Festival was an enormous success but Peter lost financially on it. However the presence of such notable therapists in the country was an enormous stimulus and Peter has continued to explore ways of bringing different healing techniques to the notice of the Australian public. For example, he helped to organise the first and second Mind, Body and Healing Festivals. These days he practises as a qualified physiatrist specialising in ten different types of massage and holds neo-Reichian workshops, although his interests are of course much broader.

In 1977 he met a man in Australia whom he considered to be a Zen master. This person has had a considerable influence on Peter's personal development since that time and has guided him towards a more intuitive level of spiritual growth. One of Peter's major interests now is mutual depth meditation between teacher and pupil for inner development. While Reich remains a major influence, Peter's approach now is to apply a synthesis of all he has learnt.

ROLFING

Rolfing is a technique devised by Dr Ida P. Rolf, who graduated from Barnard College, New York, in biological chemistry and subsequently worked for the Rockefeller Institute. Although Rolfing was developed in the 1930s it did not achieve widespread recognition until the rise of the humanistic growth potential movements of the 1960s.

The Rolf Institute of Structural Integration defines the process as 'a technique for reordering the body, to bring its major segments – head, shoulders, thorax, pelvis and legs – toward a vertical alignment'. Essentially Rolfing uses deep massage and manipulation to restore the body to its normal 'integrated' position. Like Wilhelm Reich and Moshe Feldenkrais (author of *Awareness Through Movement)* who have influenced her, Ida Rolf believes that the body itself reflects mental and emotional attitudes. Her special type of physical therapy has been developed to release the body from accumulated tensions and 'armouring'.

Like chiropractors and practitioners of the Alexander Technique, Rolfers place considerable emphasis on posture and the role of gravity on the body. The fact that man can walk on two rather than four legs has given him more flexibility and independence than most animals but efficient movement depends upon the body alignment around a vertical axis – a fact often neglected in the human lifestyle. According to Ida Rolf gravity accentuates any distortions that occur and therapy must remove these patterns by aligning the posture with earth's gravity field. 'Gravity', she writes, 'not only upholds a man, it feeds him . . . thus in an erect man it should be possible to draw a straight line through the ears (bisecting the external meatus), the shoulder (head of the humerus), hip-bone (head of the femur), knee and ankle (external malleolus).'

People often allow the weight of their bodies to produce distortions – perhaps the head slumps forward, the body may have twists, the back may be arched – in short, the body has become unbalanced.

The Rolfing technique involves applying force to loosen and lengthen specific muscles and fascia. The latter – the envelope of connective tissue encompassing the muscles, tendons and ligaments and so on – essentially unites the body. The role of the therapist is to loosen the fascia and muscles, allowing the fibres to return to their proper position. Ida Rolf compares her technique to 'rebuilding a sagging or bulging wall, rather than trying to prop it up by artificial means'. Through a series of manipulations the bodily distortions are reversed and the tissue is moved back towards the natural pattern of symmetry and balance.

Rolfing generally requires a series of ten sessions lasting about an hour each and spaced over five or ten weeks. The therapy proceeds from the surface of the body towards deeper levels. The first session, for example, opens up breathing functions through the chest area and unlocks the hips, while the second focuses on the feet and ankles. Gradually tension blockages are removed and the final sessions integrate the loosened body into 'new patterns of movement'.

After Rolfing sessions the body often acquires a new sense of lightness, the head and chest are lifted and the trunk is lengthened. The body joints tend to have more freedom and body movement is more fluid. Rolfing seems to allow more efficient use of the muscles with less expended energy : the body is indeed 'structurally integrated'.

SEXUAL THERAPY

Attitudes to sexuality have changed dramatically in Western society in the last thirty years. Until quite recently the dominant mores in the West have still demanded that sexuality remain if not a taboo subject then still an essentially private affair. Since the stereotype has survived that on the whole man is the provider and woman the child-bearing nurturer, sexual relationships have been regarded predominantly as the basis for developing strong family bonds, reinforcing a deep sense of commitment between partners and, pragmatically, for perpetuating the human race. The Victorian sense of 'woman's duty' has passed but until the decade of the Human Potential movement, sexuality had not been seen as a form of self-expression or specially valued for its aesthetic and sensory aspects.

This has not always been the case with all cultures, of course. While sexuality has been a Western 'hang-up', in Indian Tantric thought women have had a very special role which elevates rather than represses them. According to the *Cina-Cara-Sara* text attributed to the Buddha, 'women are the gods, women are life . . .' and semen, or *bindu*, is the elixir of life. An important aspect of sexual intercourse in Tantra is the exchange of positive and negative

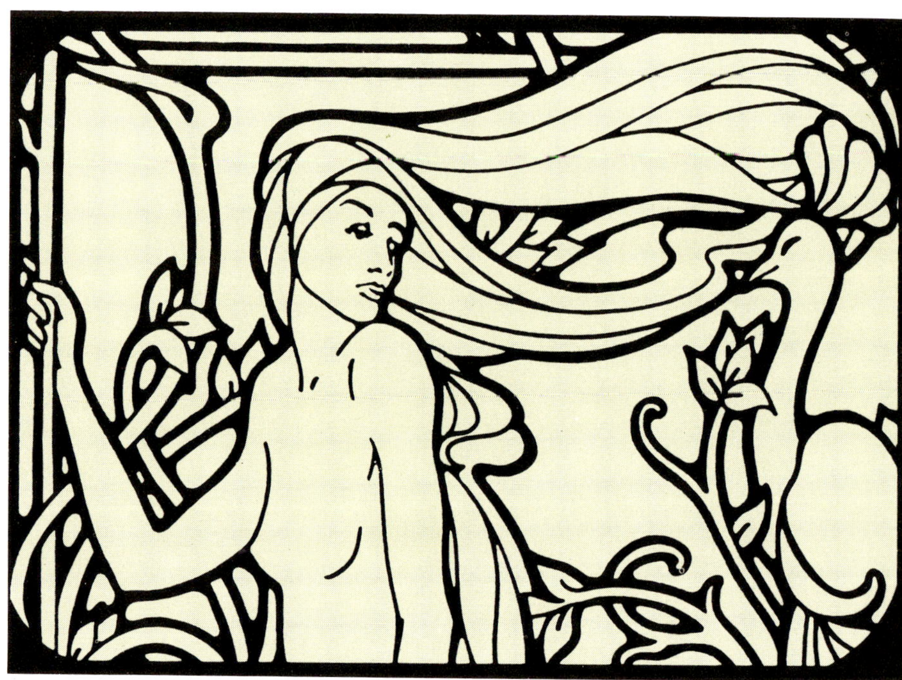

prana – the subtle energies of life. Tantra also posits the view that sexual experience arouses the *Kundalini*, the energy of mystical illumination. Yogic authority Dr Jonn Mumford explains this process lucidly as follows:

The woman's body represents the psychic tube ida *and is a natural channel for negative* (apanic) *moon* (chandra) *energy. The man's body functions as* pingala, *a psychic conduit for positive* (pranic) *sun* (surya) *power. At the moment of orgasm, two bodies fuse momentarily on a psychic plane, the energy of which fusion is focused in the middle channel* shushumna, *and the ascent of Kundalini commences, accompanied by the mutual opening of the* chakras, *or autonomic nerve plexuses in each participant.*

During the sixth International Transpersonal Conference, Esalen Institute teacher Christina Grof described how in her own experience, *Kundalini* could also be unleashed by natural child-birth. She felt a surge of 'sky-rocketing' white light as the *Kundalini* energy soared into her head.

If sexuality is such a potent source of energy why has it been largely ignored in the West?

With the advent of psychoanalysis sexuality was more openly considered. The ground had been laid by Krafft-Ebing whose collection of sexual case histories, *Psychopathia Sexualis*, had been published in 1886. Sigmund Freud recognised two basic drives in the human species which he called Eros and Thanatos: the first the urge to love and the need for sexual gratification, the second a drive towards death and self-destruction. In practical life these drives tended to fuse so that human behaviour reflected both possibilities. Freud noted the role of instincts as channels for the flow of energy. In a series of lectures published in 1933 he said:

The sexual instincts are remarkable for their plasticity, for the facility with which they can change their aims, for their interchangeability – for the ease with which they can substitute one form of gratification for another, and for the way in which they can be held in suspense . . .

The concept of energy flow and sexuality was developed further by Wilhelm Reich, the Viennese psychoanalyst who for a time worked closely with Freud. Reich similarly recognised the twin forces underlying sexuality and wrote:

'I say on the basis of ample clinical experience that only in a few cases in our civilisation is the sexual act based on love. The intervening rage, hatred, sadistic emotions and contempt are part and parcel of the love life of modern man . . .'

However he also recognised more completely than Freud the vital role of sexuality in releasing tension and combating neurosis. He encouraged his patients to develop what he called *orgastic potency* . . . 'the capacity for surrender to the flow of biological energy without any inhibition, the capacity for complete discharge of all damned-up sexual excitation through involuntary pleasurable contractions of the body . . .' Reich discovered that as a result of such self-expression, his patients also learned to develop tenderness and sensitivity in their sexual relationships and no longer considered sexuality in a furtive or repressive manner. Reich regarded sexual energy as the centre of the inner life of an individual and an essential ingredient of health. The capacity for a thoroughly satisfying orgasm was vital to a well balanced existence and he valued highly the sense of sexual freedom.

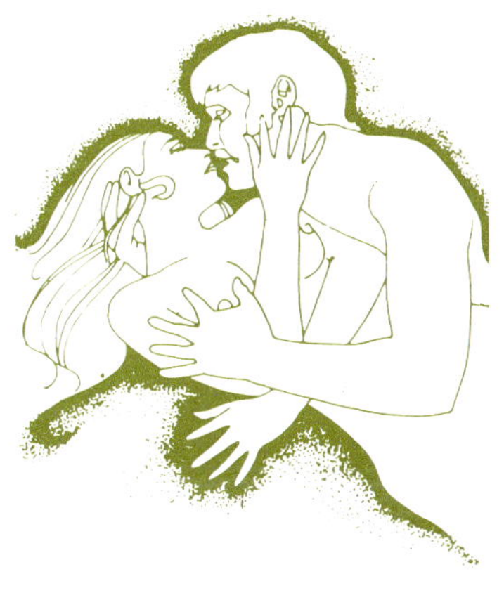

Reich isolated four factors in the ideal 'orgastic experience' : 1) Tension, 2) Charge, 3) Discharge and 4) Relaxation. On a purely physical level the sexual organs would periodically fill with fluid producing tension. Then there would be mounting excitation (bioenergetic charge) followed by sexual excitation and the muscular activity of sexual intercourse (bioenergetic discharge). The process culminated in orgasm and physical relaxation.

Reich believed that blockages in any part of the *orgasm cycle* would lessen its expression and lead to tensions and other physical and mental manifestations of stress. What he called *character armouring* – frozen patterns of behaviour – derived from blocked sexuality. On the other hand an integrated person literally went with the flow and demonstrated an unblocked energy pattern uniting mind and body. Reich subsequently directed his attention to *body armouring*, in which neurotic tendencies affected the muscular patterns of the body, and his therapy would initially focus on physical body tensions before leading up to developing the capacity for sexual release.

However while Reich's therapy was individually based, popular notions of sexuality have been strongly influenced by a variety of 'sex reports' that have been publicised through the media. Such works as Shere Hite's *The Hite Report* and the writings of William Masters and Virginia Johnson *(Human Sexual Response; Human Sexual Inadequacy* and *Homosexuality in Perspective)* have been enormously influential and underlie the practices of many contemporary sexual therapists. Other notable sexologists include Alfred Kinsey, Morton Hunt, Helen Singer Kaplan, Anthony Pietropinto and Jacqueline Simenauer.

The trouble with most sex reports is that they tend to be dominated by statistics and alleged medical 'facts' about sexuality. In 1948, for example, Kinsey reported that at the age of 29, 5.3 per cent of American men were without sexual experience and that 75 per cent of all males reached orgasm within two minutes of 'intromission'. Morton Hunt reported in his 1972 survey that 72 per cent of all young husbands still masturbated, while Shere Hite claimed that only 30 per cent of the women she surveyed could have an orgasm regularly in intercourse.

Such analyses have attracted strong criticisms from other social scientists and thinkers who value the *quality* of the sexual relationship rather than its statistical referents. Foremost among these critics is Thomas Szasz, a practising psychiatrist and professor, who is opposed to the allegedly scientific reporting of Masters and Johnson. According to Szasz they forget that

'... after nursing, sex is the most basic social arrangement for satisfying the pervasive and powerful human hunger for being needed/wanted and loved/satisfied. That experience – called love – ... so transcends the physiological need for tension-relief that it can be spiritually satisfying even in the absence of providing relief of sexual tension. But love is a profoundly personal experience ...'

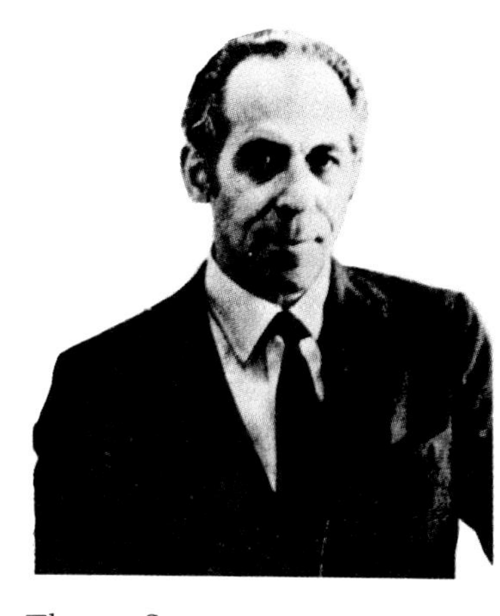
Thomas Szasz

Dr James Lynch, an authority on human relationships, echoes this view. In *The Broken Heart* he writes:

Human love involves much more than an orgasm ... The covert, nonspecific agenda of sexual intercourse – or for that matter, of any other human relationship – often involves more than sexual pleasure or sexual exploitation. One of the agendas is companionship – real, live, honest-to-goodness companionship.

The upshot of this is that sexual therapy must be individually assessed according to the perspectives it offers, and it is certainly preferable for treatment to extend beyond purely physical considerations. The situation is complicated by the fact that the leading sexual therapists do not necessarily agree among themselves who is worthwhile and who isn't. In 1975 Dr Masters said publicly that only one in a hundred sex clinics in the United States were legitimate. 'The vast majority', he claimed, 'offer little more than a superficial sex education at best and dangerous quackery at worst'.

In the final analysis we are all responsible for our own sexuality and any therapist should recognise personal needs of both a physiological and an emotional nature. The choice is up to us!

SHAMANIC HEALING

Shamanism traditionally is a technique of ecstasy or dissociation that originated in the religion of ancient Siberia but is also found among many other cultures in North and South America, Indonesia, Japan and Australia.

The shaman is a magical practitioner who through an act of will can enter into a state of trance and journey to the land of the gods. The Wiradjeri aboriginal medicine-men have a high god known as Baiame who is described as a 'very old man, with a long beard, sitting in his camp with his legs under him. Two great quartz crystals extend from his shoulders to the sky above him'. Baiame sometimes appears to the aborigines in their dreams. He causes a sacred waterfall of liquid quartz to pour over their bodies absorbing them totally. They then grow wings replacing their arms. Later the dreamer learns to fly and Baiame sings a piece of magical quartz into his forehead to enable him to see right into things. Subsequently an 'inner flame' and a 'heavenly cord' are also incorporated into the body of the new shaman.

We can see from this account that the shaman acquires new magical powers by encountering the gods as a result of a special dream journey. The transformations which follow such an encounter are regarded as initiatory.

However the shaman is not necessarily working only on his own behalf. When he ventures on his trance journey the gods may reveal to him the nature of disease on the inner planes. The anthropologist A. A. Popov recorded trance journeys among the Nanay people of the Tungus region of Siberia. Typically the shaman would descend into the 'lower world' and would meet magical animals, usually an ermine or mouse, that would act as his guides.

The Nanay shaman is suckled by a cosmic deity known as the Mistress of the Water and then with his animal guides is shown a community of spirits responsible for sickness in the world. Later he flies in spirit form to the top of an enormous tree which later explains to him: 'I am the tree that makes all people capable of living'. The tree-spirit gives the shaman a branch with three offshoots for the construction of three drums: one for performing shaman rituals over women in childbirth, the second for the sick and the third for those who are dying. Inherent in the Nanay folk-beliefs is the view that sickness and disease originate from the 'inner planes' of reality. The shaman or medicine-man is the person who is able to bridge the different levels of the universe and communicate with both mankind and the gods.

The Mazatec Indians of Mexico are unusual because they have included elements of Christianity alongside their shamanic deities; the same process

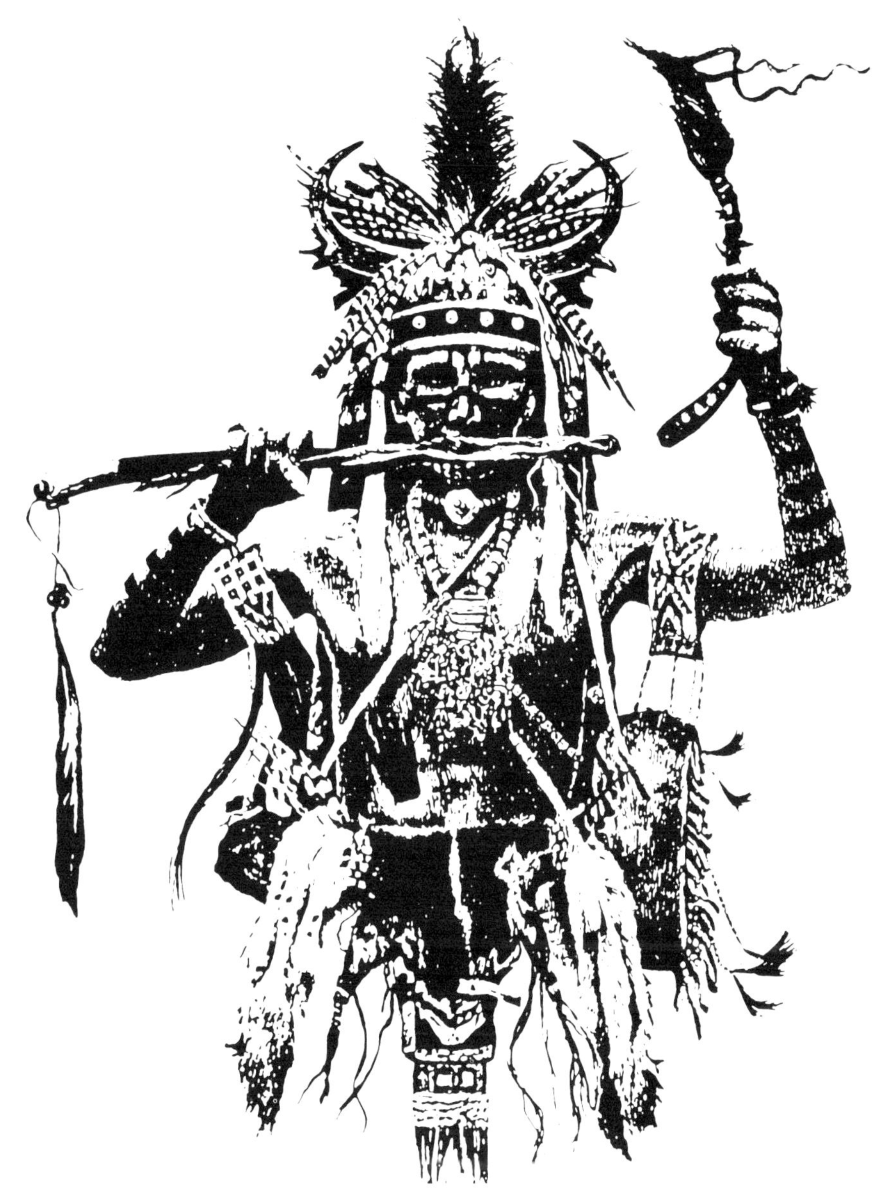

The healing journey of the shaman – an American Indian medicine man

of inner-plane contact for healing nevertheless remains. The Mazatecs make use of psilocybe mushrooms and the female shamans use the altered state of consciousness which the drug produces to determine the causes of sickness. Both the patient and the shaman take the sacred mushrooms so that the sick person can also hear the healing words which come from the spirit world. Henry Munn reports that as the female healing shaman sinks deeper into trance she seems to go on a journey. Spiritual rays of light appear:

The aurora of the dawn is coming and the light of day. In the name of the Father, the Son and the Holy Spirit, by the sign of the Holy Cross, free us Our Lord from our enemies and all evil . . .

I am he who cures. I am he who speaks with the Lord of the World. I am happy. I speak with the mountains of peaks. I am he who speaks with Bald Mountain. I am the remedy and the medicine man, I am the mushroom. I am the fresh mushroom. I am the large mushroom. I am the fragrant mushroom. I am the mushroom of the spirit . . .

Shamanism has been a remote and archaic religion for most people and as such has primarily belonged to the domain of academic anthropology. However in very recent times the healing techniques of shamanism have been formulated and explained for a Western audience by Professor Michael Harner, one of the world's leading authorities on the subject. Harner is affiliated with the Human Potential and Transpersonal movements and has recently published a new book *The Way of the Shaman* which explains how even modern Western city-dwellers can learn how to heal shamanically. Harner is best known for his account of the Jivaro who live in the Ecuadorian Andes. He experienced their psychedelic initiation near a sacred waterfall, where he had a victorious encounter with two spirit-snakes in an awesome, revelatory vision. However he has also studied the shamans of the Wintun, Pomo,

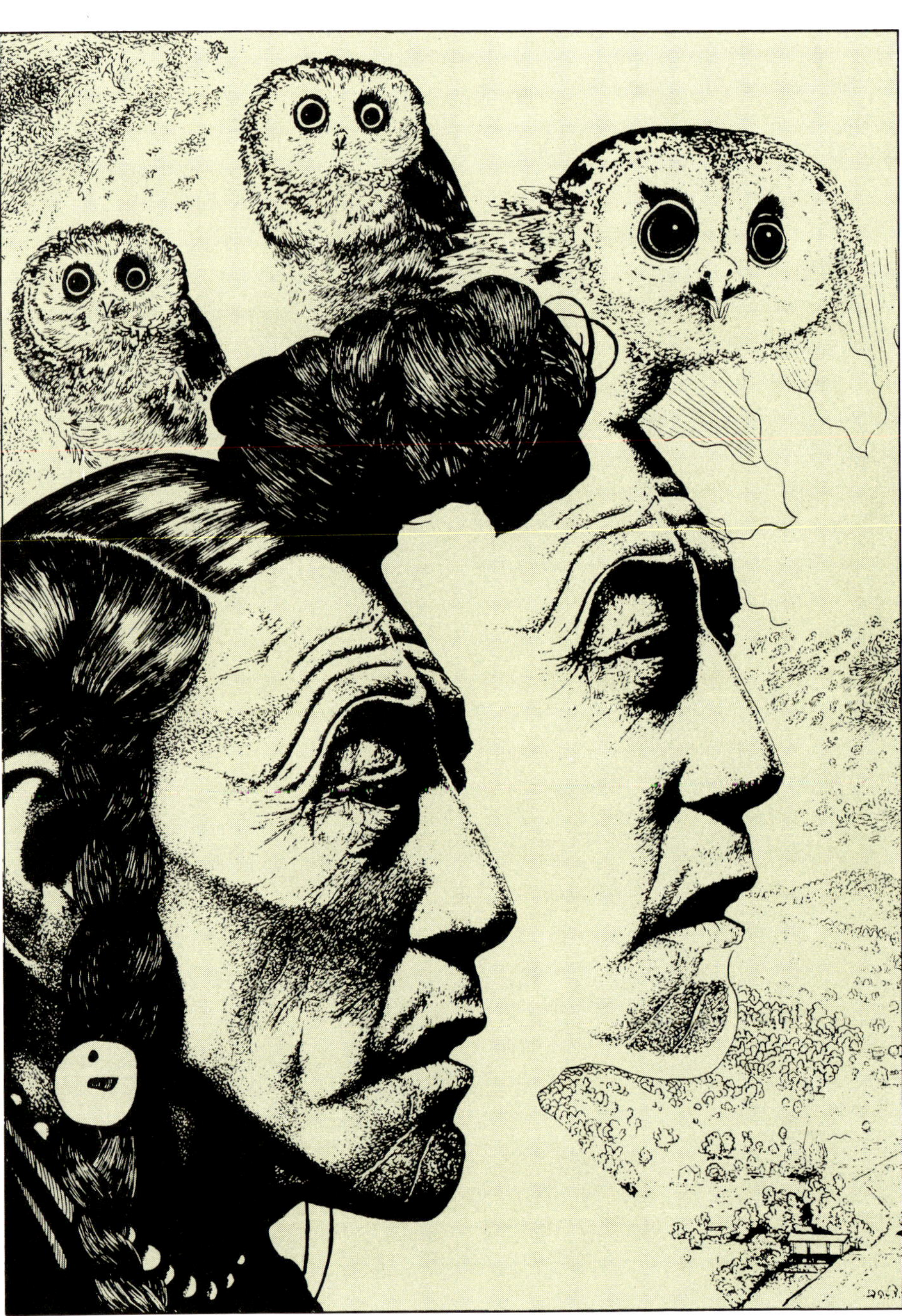

Shamanic power animals – from an illustration by Martin Carey

Coast Salish, Conibo and Lakota Sioux Indians and over the years has assimilated much of their teaching into his own practice.

Harner's workshops feature the beating of a large drum which the would-be shaman (the Western student) uses to travel imaginatively into the inner world. The technique resembles the active imagination or 'mind game' methods of Robert Masters and Jean Houston and produces a light trance state condition. The shaman travels mentally through a crack in the ground, a gateway, or down the root system of a large tree to meet a force in the underworld that is the power animal. The underworld in shamanism is a dimension filled with light and is in no way demonic or evil. The shaman may discover in the form of his power animals his own source of vitality and health; indeed Harner notes that the Jivaro Indians believe it is not possible for human beings to survive for an extended time without them.

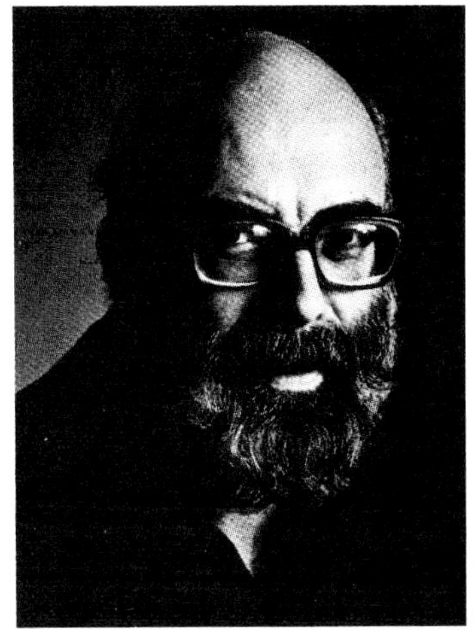

Dr Michael Harner – bringing traditional shamanic methods to a Western audience

Quite aside from personal revelations, the power animals can be used for healing purposes. If there is a person in the workshop who is feeling 'dis-spirited' Harner or one of his more advanced students travels down to the underworld to seek a power animal that will be willing to live in the body of the sick person and fill them with new vitality. The animal must reveal itself four times in the trance world and the shaman then seizes it and brings it back to the upper world where he transfers it mentally by breathing it into the crown and chest of the person requiring it.

Harner also claims he is able to assist sick people from a distance by visualising and willing power animals to enter their bodies, restoring them to health. He has been able to confirm the spirit-contact by subsequently asking such persons whether their dreams have revealed any special 'symbols' and has often been pleasantly surprised when they describe the power animal that had been sent!

Shamanism uses the descriptive symbolism of mythology to explain its meaning but it appears possible to grasp its healing potential in psychological terms. Harner believes the monotonous drum rhythm simulates theta brain activity and produces creative, dream-like imagery. It may be that the brain reveals facets of consciousness which relate to psychosomatic illness. The shaman in a sense is travelling into the unconscious mind when he undertakes his trance journey. The sacred symbols of his culture are in some degree archetypal representations of wholeness and totality and reflect a very profound relationship with the cosmos. It is not surprising that personal revelations from such a deep level of consciousness can have a special bearing on health. Shamanism may be seen as somewhat similar to meditation . . . an activity which links the inner experiential domain with the outer one and leads to new possibilities of self-realisation and psychological integration.

SHIATSU AND ACUPRESSURE

Shiatsu *(finger pressure)* is a type of physical manipulation developed in Japan this century but derived from the ancient Chinese Do-In techniques. Although Shiatsu is a healing art it is also a means of seeking harmony and stability, a combination of intellect and action; mind and body. It should be distinguished from *Anma*, Japanese massage, which came to Japan from China around a thousand years ago and has been part of Japanese medical treatment for at least three hundred years. Anma has traditionally been used to treat stiff shoulders and back tension while Shiatsu has more far-reaching uses. Shiatsu is officially defined by the Japanese Ministry of Health and Welfare as 'a form of manipulation administered by the thumbs, fingers and palms without the use of any instrument, mechanical or otherwise, to apply pressure to the human skin, correct internal malfunctioning, promote and maintain health and treat specific diseases'. Shiatsu involves 'one point' pressure and endeavours to heal by working with the natural regenerative powers of the body to remove abnormalities and disease.

While Anma, like Western massage, stimulates blood circulation, Shiatsu reinforces joints and muscles and focuses on the efficient flow of energy through the meridians and autonomic nervous system. Many Shiatsu practitioners say they prefer it to acupuncture because it can be performed by a person on himself, with complete safety, whereas acupuncture, of course, has to be administered by a specialist. The meridians in the body — its channels of living, magnetic energy — can be felt by pressing on the correct *Tsubos*, or acu-points. These number 365 and occur in such locations as the depressions at the junctures of muscles, the trunks of muscles and nerves and at spaces between wrinkles in the skin. There are 12 meridians in the body which connect the arms and legs and pass through the back, neck and head. It is also important to note that there is a direct flow of energy between the outer extremities and the inner organs. Each arm and leg has three yin and three yang meridians and when a person is in a state of good health the energy flow is evenly balanced between them. However in ill-health the energy flow stagnates in those meridians which are producing the sickness. The role of the Shiatsu healer is to diagnose the location of the stagnation and stimulate the appropriate meridian.

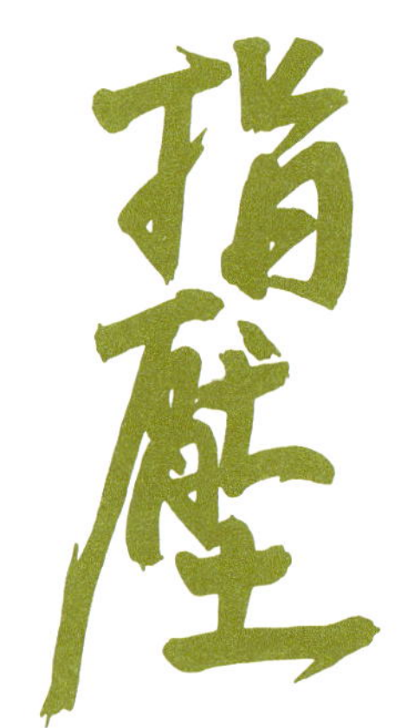

Shiatsu

In Shiatsu such diagnosis may involve considering such factors as facial characteristics, colour of the skin, posture, quality of voice, tongue, pulse-beat and body temperature. The crucial aspect is the nature of energy flow — called in Japanese *Ki* — and two polarities or extremes are recognised. *Kyo*

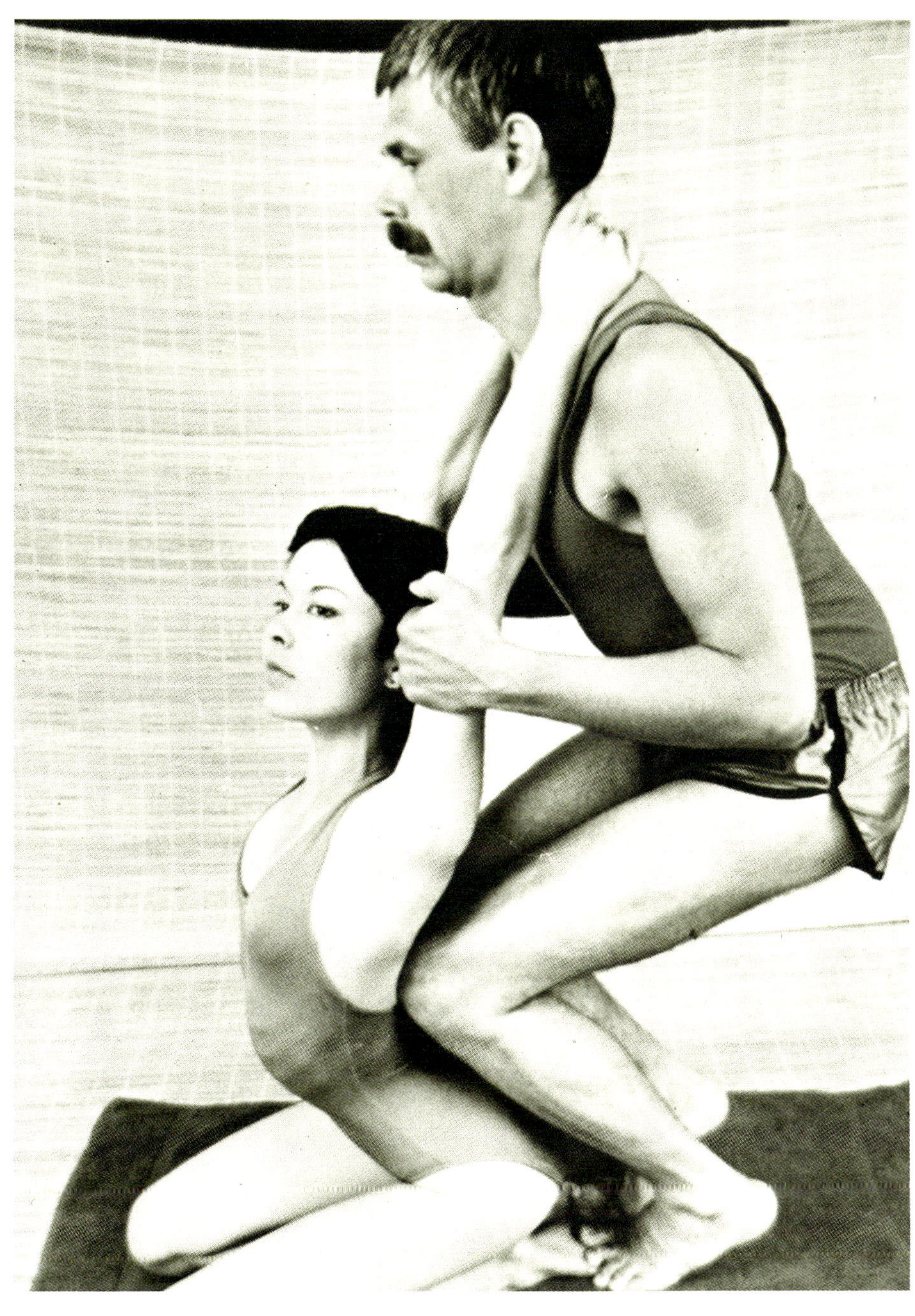

Shiatsu technique demonstrated by Daniel Weber

is depleted energy and *Jitsu* excess. To normalise Jitsu points the healer uses sedation while Kyo points receive toning. Jitsu areas are relatively easy to treat but Kyo regions require energy to be transferred to them which takes longer to build up. It is important in the healing process that the Kyo areas be located first since accidental sedation to these regions could lead to increasing the existing imbalance. The Shiatsu practitioner tries initially to isolate the meridians which show the most pronounced divergence of Kyo and Jitsu and provides counterbalancing energy to those. There are 120 combinations of Kyo and Jitsu in the body's meridians and Shiatsu treatment is applied to the body as a whole, rather than focusing on specific disease symptoms. Shiatsu helps a patient to heal himself by highlighting areas of imbalance in the body.

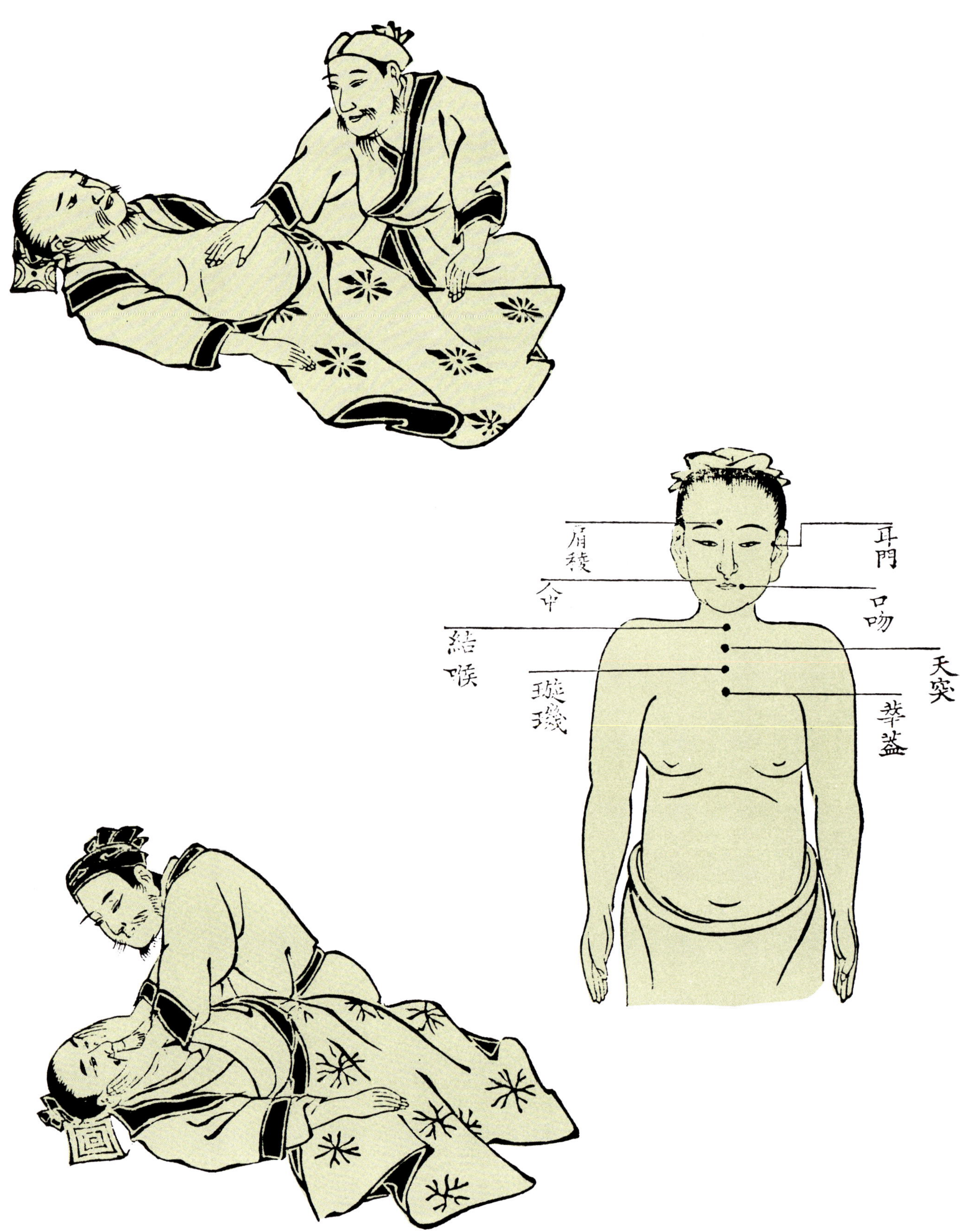

Traditional Shiatsu source material

Shizuko Yamamoto, a leading authority on Shiatsu has written of the underlying techniques used in oriental medicine. In her book *Barefoot Shiatsu* she notes:

The human body responds to three types of stimuli. When struck by some object it has a pain response. When exposed to heat or cold it has a thermal response. When touched in some manner the body has a tactile response. These three responses can be employed in treatment. Acupuncture uses the first type in the hope of producing a response to an object. Moxibustion employs the second type in its use of heat to produce changes in the body. Shiatsu and massage use the stimulus of touch pressure to alter energy flow within the body.

There are several Shiatsu techniques, including rubbing, kneading, pressing, tapping, shaking and stretching. The most common approaches involve the use of the palm, thumb and fingers. According to Shizuko Yamamoto, Shiatsu is most effective when the energy flow comes from one's centre of vitality, known as *Hara*. The sense of inner balance is vital to achieving health.

Palm Technique

This is a very penetrating form. The palms and fingers of the practitioner should be relaxed with the arm supporting the body weight. The palm and fingers follow the curvature of the body surface and the healer uses both palms simultaneously; one remains stationary, the other slides along the body providing sedation. While pressure is applied, muscles can be 'rubbed down' by moving along them vertically or else light pressure can be applied in a circular, clockwise motion, relaxing them.

Thumb Technique

Pressure may be applied to the *Tsubo* points by the thumb in a handshake-type grip or by extending the tip of the thumb while clasping the other fingers in a fist. Pressure is applied by both the thumb and fist in this instance.

Alternatively, pressure can be applied by using two, three or four fingers in different configurations either to sedate or tonify. Shiatsu practitioners learn to apply sustained but not forceful pressure vertically to the body surface, usually for around 2–7 seconds, although some treatments require longer.

Modern Shiatsu has been strongly influenced by both Shizuko Yamamoto referred to above and also Shizuto Masunaga.

Shizuko Yamamoto first visited the United States in 1965. She was associated at that time with George Ohsawa and the Macrobiotics movement. She stayed for a time with Michio Kushi in Boston and then went on to New York. Since her arrival in the United States she has treated more than 20 000 people with her Shiatsu techniques.

Shizuto Masunaga is also one of the leading figures in the field of Shiatsu. Born in Hiroshima, he worked in the area after graduating from the University of Kyoto and gave instruction for ten years at the Japan Shiatsu Institute. He was probably the first person to establish a theoretical basis for the subject and at present is the chairman of the Iokai Association for Shiatsu Therapy.

Shiatsu is attracting increasing attention in Western countries as a useful adjunct to acupuncture and massage.

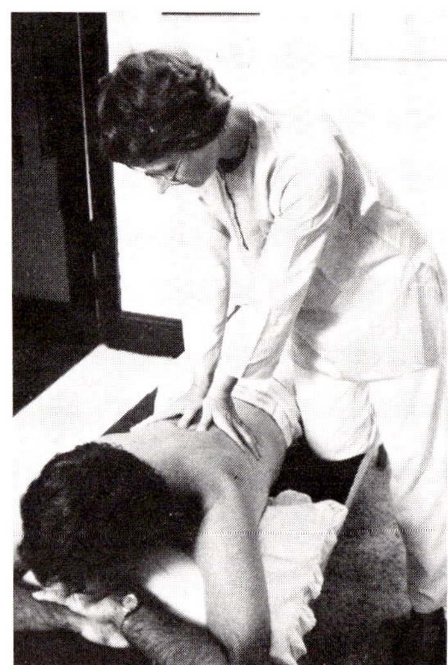

Ann Skea demonstrating acupressure

Acupressure is essentially similar to Shiatsu except that its terminology derives from acupuncture. Needles of course are not used and the practitioner applies finger pressure to the same locations where the traditional Chinese doctor places needles.

The energy flow is termed *Chi* rather than the Japanese *Ki*, and acupressure is similarly used to unblock the vital flow through the body.

Most acupressurists apply pressure with the thumbs although sometimes the index finger is used with the middle finger doubled up on top, reinforcing the pressure.

The following is a brief sample of Chinese acupressure points that can be stimulated to relieve certain symptoms. They are each illustrated in accompanying diagrams:

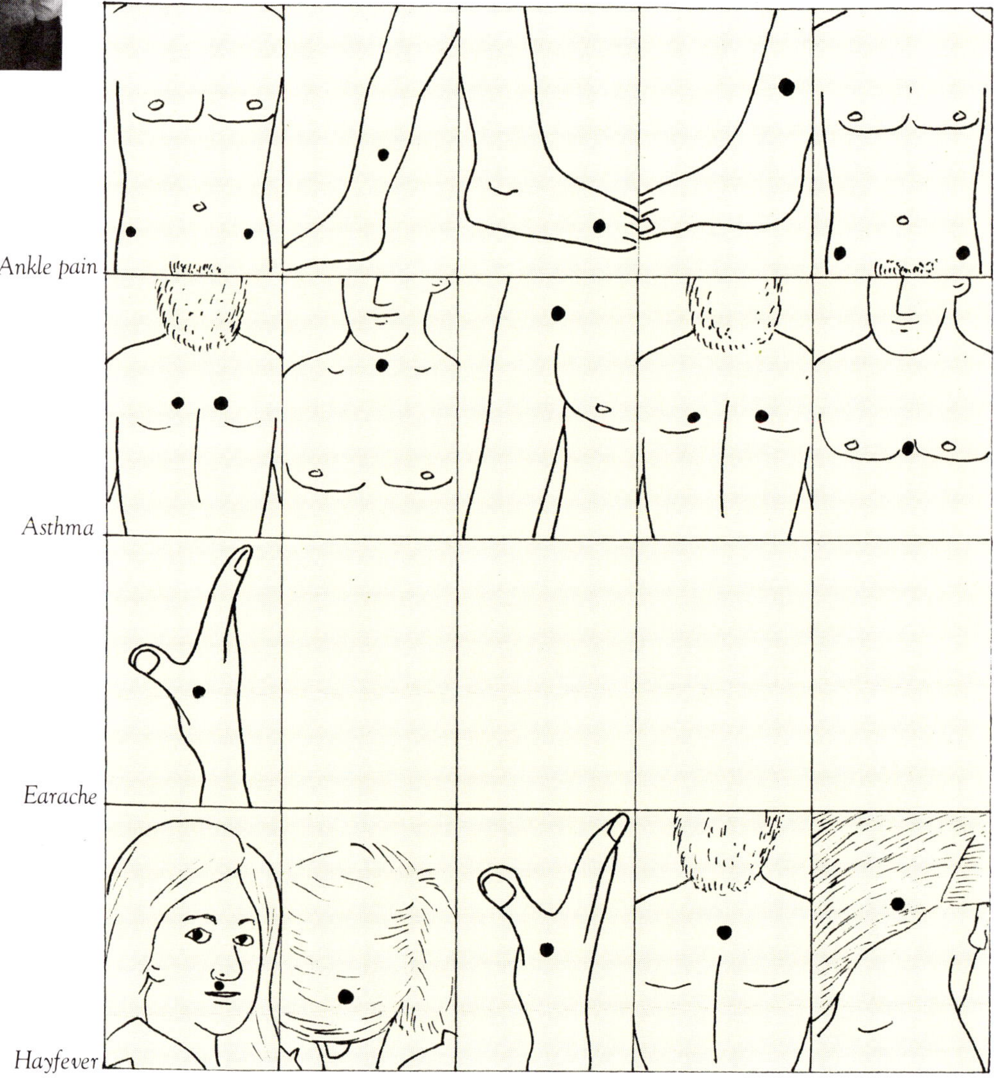

	TRADITIONAL NAME	LOCATION
Ankle pain	Five Pivots Leaking Valley Foot Coming to Tears Crossroad of Three Yins Protecting Path	Near hip bone Near ankle bones Near fourth toe Near inner ankle bone Near hip bone
Asthma	Lung Locus Sky Prominence Central Prefecture Superficial Tortuosity Upper Epigastrium	Upper spine near neck Throat region Arm shoulder fold Upper back Between nipples
Earache	Connecting the Valleys	Between thumb and index finger on back of both hands.
Hayfever	Stalk Bone Super Star Connecting the Valleys Seeking Path Windy Prefecture	Upper Buttock Forehead, near hairline Between thumb and index finger on back of both hands Upper spine near neck. Hairline, back of head.
Influenza	Outer Pass Delivering Message Big Vertebra Great Slaughter	Back of wrist Above inner ankle bone Upper spine near neck Spine knob near neck
Sciatica	Circular Jump Organ Gate Orderly Edge Stomach Granary Supporting Hill	Upper buttock Below buttock on leg Back of knee Immediately below buttock Above ankle bone

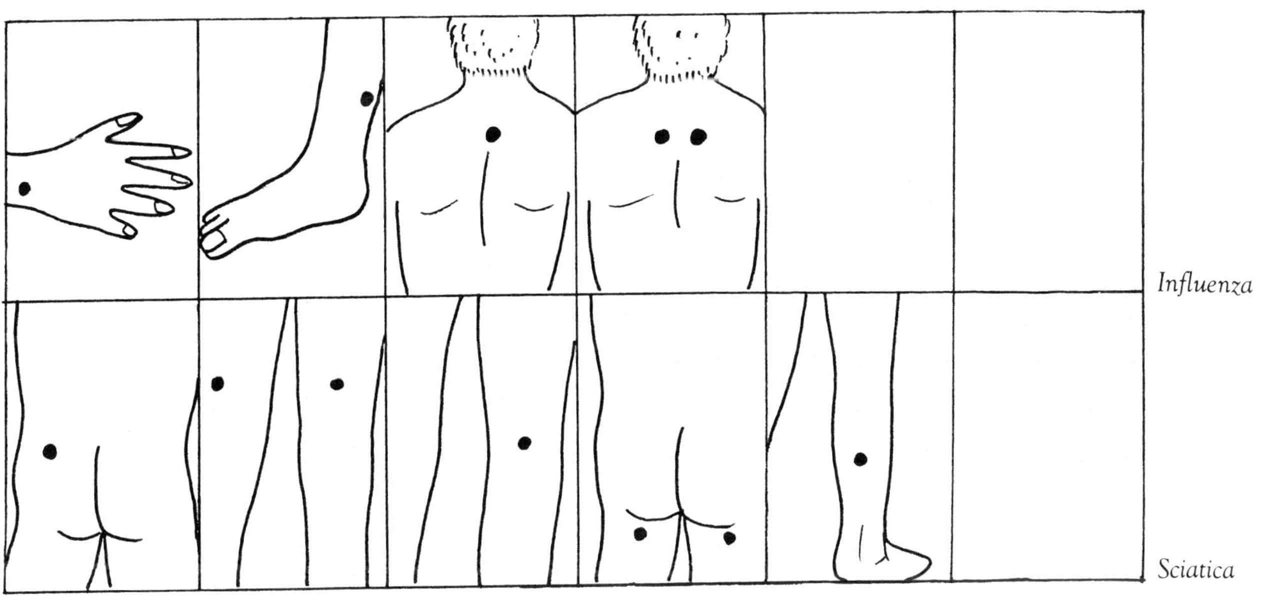

Influenza

Sciatica

DANIEL WEBER

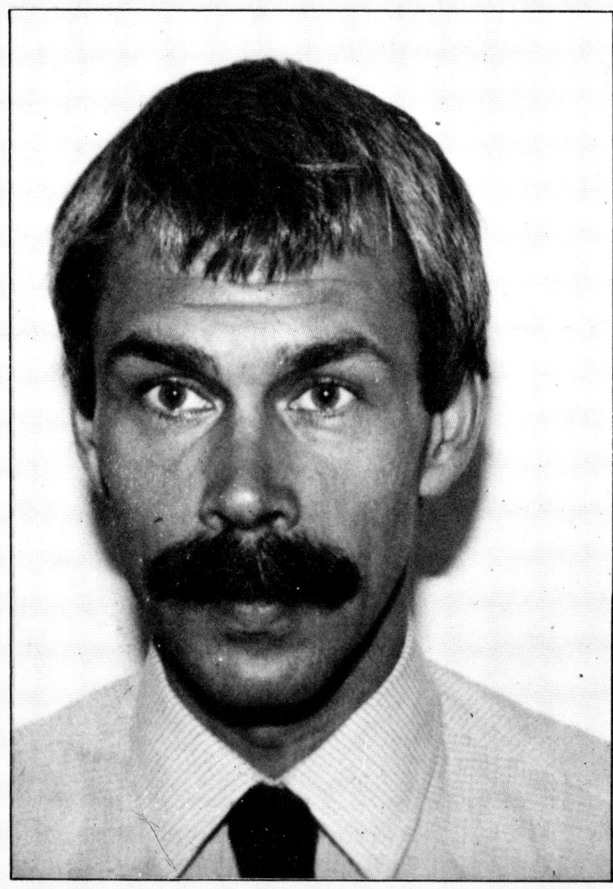

Daniel Weber heads the Australian East-West Foundation, a centre for oriental and traditional therapeutics affiliated with other branches of the Foundation in Europe, the United States, Japan and Brazil. The centre offers seminars and classes in Shiatsu, Oki (or 'Zen') Yoga, whole-food cookery and Macrobiotics, and presents an overriding philosophy of spiritual integration and emphasis on the balance of man and nature.

This is quite in contrast to the environment Daniel himself grew up in. Born in Minnesota in 1942 he was raised in what he terms a 'cultural desert' of white bread, mash potatoes and television. He rejected Western-style education, attending college for just three days before dropping out. However in the 1960s he became interested in oriental medicine and philosophy. He was also reading existentialists like Camus and Sartre and working in experimental theatre.

It was while training to be an actor in Boston that he met the Japanese teacher Michio Kushi of the East-West Foundation. The encounter was to be a fruitful one. Daniel eventually stayed with Kushi for five years, absorbing his remarkably unified Eastern philosophy and learning to understand essential patterns of life.

Eager to study techniques of acupuncture, Daniel looked for appropriate schools on the East coast but was unable to find one. In the early 1970s he went to England for two years and studied with Dr J.R. Worsley and Dr Van Buren at the College of Acupuncture, outside London. They were impressive teachers and a solid grounding in acupuncture was achieved. (Daniel now holds a Doctorate of Acupuncture from Singapore.) Later he worked as a practitioner of oriental medicine at the Hillside Clinic and helped establish the East-West Foundation in London.

From England Daniel travelled to Japan where he studied with the remarkable Zen Yoga teacher Masahiro Oki, a Samurai-educated doctor of medicine who was equally conversant in haiku, flower arrangement, martial arts and meditation. Daniel was impressed by the man's essential simplicity of vision — an unerring ability to see to the cause of things. Oki was able to lift his pupils away from central misconceptions, hone in on their weak points and fortify them by presenting them with personal challenges. His *dojo*, or study centre, in Mishima was always full but Oki, who was keen to present his Eastern philosophies to Westerners, made special concessions to Daniel and his wife Marcia who both found the experience extremely rewarding. The Webers have been in Australia for four years and are impressed by the high standard of Chinese medicine in this country. Although he makes regular overseas trips to Taiwan, Japan and the United States, Daniel feels that he has established a worthwhile base in Sydney.

He is keen, however, to point out problems which seem to be arising in some aspects of the local holistic training. Some students seem intent on focusing on a quick-cure 'technique and remedy' philosophy similar to the pill-popping notions of Western medicine. Daniel feels that therapies like Shiatsu, Oki Yoga and Herbalism are in themselves only techniques. What is really important is the self-realisation potential underlying them.

Although he has been working recently with psychotherapist Roger Dunstan, Daniel resists comparisons with Western 'equivalents' of Shiatsu like Polarity Balancing, Zone Therapy and Touch for Health, and stresses that rather than intellectualise his subject he likes to communicate it simply, on a practical level. His Shiatsu therapy is modified to suit the individual requirements of the client. 'Even though a problem may appear to be the same,' he says, 'each person will require a different treatment'. In essence, he works initially with symptoms, probes deeper to the immediate cause of the problem and then seeks to discover the actual origin of the disease. An implicit assumption is that man creates his own ill-health and is finally responsible for rectifying balance and harmony. Daniel's Shiatsu techniques involve working on the body as a whole, relating positive and negative meridian connections to specific organs and stimulating vital energy flow: harmonising the forces by applying pressure to the 365 main points of the body.

It is absorbing work and Daniel feels privileged to be working in a field he thoroughly enjoys.

ANN SKEA

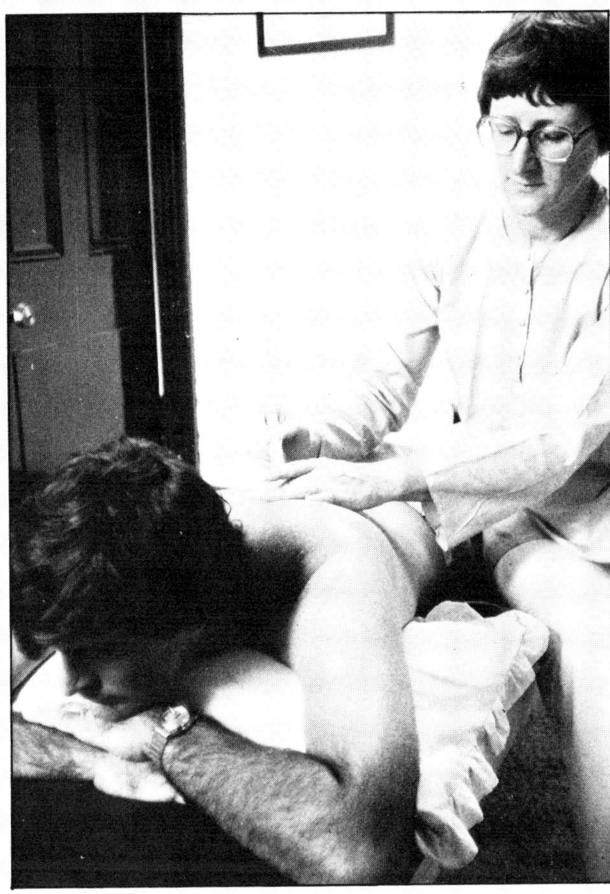

Ann Skea works as an acupressurist at Dorothy Hall's College of Herbal Medicine and also in Sydney's Alexander Street Herbal Centre at Crows Nest – an attractive older-style cottage which has been converted into offices amidst a flurry of modern civic developments.

Trained originally in Brighton, England, as a pharmacist, Ann went with her husband in 1976 to live in Hong Kong. There the life for a European woman seemed to be an endless stream of bridge parties and other neo-colonial pursuits so she quickly sought an alternative interest – and found it in Chinese medicine. She became absorbed by the possibilities offered by both acupuncture and acupressure and took Diploma studies in both, with Chinese doctors. She prefers acupressure because she can feel its effects through her fingers, but employs the same points and meridians in her work as those used by a traditional acupuncturist.

In Hong Kong – where acupressure is less popular than in other countries, for example, Korea – Ann found that Chinese doctors were inclined to present acupuncture as a universal cure. She believes, however, that bacterial and viral infections are not reached specifically by such methods but that acupuncture does affect the symptoms and body energies. By the same token she feels that acupuncture and acupressure also have different applications. Since with finger pressure one reaches a broader surface area than with a needle, acupressure seems to be more effective in treating such structural ailments as misalignments of the spine, while acupuncture appears to be a quicker method for remedying specific organic problems.

Ann finds the process of acupressure often physically tiring since it involves intense concentration. However it can also be relaxing and, at times, meditative. During an effective treatment she is consciously aware of energy transfer, and each of her patients receive special and individual attention : she sees only between six and ten people a week in the two days she practises. She also works part-time as a science teacher in a private school.

Like many traditional Chinese doctors, Ann uses moxa frequently during her healing sessions and finds it is extremely effective in stimulating a specific pressure point. However, while a few practitioners still rest a piece of moxa on a slice of ginger on the skin, or on the tips of acupuncture needles, she feels this is often painful for the patient – which defeats the purpose. Having ignited the moxa stick she holds it close to the skin without touching the surface, and finds this more effective since patients invariably find it very relaxing. Although there is no conclusive evidence on how moxa works, French research indicates that it increases the white blood cell count, and it is these cells in the body which are effective in clearing away infection. Moxa is used primarily to treat muscle tensions and some cases of spasm, but is never used with 'hot, excess' conditions like fevers. Since one of its notable effects is inducing relaxation it is not surprising that some of her patients have actually fallen asleep during an acupressure session.

Over the years Ann Skea has used acupressure techniques to effectively treat cases of chronic backache, spinal misalignments, swollen joints, rheumatic conditions and stress-based ailments, as well as bronchitis, high blood pressure and digestive disorders. However she points out that acupressure is not only a treatment and a diagnostic aid, but also a form of soothing relaxing massage aimed at keeping the body healthy. In ancient China the mandarins paid their doctors to keep them healthy. When they fell ill they stopped payment until they were cured. There is a clear message inherent in this approach for in a holistic sense we are all finally responsible for our mind and body functioning : 'Curing is not as good as preventing, and preventing is not as good as taking care of yourself'.

SPIRITUAL HEALING

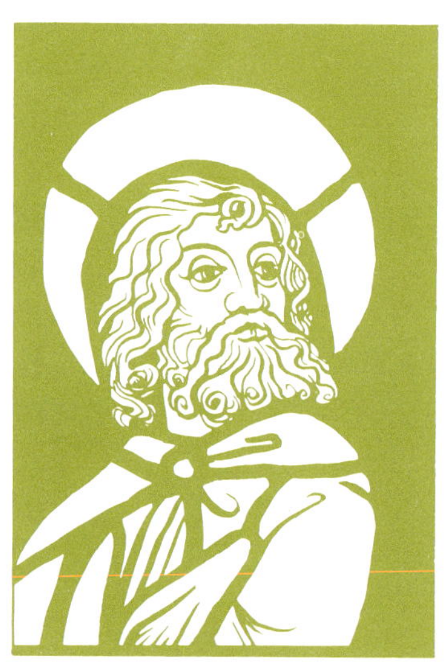

Spiritual or 'faith' healing is an ancient tradition and has embraced many different religions. In modern times it has been associated more with Christianity than any other faith although it has also been practised by certain spiritualist and non-denominational groups.

The essence of faith healing is an appeal to a higher spiritual source – a God or spirit – to participate in healing the sick. Sometimes the God is believed to manifest in a divine presence; on other occasions a healing energy is transmitted through a medium to the patient and the cure effected. Consequently the technique of 'laying on of hands' is a form of spiritual healing.

Appeals to healing gods abound in ancient history and can be found, for example, in the records of Egypt, Mesopotamia and classical Greece.

In Egypt there were famous healing temples at Philae, Karnak, Heliopolis and Memphis, associated with different deities. At Hermopolis, Thoth was believed to give healing remedies. The walls of the sanctuaries contained inscriptions commemorating miraculous cures and statues were erected by grateful patients. The *Leyden Papyrus* shows that the ancient Egyptians believed that the body could be divided into 36 parts and that there was 'no limb without a god'. These gods were invoked to heal specific diseases of the body. The *Ebers Papyrus*, meanwhile, includes an invocation for remedying cataracts of the eyes:

Come verdigris ointment! Come verdigris ointment! Come thou verdant one. Come afflux from the eyes of Horus. Come thou effusion from the eyes of the god Turu! Come ye stuffs, ye who proceed from Osiris! Come to him (the patient) and take from him the water, the pus, the blood, the pain in the eye, the chemosis, the blindness, the flow of matter, which are worked there by the god of inflammations . . .

The Assyrian Library of Assurbanipal included similar invocations as a remedy for diseases caused by demon-possession:

By Heaven be ye exorcised! By Earth be ye exorcised! . . . Depart, Namtar, black demon! I am the beloved of Bel, depart from me . . .

In Babylonia, the water deity Ea was the supreme healing god and appeals were made to him through prayers, hymns and incantations. The priests of Ea dressed in robes resembling fish-skins to symbolise their deity and sprinkled water from a sacred stream over the body of the sufferer.

Spiritual healing was also practised in ancient Greece. While the intervention of the gods could cause disease and death for the unfaithful or unjust, deities could also be called upon in prayer or through rituals or hymns of praise to bestow their healing gifts. They would manifest through divine visions, mediumism or the laying on of hands. In Greece, as with many contemporary alternative healing therapies, the right hand was considered to be the source of positive power, the left negative. Suidas reports that Asklepios healed the writer Theopompos with a laying on of hands and the event was depicted in Attic relief – an interesting circumstance since Asklepios was originally an earthbound hero from Thessaly who was later 'placed among the stars' by Zeus. Healing sanctuaries sacred to Asklepios were established at such locations as Athens, Epidaurus, Kos, Kleiton and Aigion and in due course he became the main healing divinity of the ancient Greeks.

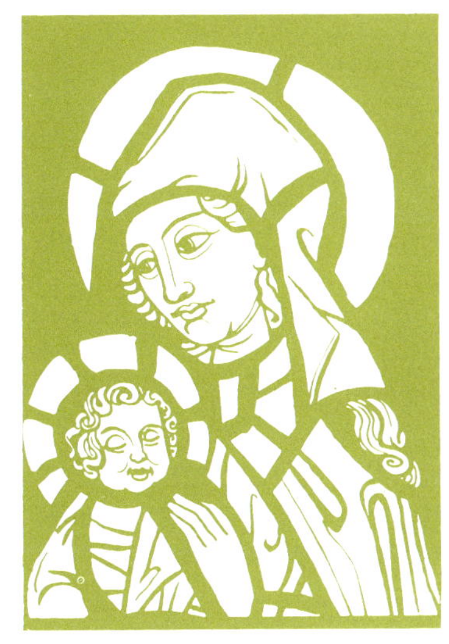

Christianity also has a strong healing tradition and has its very foundations in Jesus' spiritual powers. During his lifetime around forty healing miracles were recorded. In the Middle Ages the Church encouraged recognition of the shrines of saints and claimed that their relics could transmit a healing power. More recently Lourdes in France has become established as a sacred healing site as a result of a series of visions experienced by a young shepherdess, Bernadette Soubirous. In 1858 Bernadette, who suffered from asthma, claimed to have 18 visions of the Virgin Mary and was instructed to bathe in a spring near the River Gave. Later she became a nun. Bernadette's asthma continued to recur and she also suffered from rheumatism and a tumour. Notwithstanding that she died prematurely at the age of 35, Lourdes began to acquire a mystical healing aura and the Roman Catholic Church established the Bureau des Constatations Medicales to authenticate miracles said to occur there. One of these concerned Francis Pascal of Beaucaire, who was apparently cured of total blindness and paralysis in the arms and legs caused by meningitis. A report to the Bureau by twelve doctors stated

There can be no doubt concerning the reality of the illness. It was an infection involving the meninges, nervous system and optic nerve, associated with papilloedema, flaccid paralysis of the lower limbs and incoordination of the upper limbs. Symptoms of cerebellar disorder were also present. Symptoms cleared up suddenly when the progress of the disease gave no reason to hope for improvement . . . No medical explanation appears possible.

The Christian Church in general has encouraged the healing aspects of ministry although this does not always extend to laying on of hands. In 1936 the noted Methodist psychologist Dr Leslie Weatherhead opened a clinic in London to treat psychosomatic illness and neurosis through 'Christian love and good will', and a similar healing function is achieved through special Masses held weekly at St Joseph's Church in Woollahra, Sydney. Originated by Father Luke, the services include laying on of hands and have reportedly resulted in the healing of such ailments as migraine, backache, arthritis, asthma and blindness. Father Luke concedes that psychosomatic factors could be involved. 'There seems to be a connection between bitter, resentful feelings and arthritis', he says, 'and we know hatred can be a cause of cancer'.

In 1975 the former Congregational minister Dr Mario Schoenmaker founded the Church of the Mystic Christ in Perth and began to conduct spiritual healing services. He had acquired 'psychic gifts' after meditating on the cause of suffering, following his mother's death. Reverend Schoenmaker

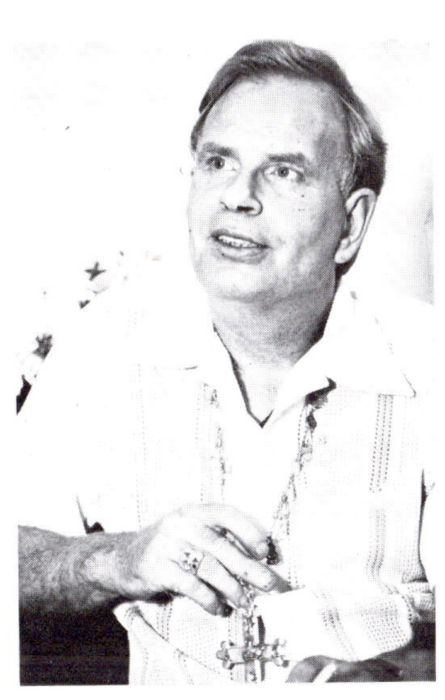

Dr Mario Schoenmaker

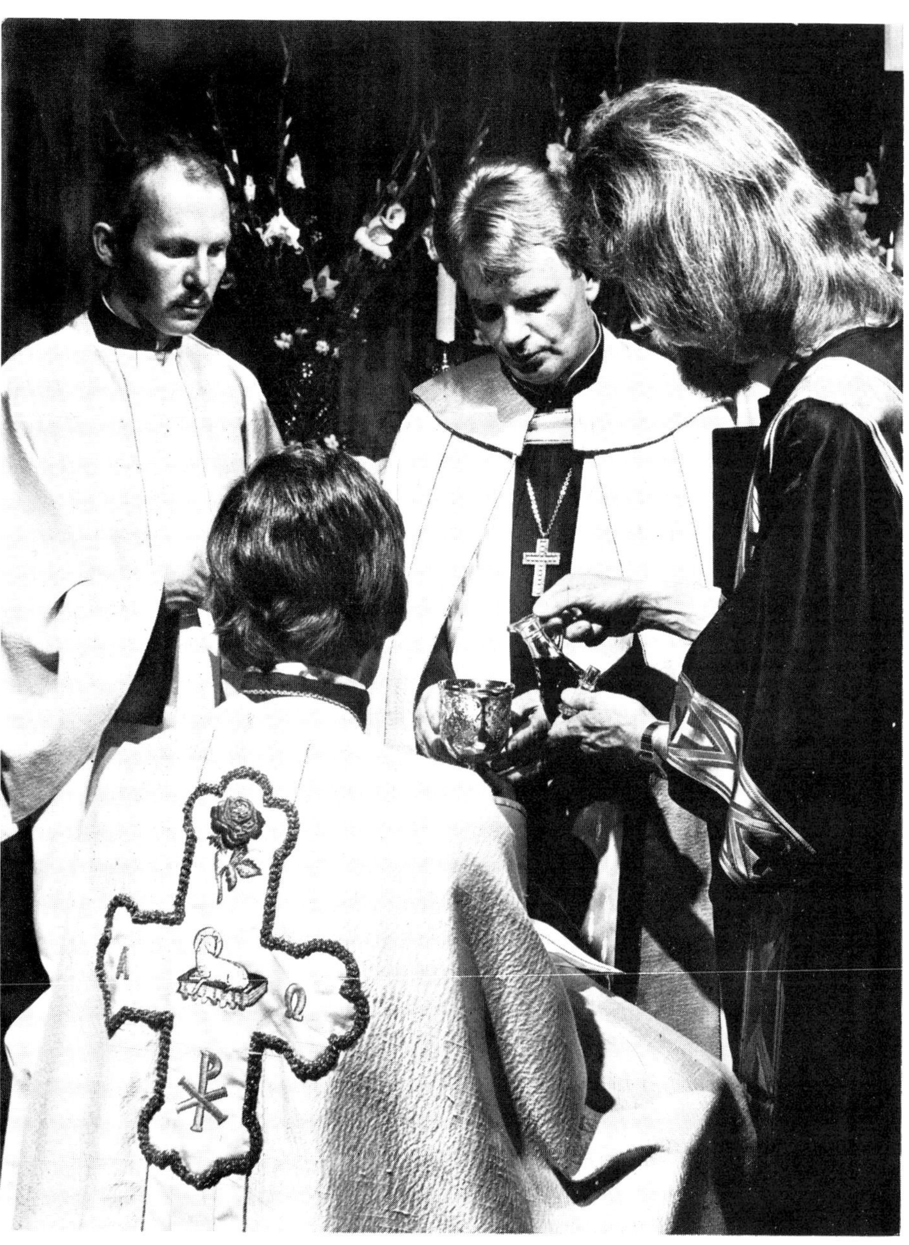

Dr Schoenmaker conducting a healing service

began to practise as a spiritual counsellor, analysing aura readings relating to the subject's state of health and energy. He also 'reads' the vibrations given off by an object habitually worn by the person — thus linking his spiritual healing techniques with psychometry. Reverend Schoenmaker emphasises the strengths and weaknesses of the personality as a major factor in regaining health.

In Britain there has also been a tradition of spiritual healing outside the Church.

Between 1662 and 1667 Valentine Greatrakes, an English magistrate living in Ireland, acquired a reputation for healing patients by gently stroking their limbs 'in order to squeeze the illness out of them'. Greatrakes impressed diarist John Evelyn and the noted chemist Robert Boyle and claimed his powers came from God. He did not earn the acknowledgment of the Church, however, and gave up the practice after he felt his powers were waning.

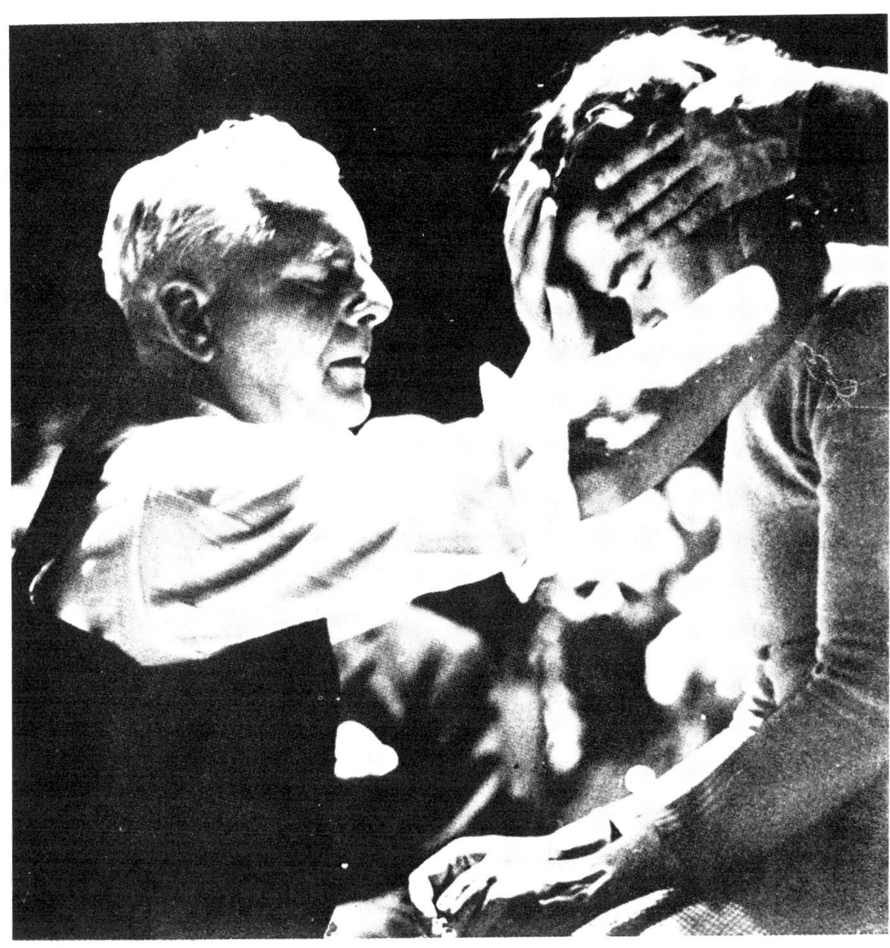

Spiritual healer Harry Edwards

More recently the faith healer Harry Edwards acquired an international reputation for 'miraculous' cures using medium controls – among them the 'spirits' of Pasteur, Lord Lister and a number of Red Indians. Edwards, who died in 1976, claimed that his healing gift first showed itself in Persia during World War One, when he healed a woman who had been bitten by a scorpion by spontaneously laying on of hands.

Edwards established his Spiritual Healing Sanctuary at Shere in Surrey and consulted many leading politicians, public figures and members of the Royal Family.

What is to be made of faith healing? Are the claims genuine or is the whole domain of spiritual care simply a delusion fostered by religious enthusiasm?

Edward Barker, a psychotherapist and author who was formerly a Methodist minister, believes that miracles and faith healing are simply psychosomatic cures. In an illuminating book titled *The Church's Neurosis and Twentieth Century Revelation* he writes:

In an age when modern medical practice was unknown, Jesus penetrated to the emotional quandaries of the individuals who sought healing and it was as he diagnosed their emotional distresses and subterfuges that he was able to bring healing to their bodies.

Barker goes on to cite the example of the healing of a deaf man, described in the Gospels of Mark, Matthew and Luke. Mark's account – the earliest

– suggests that the man suffered from deafness associated with aphasia and disturbed emotions. Jesus took the man away from the busy crowd to talk with him more privately. 'It was only when Jesus had diagnosed the man's troubled mind', writes Barker, 'that he implemented measures to suggest healing'. It is interesting that the later accounts in the other gospels embellish the incident and suggest that the man was suffering from demon possession – making the healing miracle seem more dramatic than it perhaps deserved to be.

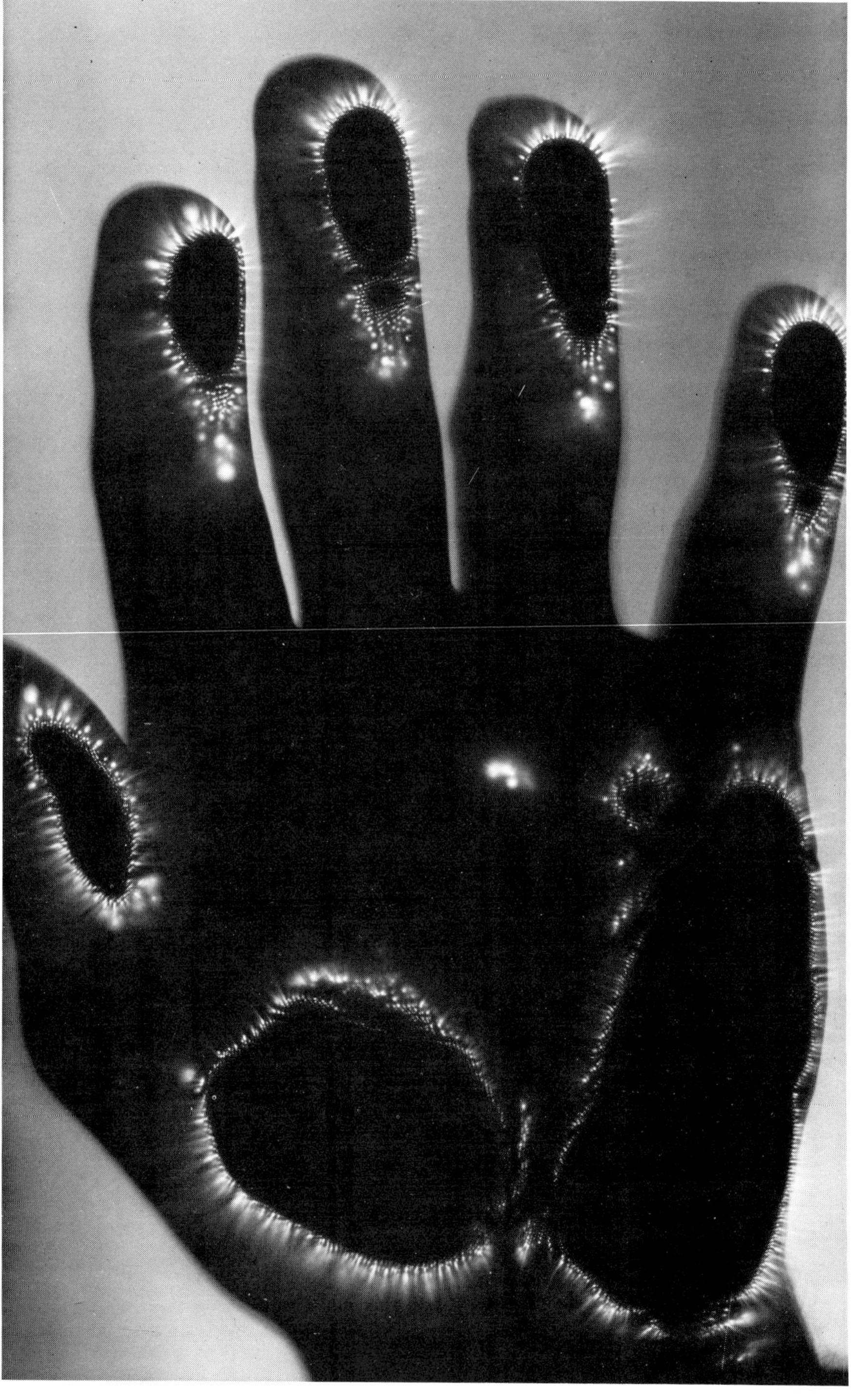

Kirlian photograph by Graydon Rixon: the hands of a healer

Psychological tests and surveys of the faith healing phenomenon have produced mixed results. Dr Louis Rose, a clinical psychiatrist, investigated faith healing over a 15-year period and summarised 96 cases in *The Journal of the Society for Psychic Research*. Part of the trouble lay in identifying the ailment the patient claimed to be suffering from, quite aside from any question of cure. In 58 cases, no medical records could be obtained and 22 had contradictory records and claims. In only one instance was 'demonstrable organic disability' relieved or cured by a faith healer alone. In five other cases involving substantial improvement, subjects were treated by both faith healers and doctors.

Somewhat unusual experiments aimed at testing laying on of hands (LH) have been conducted by Professor Bernard Grad of the Department of Psychiatry at McGill University, Montreal. The tests did not involve human subjects but mice! A noted healer was asked to place his hands on mice located in the compartments of a galvanised iron box for 15 minutes twice daily for six weeks – under experimental test conditions.

In one test with two control groups, the mice were subjected to a deficiency of iodine resulting in the induced enlargement of the thyroid gland. Grad found that the LH group did not register the iodine deficiency to the same extent as the control group mice. In another experiment designed to test the healing of a wound, there were three separate groups of mice: a control group, the LH mice and a group given electrothermal heat treatment.

Each animal was put to sleep temporarily and a coin-size section of skin removed from the back. The wound area in each case was traced and recorded. After 14 days it was clear that the LH mice were healing faster than the other groups.

Professor Grad believes that laying on of hands works by a transfer of energy from healer to patient. He notes that some healers claim to be able to diagnose sickness in patients by their resistance to the flow of energy from the healer's hands. The idea of energy transfer is often referred to in holistic healing and practitioners of acupressure, deep massage, polarity balancing and reflexology, often report the same sensations. It would seem that faith healing probably draws on similar energy resources and involves a re-balancing of the energy fields of the patient through the active involvement of the healer.

DIANA CRAIG

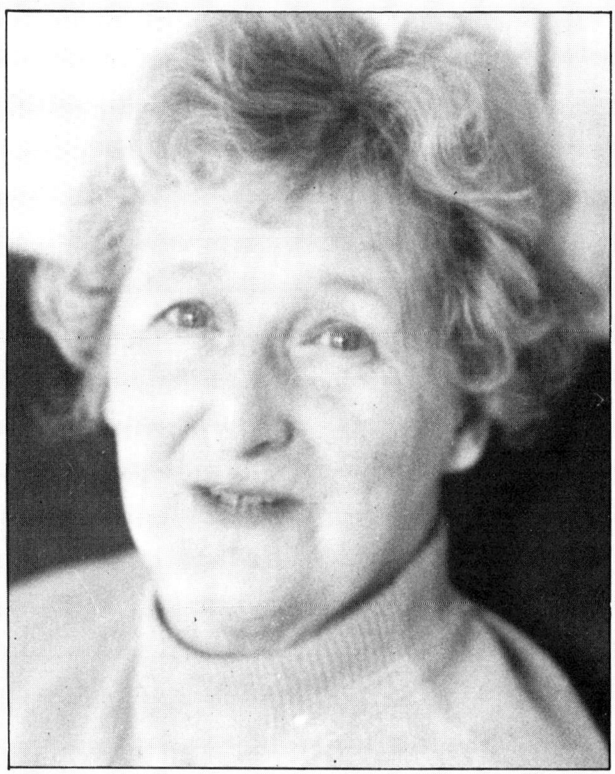

Ask Diana Craig about spiritual healing and she offers a simple recipe – 'a little sprinkle of healing, a little sprinkle of love and there you are'. A typically warm and human answer from a woman who radiates love, humour and vitality. Elected the first woman President of the National Federation of Spiritual Healers in 1979, she is herself a highly successful healer and in her sixties lives a full and intensely active life that would do credit to someone twenty years younger.

How did her healing work begin? She says that she always had the desire to help people. 'If I was washing up or doing something in the house and someone in trouble rang up, I would drop everything and go and help them. I used to adopt "lame ducks".' When she was in her thirties she worked with her husband's film company but she felt that this wasn't what she was meant to be doing. 'I felt lost, I was looking for something.'

Across the road from where she lived at the time, at St. Margarets, near Richmond, there was a healing sanctuary called St Francis of Assisi. Her interest in it led her to read the life of St Francis. 'That had the most enormous impact on my life,' she says, 'I loved the way he healed lepers, the way he lived in poverty, wanting nothing for himself'. At the sanctuary, where she became a probationer, a medium told her she was a born healer and that one day she would have all the gifts.

She recalls the time when she decided to try for herself. It was when she was taking her dogs for a walk in Richmond Park. A dull day, and as she walked along she prayed out aloud for someone in deep trouble. She said 'Oh Father, help this one' – and flung out her hand as she spoke. She describes the feeling she had at that moment. It was as if a burning sun came into her hand. In fact, she says, I looked up thinking the sun had come out, but there was only rain and cloud. She believed that she would become a healer when she felt the same power in the other hand as well. There was further training at the College of Psychic Studies in London, where Paul Beard, its Head, was a major influence in her life and work and she conducted healing classes and ran her own healing sanctuary.

For Diana Craig, a sanctuary is a room, however big or small, where nothing takes place except spiritual healing. It is somewhere where people in trouble, people in pain and sorrow can come into quietness. 'In a sanctuary, a room that is kept solely for peaceful projects, you can feel the power that builds up, the atmosphere. People would come in and say "What a beautiful feeling in here".' What of healing itself, is there a way to define it? 'For me,' she says, 'it is an attunement between myself, the person I am working with and a "higher source of supply". It is completely founded on love, a combination of human and spiritual love. It flows through you.'

Among all her activities, one that has given her great satisfaction is the work she has done helping to build the spiritual healing movement in Germany, where she has been lecturing and healing since 1975.

In 1979 she took part in a German television programme, together with Tom Johanson, secretary of the Spiritualist Association of Great Britain. This resulted in 1500 requests by letter in one week for healing and a studio switchboard jammed with enquiries. On another occasion, at a healing conference held at a German Roman Catholic monastery, a monk told her afterwards, 'We have many conferences here and after them we feel spiritually drained, but you not only brought your own light, you have added to ours'.

Much of her time is taken up with her work as President of the National Federation of Spiritual Healers which advances the work of the various healing organisations that have grown up spontaneously in various parts of Britain. Since 1965, under an agreement with more than 1500 National Health Service hospitals, Federation members may attend patients in hospitals who request the services of a healer. An important development took place in 1977 when the General Medical Council agreed to allow doctors to recommend spiritual healing to their patients. Diana Craig is a firm advocate of cooperation between doctors and healers. In the early days, she explains, there was conflict between doctors and ourselves because they thought we wanted to interfere and make claims about healing people. Now they are coming to trust us. She looks forward in the future to an intermingling of therapies when healers will be approached to act in conjunction with doctors. Her down to earth manner, her enthusiasm and her warmth are likely to bring that day nearer.

JOSEPH MARTIN

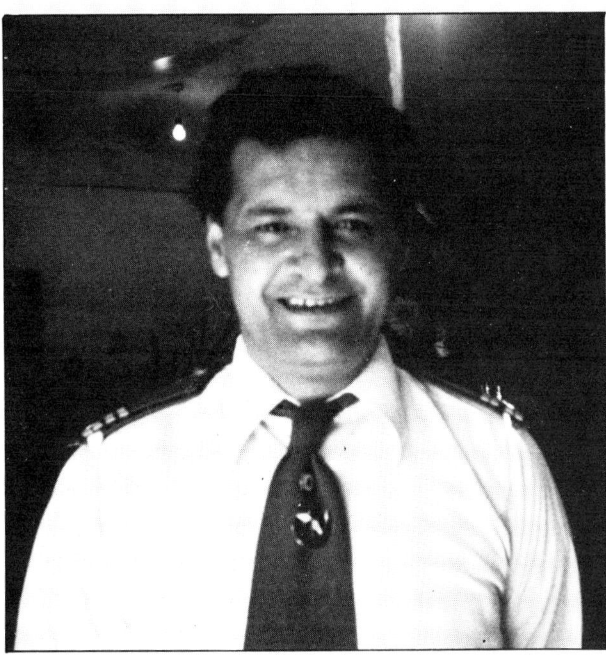

Throughout the western world, there is a swing toward spiritualism, very often combined with religion and spiritual healing. Generally, we associate this with white people of British or European descent, although the spirit guides of mediums are often of other races.

It is rare to find an ethnic group which combines parts of the culture and religion of the white races, together with their own rich traditions. Where this does happen, it tends to be divisive: the rituals can be understood only by the initiates.

A movement was started about six years ago, and led by a young Maori man steeped in the traditions of his people, a young man who, at an early age, had been separated from his peers, partly by his own tendencies and partly by decree of the elders of his Taranakei tribe who observed this unusual child and decided to teach and drill him in the arts of the *tohunga* (priest) and many other facets of an old culture.

Joseph Martin is seen by his followers as a healer and their spiritual leader. They call themselves Maramatanga (Children of the Light), and follow a philosophy based on peace and love and healing. The ritual is a fascinating combination of Roman Catholicism, Ratana, western spiritualism, and Maoritanga, including great reverence for the ancestors. Elements of other Christian faiths are also included. Maramatanga reject no beliefs, and demand none other than peace and love. The headquarters in a house in Otahuhu, Auckland, is filled with the symbols of many faiths.

Central to the several hundred strong group is the belief in spiritual healing. Unlike many who call themselves healers, Maramatanga healers undergo rigid training in the practice and control of the art. None is permitted to work alone until he or she has served a rigorous seven year apprenticeship, working only in supervised groups. Joseph is adamant that this is necessary, that it takes those years for a person to learn to use and control the power without 'making mischief'. (Also, perhaps, because seven years was the length of time during which, he says, he was visited and trained by the spirits of the ancestors.) He is as severe with his students as the ancestors were with him.

Joseph believes strongly that people are not healed by healers; they heal themselves. The healer is merely a channel, bringing extra energy to help a sick person to make him or herself well. 'At first I thought I was God, waving my arms around. I thought, "This is great!". But I soon got slapped down.' He laughs. This is one of the many things he teaches the students – that healers do no more than open themselves to direct the power to where it is needed. They do not create it; it comes from a kind of universal pool to which every living thing contributes, and from which all have the right to take. Joseph and his healers simply make it easier for the energy to be tapped.

He is adamant that touching is unnecessary for healing to take place, and is suspicious of those who insist on stroking or other forms of touching. He says this is quite unnecessary and can make people feel uncomfortable, which makes them less receptive. He prefers, and says he gets his best results from, absent healing. The concentration is better, there are fewer distractions, and healing can be done at a time when his own energies and abilities are at their peak.

Maramatanga healers are forbidden to try to diagnose illness. 'That is the job of the doctors, and we are not doctors.' Attempts at diagnosis are also seen as dangerous because they leave open the possibility for a healer to try to be clever.

Joseph sees healing as an intensely personal and private thing, not to be played with or exploited. It should be carried out with great humility and sensitivity, and with a constant awareness of the need for discipline and direction, in the knowledge that power has two sides – bad as well as good.

No healer in the movement may take payment for his or her work. It must be done in the spirit of peace and love that are at the heart of Maramatanga.

The Maori race has a long tradition of healing, and Joseph has incorporated his cultural heritage into the more European form of the art. He learnt the European way through association with the Spiritualist Church and through individual healers and mediums.

In addition to the two ancestors, a man and a woman, he says he has three spirit guides: Indian Red Cloud, Chinese Ching and English John, each with his own personality.

The Maori way is very strong in Maramatanga whose members believe that Joseph has been chosen to carry on the work of Ratana, the founder of a church which still flourishes among many of the Maori people. Ratana is said to have prophesied that 'a young man will be born to take over and carry on the work I have started'. Aunty Queenie remembers this. She knew Ratana and was brought up in his faith. She remembers that the prophecy was accepted by her people who spoke of it freely more than forty years ago. She has no doubt that Joseph Martin is the fulfilment of that prophecy.

This was confirmed for her six years ago, when, very sick, she was taken to a healer – Joseph. Luckily, at the time, she did not know he was her nephew (this can happen in Maori families). 'Relations don't know anything. I would never have gone to him if I had known. My uncle was a doctor and I wouldn't go to him. How could he know anything? He was my uncle!' She chuckles at the joke against herself because, in the event, she did get well.

At her healing, the people sang *Kua Whanau nei he Mangai* – Ratana's theme. From that time, she says, she knew. This was confirmed for her when she saw in the sky two stars that Ratana always referred to as Alpha and Omega. Joining the two together, she saw the shape of a pipe – Ratana's pipe. There have been other signs to confirm her belief further.

Aunty Queenie has become Joseph's confidante and guide, helping him to learn to share and to realise that no single person can take all responsibilities or be all things.

Joseph himself is a combination of childlike naivete, a very Maori calm fatalism, steely strength and maturity, and occasional flashes of fun. A part of him stands off and watches himself all the time, scoffing when he does silly things or gets 'too big in the head'. He tells the story of how he joined the army by mistake. He really meant to join the navy, thought he was only enquiring at the army office, but found the papers he had signed committed him to the army. He lasted about five years in his accidental occupation.

Joseph was brought up a Roman Catholic. He was always fascinated by the ritual and the robes of priest and altar boy, so much so that he entered a seminary and began training as a Brother. When it came to taking his final vows, he found he could not. He felt his work was on the outside. But the vow he made then to the Virgin Mary has stayed with him. He promised to keep the three vows of the priesthood: poverty, chastity, and obedience. His attempt at marriage failed dismally. His wife did not stay because she said she could not live with a *tohunga*.

Joseph may be one of the last of the fully initiated *tohunga*. The traditional form is something he will not pass on because, he says, he does not want to give to others the *tohunga* power of revenge and death. His grandfather gave his life so Joseph could fulfill all the initiation requirements. One of these was to kill another human being, using the power of the mind. When the old man was dying, he called Joseph to his side and offered his life so his grandson would not have to take a life that was not yet ready to end. 'We cheated a little, but I believe my grandfather arranged it with the elders'.

Joseph's life is peppered with such incidents, on both the physical and spiritual planes. He has been chosen by his followers as their spiritual leader, teacher, and healer. Although he is still young, in matters of the spirit, he takes precedence over the elders.

All people, of all colours and races are welcome. None is turned away.

And the spirit of *aroha* (love) extends beyond the congregation into welfare and other areas, especially among young people. Joseph's and Aunty Queenie's home has, over the years, been a haven for many young people who need a loving family. It is not a very big house, but they say that even if it were huge it would still be bursting at the seams.

During the six years of its life, Maramatanga has spread to centres on Otara (Auckland), Papakura, Rotorua, Taneatua, Palmerston North, Kakariki (Marton), Wellington, Christchurch, and Reporoa. There is also a group in the Brisbane area. In their search for healing, people have come from as far away as the United States, sometimes setting off with little more than a few clues as to where to find the Maramatanga healers.

TAI CHI CH'UAN

Tai Chi is motion, unity, dance – a surrendering to the natural flow of energy in the universe. The Chinese expression 'Tai Chi' itself approximates to 'supreme ultimate' and has some of the same connotations as Yin/Yang. 'Ch'uan' means a 'fist' or 'boxing' and demonstrates the links between the oriental martial arts like Kung Fu and Karate, and the more contemplative practice of Tai Chi. The latter replaces aggression and hostility with sensitivity and the capacity to yield to an overriding calm.

Tai Chi is a means of exploring the processes of mind and body through creative movement and reflects the view in the *I Ching* that 'Nature is always in motion'. A person learning the basic movements of Tai Chi – which soon become very much an individual expression – begins to experience transformations, inward and outward polarities, and the sense of energy vitalising the body.

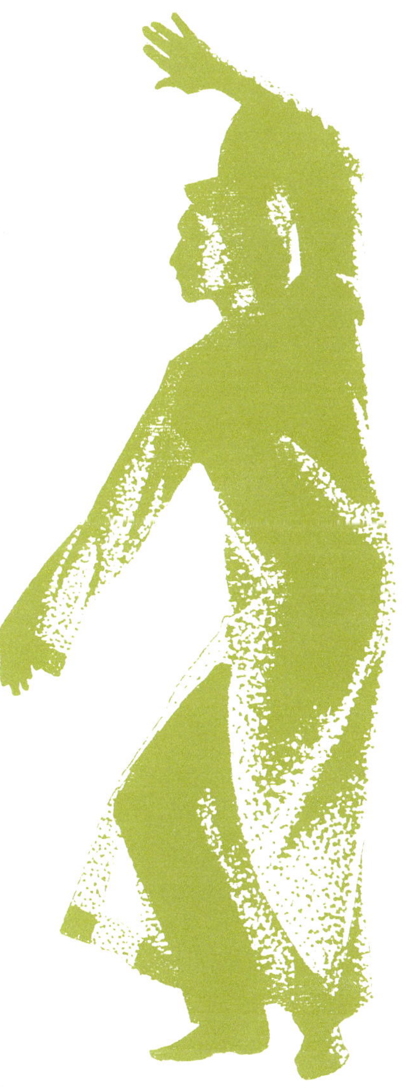

Tai Chi is said to have originated with the meditation of the Taoist monk Chang San-feng. As he looked out of a window he watched a magpie trying to attack a snake. The snake teased the bird and remained always just out of reach, writhing and curling in a spiral motion. Similar movements are now an integral part of Tai Chi.

Several symbols recur in Tai Chi: the image of *water*, to represent the flow of energy and the yielding adaptability of its form within a container; the symbol of *earth* as a 'centering' link between person and planet; and the use of circular forms of expression to show unity, containment and polarity change.

In Tai Chi all movements complement each other. According to Chang San-feng, 'the inner strength is rooted in the feet, developed in the thighs, controlled by the waist and expressed through the fingers'. All movements begin with stillness and manifest a sense of revitalisation while producing a profound feeling of serenity and well-being.

There are various forms of Tai Chi – Yang and Wu for example – but they tend to overlap. Traditionally Tai Chi techniques were passed from master to pupil but today in the West many practitioners conduct Tai Chi workshops on the art of creative self-expression, and the more formal aspects are disappearing.

One of the best known international exponents of Tai Chi is Al Chung Liang Huang, who has taught Tai Chi in many countries including the United States and the Far East. Associated with the Human Potential Movement, he visited Australia to attend the sixth International Transpersonal Con-

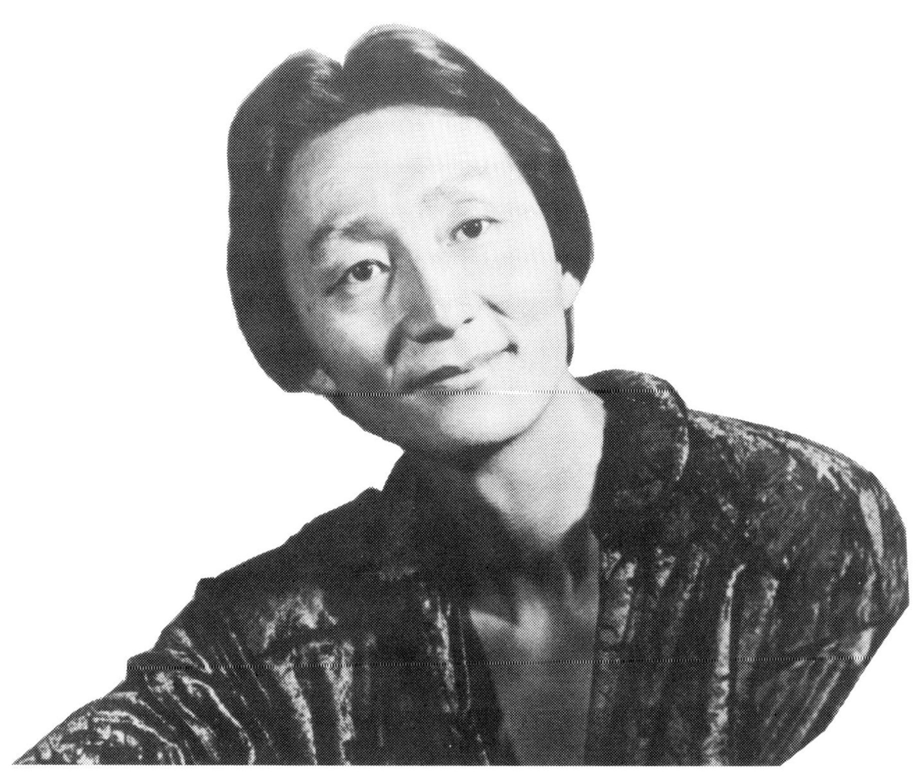

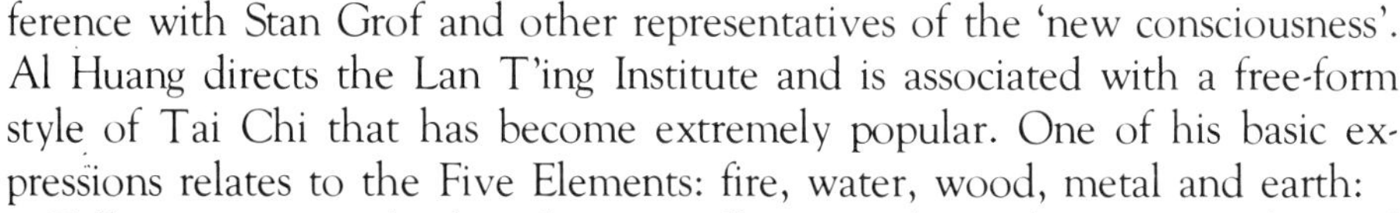

Well known Tai Chi teacher Al Chung Liang Huang

ference with Stan Grof and other representatives of the 'new consciousness'. Al Huang directs the Lan T'ing Institute and is associated with a free-form style of Tai Chi that has become extremely popular. One of his basic expressions relates to the Five Elements: fire, water, wood, metal and earth:

Following a period of meditative stillness we begin by stepping forward on the right foot. This is an energy step and *fire* is visualised shooting from the palms. Then the energy is pulled back into the body and the weight transferred to the left foot: *water* (During the Conference workshop I attended we visualised water cascading over us like a life-giving shower). Turning to the left we let the palms rotate and curve back towards the right. The arms are moved in a sweeping, circular motion to symbolise *wood*. The body continues to turn to the right with both feet fixed: *metal*. Then the left leg is brought around and we return to the centre: *earth*. All energy is focused in the body.

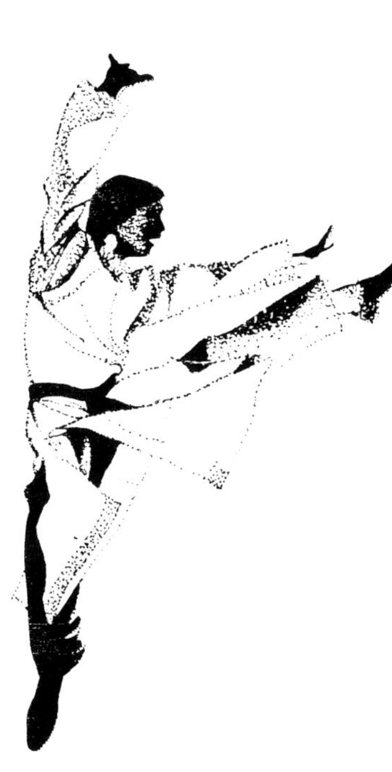

Tai Chi is a form of self-actualisation and in keeping with other holistic philosophies emphasises the inter-relatedness of mind and body and the importance of the natural and unimposed flow of energy. As Al Huang says in his famous book *Embrace Tiger, Return to Mountain*, 'Tai Chi is to help you to get acquainted with your own sense of potential growth, the creative process of just being you'.

Tai Chi is a process of self-discovery and like Yoga demonstrates the link between body movement and posture, and contemplative states of being. It has been said that 'Tai Chi seeks serenity in activity' and this captures the essential paradox. We live in both the inner and outer worlds – the inner domain of thought and reflection, the outer one of force and action. Tai Chi shows us how we can blend these worlds together and express a sense of unity and fulfilment.

NANCY TREHARNE

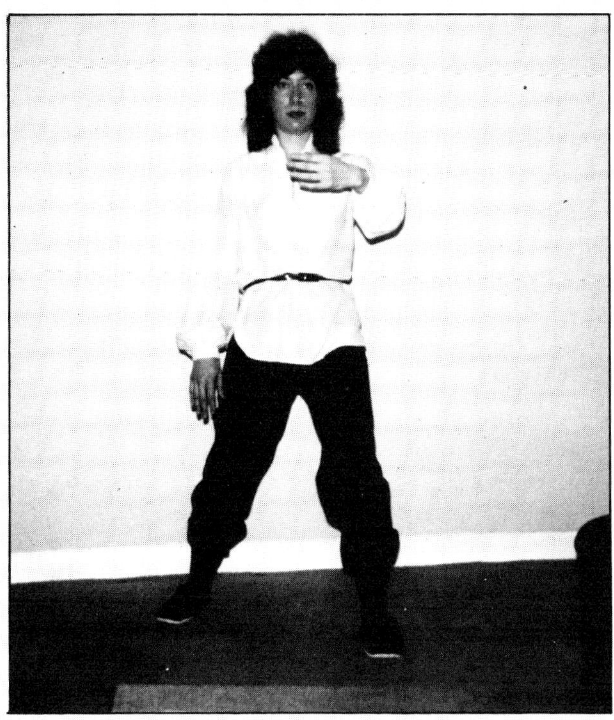

A woman member of the British House of Lords once told Nancy Treharne that just watching her demonstrate T'ai Chi made her feel relaxed. This slim young American from Massachusetts, who looks six or seven years younger than her thirty years, has that sort of effect on people. As you watch the grace and gentleness of her flowing movements you might be witnessing a classical ballet performed in slow motion. You begin to understand why this ancient Chinese exercise becomes for its devotees a way of life.

Nancy Treharne first saw it demonstrated by a group of students in New York. 'I was captivated by its beauty and the calm of the performers, each moving in response to their own inner rhythm.' She was working at the time with the Arica Institute, founded by Oscar Ichazo, the first function of whose training is go get the body in good shape so that the trainee can fully experience 'all higher levels of consciousness'. Nancy had become interested in the writings of Lao Tze, the founder of Taoism. She warmed to his philosophy and wondered how best to realise it in her own life.

T'ai Chi proved to be the answer for her. She studied with an instructor who had trained with the renowned teacher, Professor Cheng Man-Ch'ing, a Master of the 'Chinese five excellencies'. She then trained to become a T'ai Chi teacher. 'It was not long', she says, 'before it became the core of my approach to health and remains my philosophy of life'.

Nancy Treharne, who now lives in England, works with the London School of T'ai Chi Chuan. Together with her colleague and fellow teacher, Richard Royds, she teaches the Yang Family Style Short Form of T'ai Chi as modified by Professor Cheng, taking course in various parts of London.

The Beginning Form is a thirty-hour course which teaches the entire sequence of the 37 movements and the basic principles of T'ai Chi. 'It's rather like learning a dance', she explains, 'you have to memorise a sequence of movements and once you have mastered them they stay with you'. She teaches every type of person and every age. 'T'ai Chi', she says, 'is suitable for absolutely anybody, and for those who for reasons of health or age cannot take part in active sport or vigorous exercise it is the ideal activity. T'ai Chi helps you to grow spiritually. You acquire an increased awareness of yourself. You discover how your mind and body can work together to produce effortless movement'. For many it has an effect that is positively dramatic – for the first time 'their body comes to life'. The movements of T'ai Chi, she explains, help the chi (life-energy) to flow through the body uninterrupted by stress or strain. She suggests to her trainees that they practise the exercises each morning and evening for between five and ten minutes. Many of those who come to her for instruction have already become interested in disciplines such as Yoga and Meditation and find they can turn fairly easily to T'ai Chi.

Among her pupils some suffer from poor circulation, arthritis or varicose veins and find they benefit from the exercises. She tells of one young man who came for instruction on crutches, suffering from atrophy of his limbs. He began receiving instruction and within a year was able to walk unaided. She finds that people with chronic back tension and stiffness in their knees are helped. Surprisingly, perhaps, because the movements of T'ai Chi epitomise gentleness and passivity, it helps in self-defence. Nancy explains that if your mind is still and mind and body working in coordination, a state T'ai Chi produces, you can produce the most appropriate response faced with sudden attack.

She tells of a young woman who had only had a few lessons in T'ai Chi. She was in Central Park, New York when a man walked up to her apparently determined to steal her purse. She took up the T'ai Chi position of 'the push', with her elbows and shoulders relaxed her hands out, palms facing her would-be assailant. 'The push' involves no physical force or strength, it is merely a position of relaxation, and the relaxed body is a conductor of chi. The man collided with her hands, she stayed erect and he fell back so stunned by her response that he fled.

Nancy points out that T'ai Chi teaches that you don't need to meet force with force. By offering no resistance you change the nature of the situation to a non-aggressive one. That attitude can be used in many other areas of life. Nancy emphasises the simplicity of the exercises. She has learned from them that 'by small means much can be accomplished'. The benefits vastly outweigh the efforts expended.

TONING

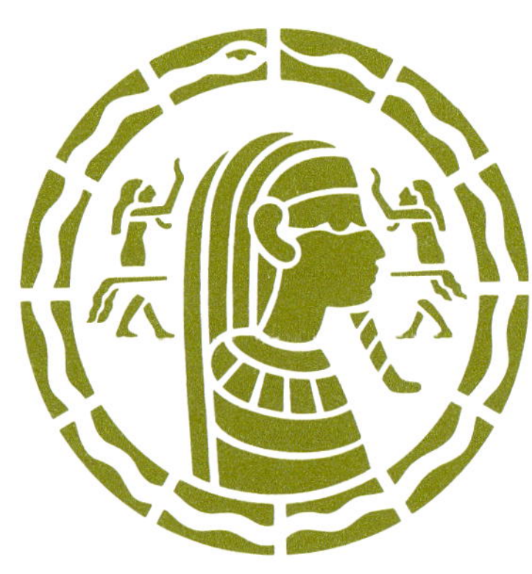

'In the Beginning was the Word . . . ' Many world religions have expressed the idea that sound is the very basis of the mystery of creation and the origin and renewal of the world. Philo, when speaking of the God-energy or *Logos*, said: 'His image is the Word, a form more brilliant than fire . . . ' The ancient Egyptians similarly believed in the power of the mystical utterance. The Egyptian Books of the Dead known as the *Am Tuat* and *The Book of Gates* describe the passage of the sun god through the underworld and relate how through words of power – *hekau* – this god of life was able to bring light into the realms of darkness and herald forth the new day.

The concept of Toning is somewhat similar. Elyse Betz Coulson has written: 'There operates within the body vehicle a musical scale, and when it is allowed to "sing" forth in total freedom, then we are attuned to "the music of the spheres" . . . that vibrational movement of our own creation'.

Probably the leading exponent of Toning is the American healer Laurel Elizabeth Keyes, who has been exploring the integrative powers of sound since the 1960s. A student of comparative religion and philosophy she has conducted several spiritual retreats for different religious groups and is well known as a lecturer on transpersonal subjects. She is a Director of the 'Restorium', a chapel and retreat in the mountains near Denver, Colorado, and has also founded a non-profit group known as the Order of Fransisters and Brothers to study the effects of meditation, Toning and chanting.

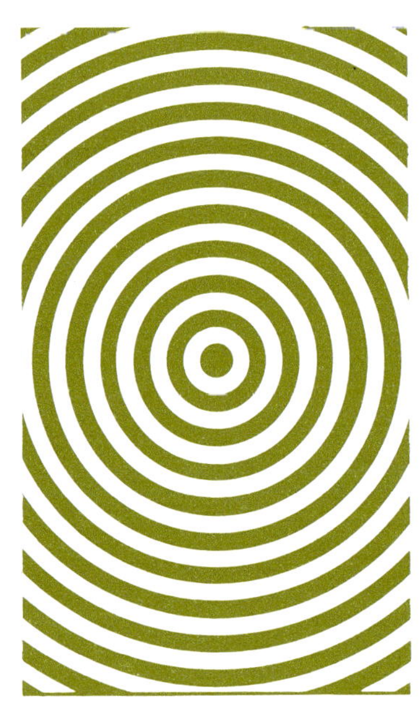

Laurel Keyes has conducted a meditative study group for some years. It was after one of these meetings that the techniques of Toning came to her:

I was standing alone in the room, enjoying the stillness and the charged atmosphere which remains after such a meeting. I noticed a sensation in my chest and throat as though a force were rising, wanting to be released in sound . . .

I found my lips parting and my mouth opened very slightly in an easy relaxed manner so that the teeth were just barely parted. Unexpectedly, a sound bubbled up, like something tossed up on a fountain spray. A single syllable emerged: 'Ra'.

Laurel Keyes was surprised by this since she did not use Egyptian terms in her study group. She has emphasised that she did not feel the voice to be extraneous manifesting through her body like a trance medium. Rather the sound seemed to well up from her body itself.

Since that experience, Laurel Keys has developed Toning as a means of activating the creative energy which she feels lies dormant in everyone, awaiting release. It is almost as if creativity is naturally rebellious, waiting to be freed from the inhibitions of our patterned behaviour.

Laurel Keyes asked a psychic friend to watch her while she Toned. The latter reported a swirling force rising from the reproductive organs and solar plexus, then attracting magnetic currents from the earth through the feet and limbs before rising in a spiral of light to the throat. This process produced a wonderful sense of balance and well-being in the body.

Laurel Keyes has since come to believe that Toning is a way of letting the body speak. The body is satisfied when it manifests the perfect tone, 'the jewel which it offers in reverence to Life'. There are vibrationary notes also which resonate with pain and relieve tension – Toning is a means of bringing new life energy to inhibited or unbalanced parts of the body in an act of 'inner sonar message'.

Toning may be performed in conjunction with meditation. When a person wishes to Tone for himself, he should stand erect with the feet apart and shoulders evenly aligned, the eyes closed and the body swaying slightly from side to side, inviting the life rhythms to manifest. The tone comes up from the earth through the feet, rather than emanating from the mind. Initially, according to Laurel Keyes, it doesn't hurt for the person to instinctively groan a little . . . this is a clearing process which releases tensions. Gradually the voice will rise, and there is an accompanying feeling of release. The voice is toned low from the earth, but gradually rises in exultation to the sky. As Laurel Keyes says: 'Let the body be free, let the voice be free, let health emerge'. Her research has shown that the natural range for Toning is from A to A, above and below Middle C. Toning blends naturally with meditation and slow, rhythmic breathing. After one has Toned, which is recommended as a daily practice, it is preferable to sit down in a chair, with the back straight and the head erect. One should close the eyes and breathe slowly, visualising a pure white light pouring in through the head. The light descends, moving down the spine and out through the nerve channels: 'Inhale the light . . . with each breath feel the light flooding in, filling the body. With each breath you exhale visualise this changed to a cool, violet, cleansing light . . . make a soft humming sound and feel cleansed, healed and filled with peace'.

Laurel Keyes has treated many patients with Toning over the years and claims to have produced various healing effects through her techniques. These include diminishing the effects of multiple sclerosis, relieving migraines and curing skin cancers. When she went to the Menninger Institute for research tests conducted by Dr Elmer and Alyce Green – the famous exponents of biofeedback – she found that Toning produces an Alpha brain-wave pattern almost immediately. She also produced Theta with her deep meditation. Laurel Keyes believes Toning works because it releases tensions, pressures and blockages and in that sense is a purely natural therapy with obvious beneficial effects . . . For her, Toning is a means of re-establishing the links between the body and its intrinsic life patterns. As she has said, 'Once you feel energetic and alive, you *are!*' The positive power of thought is linked to the positive power of sound and the energy which wells up from the solar plexus activates a renewed sense of harmony and well-being.

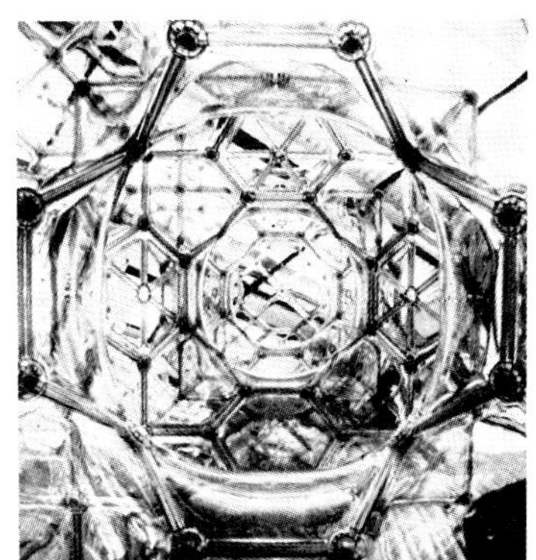

The geometry of music . . .

JULIE CHENERY

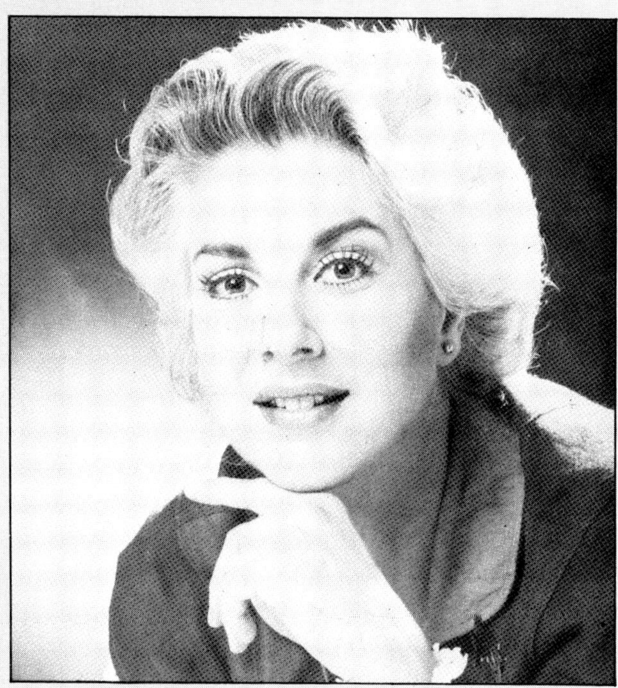

It seems natural that healers should be drawn to modes of expression which reflect their inherent talents and intuitive inclinations. Julie Chenery developed a career initially as a singer in such diverse styles as opera and cabaret and later moved towards a form of therapy which depended on the healing qualities of the voice. Today she is possibly the only person in Australia who is practising what has come to be known as Toning, a healing technique which uses harmonics to rectify imbalances in the human organism.

Born in Sydney and raised in a musical family, Julie Chenery developed an active interest in choral work while still at school. Later she took singing lessons and began acting in Gilbert and Sullivan productions. She had been discouraged by her school teachers from focusing on music when there were more 'useful' pursuits, but proved them wrong by winning an opera scholarship to the NSW Conservatorium of Music in 1967. For several years after her period of training she performed in opera, musicals and in cabaret, working for the Australian Opera, J. C. Williamson and The Australian Theatre Trust. She was soon receiving widespread recognition, and yet she still felt that in some respects she was not fulfilling aspects of her own inner potential.

In 1975, she recalls, a friend invited her to participate in a group meditation and she was surprised by the profound effects it produced in her. It was a peaceful, contemplative feeling and she warmed to it immediately.

After this introduction to meditation, Julie noticed that her life-style began to change in subtle ways and her range of experiences now seemed more integrated and meaningful. Temporarily she put her career aside — she felt drawn towards a deeper perspective that music and theatre were not providing. In 1976 she began studying herbalism with Dorothy Hall and the following year she let theatre and music slip into abeyance; the demands of touring interfered with her studies in Sydney.

Soon afterwards Julie Chenery opened a herbal clinic in Eastwood with a friend, Kim Dudley, who now has a practice in Canberra as a herbalist and acupuncturist. The clinic began to attract a constant flow of patients and Julie also branched out into related areas like aromatherapy and the activation of the chakras, or energy centres, in the human body.

In 1977 during a quiet time of personal meditation she received a communication from an inner voice which advised her to develop the technique of tuning into other people's tonal vibrations. At first she would focus this healing power from a distance, and she says that she knew when she had developed the right tone, or pitch, for a particular person because the note 'expanded' by way of harmonious response.

Today she has developed her range of healing techniques to include not only Toning but also nutritional and iris diagnosis and physical, etheric and magnetic readings.

Julie says she doesn't tone for all her patients but uses the techniques which seem appropriate to the occasion. Sometimes aromatherapy is sufficient; alternatively she might use colour therapy or hold her hands extended on either side of the patient to check the chakras and energy discharge for imbalances.

Julie finds that during Toning the quality of her voice varies according to the nature of the sickness. When patients are very ill, more healing energy seems to come through and the Toning has more intensity.

Recently Julie Chenery visited two healers in the United States who have become well known for Toning: Patricia Sun, who is resident in Berkeley, California, and Laurel Elizabeth Keyes, who is based in Denver, Colorado. Julie found the sharing of techniques to be most valuable and has returned to Sydney anxious to develop her range of approaches still further. She hopes, for example, to link music awareness to methods of creative imagination enhancement and also relate Toning more specifically to the activation of the chakras. There is still a lot of experimentation to do. Lately Julie has been listening to Sufi choir music, and there is also the possibility of working with a flautist on new combinations of voice and woodwind. Quite aside from her consultations at the Eastwood clinic — she sees around twenty people a week — and her time spent at the Village Healing Centre, there are many new avenues to follow. Despite Julie Chenery's many years of healing experience she feels she is still at the beginning. The more she discovers, the more she is aware of what still has to be learned. And Toning is very much a new therapy with frontiers still to explore.

YOGA

Yoga is a technique of self-awareness and to the extent that it integrates mind and body, it has considerable relevance to holistic models of health. The word 'Yoga' itself derives from the Sanskrit *yuj* meaning 'to bind together'. Man learns through Yoga to find union with the universal process of *being*.

The four main concepts underlying Indian spiritual philosophy are *karma*, the law of causality which links man to the universe; *maya*, the illusion of the manifested world; *nirvana*, absolute reality beyond illusion, and *yoga* the means of gaining liberation from the senses.

The basic human dilemmas of suffering, anxiety, stress and so on derive from ignorance of 'spirit'. According to Indian philosophy, man tends to confuse feelings and thoughts with 'spirit' while in fact the realm of human experience belongs to nature *(prakrti)*. A means has to be found for overcoming the limitations of the senses.

Yogis recognise the inter-relatedness of the mind and body. Hatha Yoga teaches techniques of physical control of the body through postures known as *asanas* and breathing techniques *(pranayama)*. The word 'Hatha' itself contains the polarity of opposites. 'Ha' means the sun (masculine) and 'Tha' the moon (feminine). The asanas used in Hatha Yoga make the body supple and enhance the neuro-muscular system. Each posture combines mental acuity with breathing techniques and a specific body movement. Pranayama meanwhile builds up the energy in the body. In the Yogic view, breath brings *prana* as well as oxygen into the body.

Yoga is a means of training to see things as they *are*, rather than as they seem. All bodily and mental tensions must cease if this is to be so. Accordingly one of the basic yogic techniques is meditation since this turns man's consciousness towards the inner calm and finally transcendence in *samadhi* (cosmic or 'pure' consciousness).

A basic meditative pose used in Yoga is *sukhasana*, in which the spine is held straight, the legs are crossed, the eyes are closed and the head is poised above the shoulders. The lungs are free for deep breathing and the meditator is able to focus on the rhythm of his breath while concentrating on *being*.

Although Yoga has existed as a timeless philosophy and practice, it was first formulated systematically by the mystic Patanjali who compiled a series of *sutras*, or sayings. The essence of Yoga is contained in the first four sutras which specify that one must learn to slow the movement of the mind down to a complete halt. One must be free from distraction. The mind *(citta)* is conditioned by past events and contains the contents of man's tensions, pressures, desires, likes and dislikes. The Yogi learns to disengage himself from the world of choice and duality and gradually gains an awareness of total quietitude and freedom.

Yoga is a calming of the waters of the mind. In order for this to be achieved, a number of tensions or obstacles *(klesas)* have to be overcome.

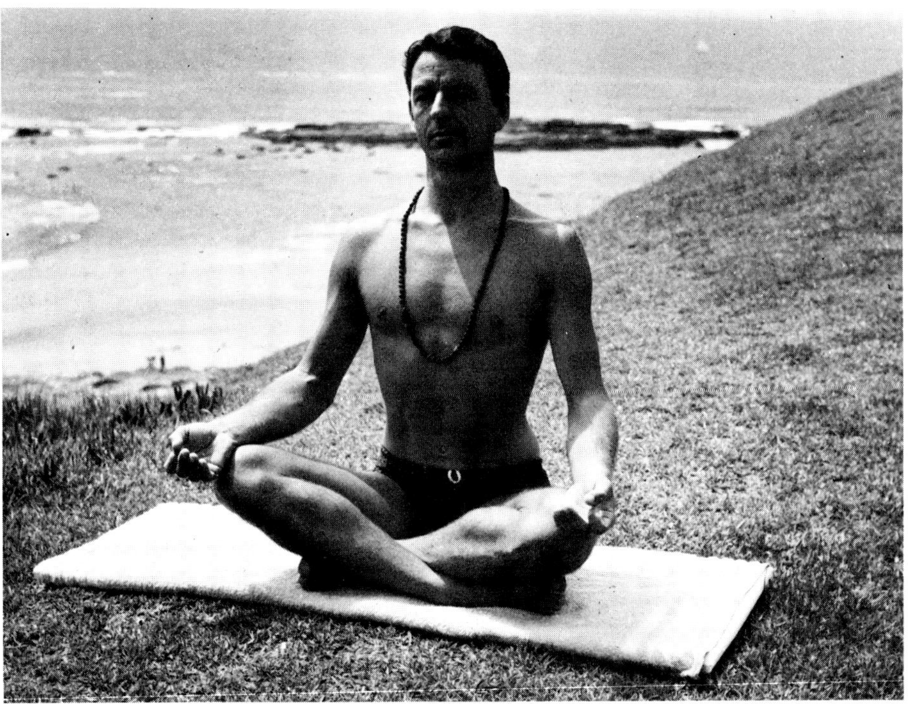

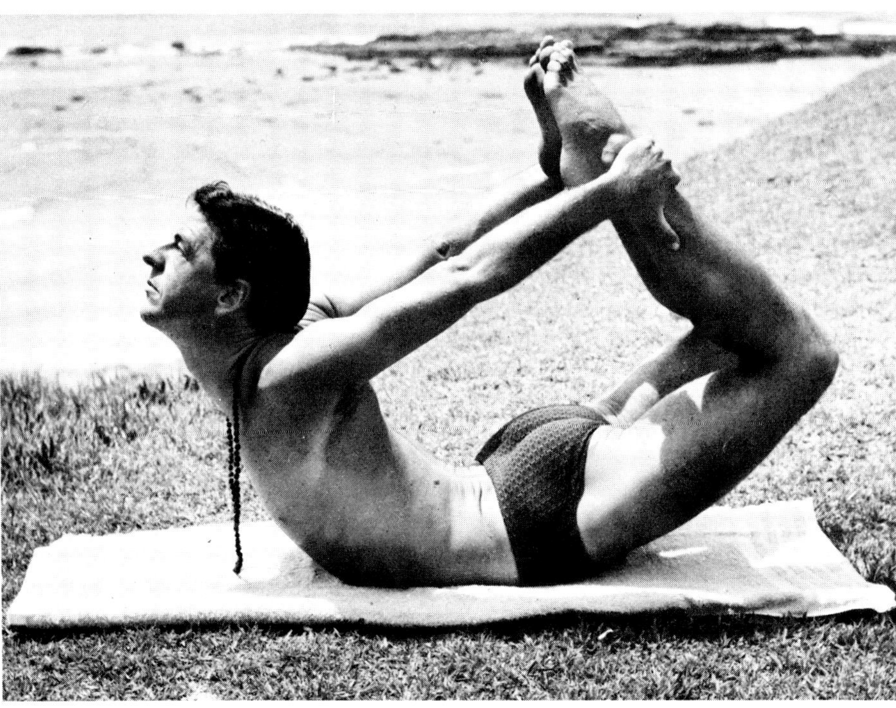

Russell Atkinson demonstrating yogic asanas: the 'easy pose' (above) and 'the bow' (below)

Basically, they are: ignorance, the sense of ego and identification with the body, attention to pleasure, repulsion from pain, and the desire for life. From the Yogic viewpoint, man is trapped in a world clouded by impure perceptions and preconceived ideas. It is this false reality that has to be transcended.

Patanjali emphasises four basic processes:

- withdrawal of attention from the external world *(pratyahara)*
- concentration of energy in a definite direction *(dharana)*
- the subsequent spontaneous flow of consciousness *(dhyana)*
- unity of consciousness *(samadhi)*

In the final attainment the yogi becomes united with the object of meditation and the separateness of self (ego) disappears.

In meditation psychic energy may be raised through the channel *shushumna* which corresponds to the spinal cord, and *ida* and *pingala* which run on the left and right corresponding to the sympathetic nerve ganglion on either side of the spine. Often the yogi raises energy by fixing the concentration on geometric designs called *yantras,* and in the case of Kundalini meditation different geometric symbols are used which represent different psychic energy locations in the body. These centres or *chakras,* are the familiar symbols shown in illustrations positioned on the body of the meditating yogi.

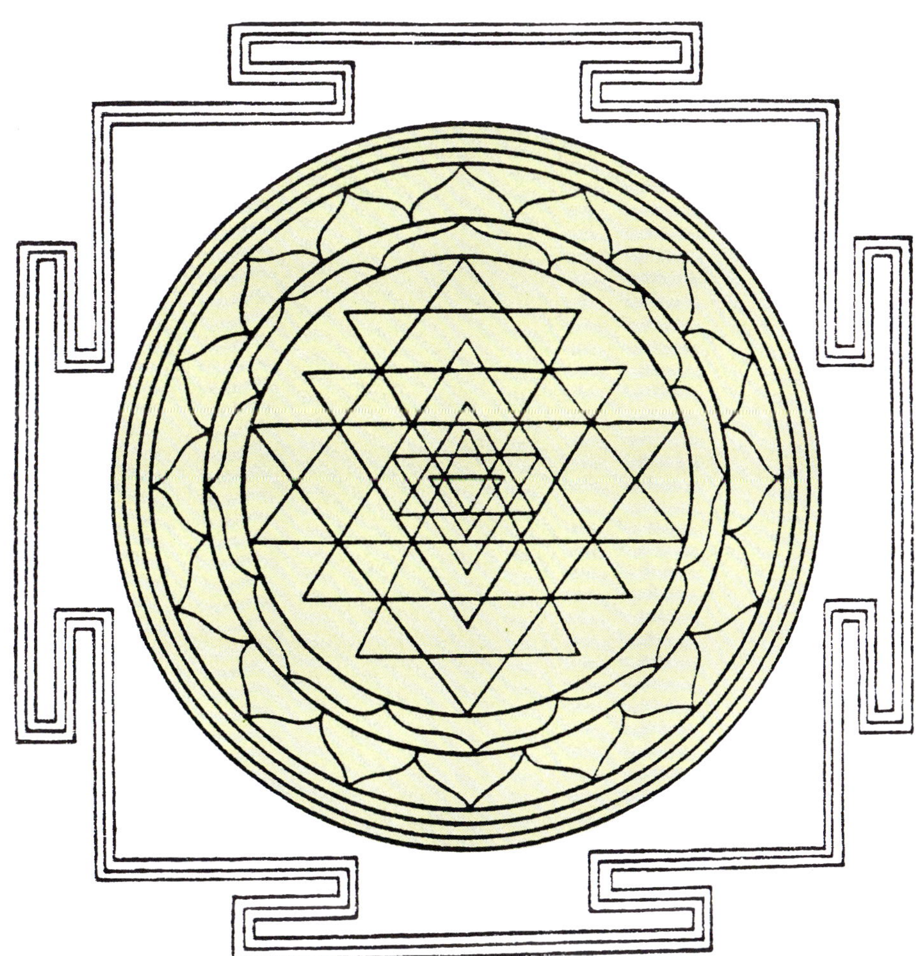

The Kundalini 'serpent energy' is aroused from the base of the spine and passes through the following levels:

Muladhara located near the coccyx
Swadhisthana below the navel in the sacral region
Manipura above the navel in the lumbar region
Anahata near the heart
Vishuddha associated with the cervical region and throat
Ajna located between the eyes
Sahasrara located on the crown of the head and associated with the pineal gland

As the yogi finds unity of mind and body he merges with the object of his perceptions and loses all sense of duality. He is finally illumined with all pervasive cosmic consciousness and is able to perceive the core reality beyond the limitations of the senses.

As the yogic philosopher Haridas Chaudhuri writes in his article *Yoga Psychology:*

On the attainment of this (cosmic) level of consciousness, a person gains enormous power for healing people and making them whole by transmitting the power of illumined and integrated consciousness. The built-in healing power of the psyche reaches the highest point of development on the activation of this centre. It is the revitalising, rejuvenating and inspiring power of perfect unity of wisdom, love and peace . . . it is the alchemy of luminous Being-energy, capable of transforming clay into gold, ordinary men into heroes and saints, as demonstrated in the lives of such great masters as Jesus, Gautama, Lao-Tzu, Ramakrishna, Aurobindo and others . . .

Yoga is *union* – union with the Source of all Being.

APPENDIX: NATURAL HEALTH RESOURCE DIRECTORY

The following is a list of organisations and practitioners dedicated to particular alternative medicine and holistic health practices. It is not possible for this directory to be exhaustive and, hopefully, any notable omissions can be rectified in future editions of this book.

The fact that a practitioner is listed here should in no way be taken as an endorsement of that person's therapeutic practices and readers are asked in all cases to investigate to their own satisfaction the quality of training and personal skills of the practitioners from whom they are intending to seek health care. Aside from chiropractic, osteopathy and acupuncture where regulatory practices apply, many holistic modalities do not have universally accepted standards. However, word of mouth recommendations are often a good sign and it is our view that since the underlying philosophy of the mind/body therapies is towards self-integration, by and large the modalities listed in this directory are safe and worthy of personal investigation as alternative health care systems.

Practitioners who have been interviewed in this book are indicated by an asterisk (*).

When writing to any of the associations or organisations listed below, it is advisable to enclose a stamped addressed envelope if you require a written reply.

ACUPUNCTURE

The British Acupuncture Association and Register, 34 Alderney Street, London, SW1V 4EV, ph. (01) 834 1012, Publishes register of qualified practitioners.
British Medical Acupuncture Society, c/o 21 Aigburth Drive, Sefton Park, Liverpool L17 4JQ, ph. (051) 728 7366, Promotes acupuncture as part of medical practice.
The British College of Acupuncture, 118 Foley Road, Claygate, Surrey, ph. 78 64171, Runs 2-year part-time courses.
College of Traditional Chinese Acupuncture, Queensway, Royal Leamington Spa, Warwickshire CV32 5EZ, ph. 0926 39347, Runs 2½ year full-time courses.

ALEXANDER TECHNIQUE

Society of Teachers of the Alexander Technique, 3 Albert Court, Kensington Gore, London SW7, ph. (01) 589 3834, Maintains register of qualified Alexander teachers.
The School of Alexander Studies, 61a Onslow Gardens, London N10, ph. 883 7659, Runs 3-year full-time course.
The Constructive Teaching Centre, 18 Landsdowne Road, London Wll, ph. (01) 727 7222, Runs 3-year full-time course

AROMATHERAPY

The Guild of Aromatherapy Practitioners, 123 Coombe Lane, London SW20 OQY, ph. (01) 946 4643, Runs diploma courses
Aromatherapy Training Centre, 4 Eltham Road London SE12, ph. (01) 852 7591, Runs 3-day intensive course for physiotherapists, nurses and beauty therapists
Daniele Ryman, Park Lane Hotel, Picadilly London W1, ph. 493 6630, Aromatherapy treatments as practised by Marguerite Maury. Personally formulated oils available by post

ASTROLOGY

Astrological Association, 36 Tweedy Road, Bromley, Kent, ph. (01) 464 3583, Runs conferences, meetings, publishes journal and newsletter
Faculty of Astrological Studies, 37 Sherwood Court, Bryanston Place, London WIH 5FF, ph. (01) 262 7543, Runs correspondence course leading to certificate and diploma examinations. Maintains list of qualified astrologers.
The Mayo School of Astrology, Piper's Wood, Leighton Drive, Beetham, Milnthorpe, Cumbria LA7 7BE. Runs correspondence course.

AUTOGENIC TRAINING

Centre for Autogenic Training, 12 Milford House, 7 Queen Anne Street, London WIM 9FD, ph. (01) 637 1586, Runs courses on group or individual basis

BACH FLOWER REMEDIES

The Edward Bach Centre, Mount Vernon, Sotwell, Wallingford, Oxon. 0X10 OPZ, ph. 0491 39489, Bach flower remedies available from Centre and advice on their use.

BATES METHOD OF EYESIGHT TRAINING

Bates Association of Eyesight Training, 49 Queen Anne Street, London W1, ph. 935 9487, Michael Ronan, Secretary and Bates practitioner, information.

BIOFEEDBACK
Audio Ltd, 26 Wendell Road, London W12, ph. 743 1518, Manufacturers of biofeedback equipment

BIOENERGETICS
Boyesen Institute of Biodynamic Psychology, Acacia House, Centre Avenue, The Vale, Acton Park, London, W3 7JX, ph. (01) 743 2437, Run short and intensive courses on biodynamic psychology, incorporating bioenergetics.
British Association for Bioenergetic Analysis, Meeting House, University of Sussex, Falmer, East Sussex BN1 9QN, ph. 0273 66755 ext 296, Run training programme for professionals in caring professions and weekend workshops and seminars.

CHIROPRACTIC
BRITISH Chiropractor's Association, 5 First Avenue, Chelmsford, Essex CM1 1RX, ph. 0425 353078, Maintains register of members (graduates of Anglo-European College of Chiropractic).
Anglo-European College of Chiropractic, 1 Cavendish Road, Bournemouth BN1 IQX, ph. 0202 24777, Runs four-year full-time course

COLOUR THERAPY
Hygeia Studios, Brook House, Avening, Tetbury, Glos. GL8 8NS, ph. Nailsworth 2150, Runs courses and lectures on environmental influences of colour, sound and form on man

ENCOUNTER THERAPY
The Open Centre, 188 Old Street, London EC1, ph. (01) 278 6783, runs classes at reasonable prices

GESTALT THERAPY
London Gestalt Centre, 31 John Ratcliffe House, Chippenham Gardens, London NW6, ph. (01) 328 9062, Runs courses.
Ursula Fausset, 7 Parliament Hill, London NW3, ph. (01) 794 6071, Runs groups and workshops.
Alive in Leeds, 8 Granby View, Leeds, 6, ph. 0532 780660, Runs classes and workshops.
Beanstalk, 128 Byres Road, Glasgow G12 5HD, ph. (041) 339 2803, Runs workshops

HERBALISM
National Institute of Medical Herbalists, 65 Frant Road, Tunbridge Wells, Kent TN2 5LH, ph. 0892 27439, Maintains list of graduates of its four-year part-time training courses
Tutorial School of Herbal Medicine, 148 Forrest Road, Tunbridge Wells, Kent, ph. 0892 30400, Runs four-year home study course, including weekend seminars, and four-year full-time attendance course.
The Herb Society, 34 Boscobel Place, London SW1, ph. (01) 235 1023, Promotes knowledge of herbs. Publishes list of herb growers and suppliers.

HOMEOPATHY
British Homeopathic Association, 27A Devonshire Street, London WIN IRJ ph. (01) 935 2163. Information including lists of homeopathic doctors, hospitals and chemists supplying homeopathic remedies.
The Society of Homoeopaths, 59 Norfolk House, Streatham, London SW16, ph. (01) 677 3260, Promotes education and research. Maintains register of practitioners.
The College of Homoeopathy (Registrar), 7a Gilmore Road, Lewisham, London SE13, runs part-time courses, diploma training.

HYPNOTHERAPY
British Hypnotherapy Association, 67 Upper Berkeley Street, London W1, ph. (01) 723 4443, Maintains register of qualified practitioners.
Blythe Tutorial College of Hypnosis and Psychotherapy, Warwick House, Stanley Place, Chester, ph. 0244 311414, Runs training courses.

IRIDOLOGY
Community Health Foundation, 188 Old Street, London, EC1V 9BP, ph. (01) 251 4076, Runs courses.
Research Society for Natural Therapeutics, 8 Stokewood Road, Bournemouth BH3 7NA, ph. 0202 25997, Runs seminars.

MACROBIOTICS
Community Health Foundation, 188 Old Street, London ECIV 9BP, ph. (01) 251 4076, Runs classes and groups.

MEDITATION
The School of Meditation, 158 Holland Park Avenue, London W11 4UH, ph. (01) 603 6116, Training in meditation. Centres in Sheffield, Basingstoke, Lincolnshire.
Transcendental Meditation, Roydon Hall, East Peckham, Nr Tonbridge, Kent, ph. 0622 813243, Runs courses. Teacher training.
British Meditation Society, 51 Aldridge Road, London W 11, ph. 229 8912, Runs structured courses.
Kalptaru, Top floor, 10a Belmont Street, London NW1, ph. (01) 485 3216, Rajneesh meditation centre.

MUSIC THERAPY
British Society for Music Therapy, 48 Lanchester Road, London N6 4TA, ph. (01) 883 1331, Promotes music therapy in treatment and rehabilitation of mental, physical and emotional handicap. Publishes journal.
Guildhall School of Music and Drama, Barbican, London EC2Y 8DT, ph. (01) 628 2571, Runs diploma course in association with British Society for Music Therapy.

NATUROPATHY
The Nature Cure Clinic, 15 Oldbury Place, London WIM 3AL, ph. (01) 935 2787, For people of limited means. Staff includes naturopaths, osteopaths and homeopaths.
The British College of Naturopathy and Osteopathy, Frazer House, 6 Netherhall Gardens, London NW3, ph. (01) 435 8728, Runs four-year full-time course.

OSTEOPATHY
General Council and Register of Osteopathy, 16 Buckingham Gate, London SW1E 6LB, ph. (01) 839 2060, Maintains register of qualified osteopaths.
The British School of Osteopathy, 16 Buckingham Gate, London, SW1E 6LB, ph. (01) 828 0601, Runs four-year full-time course.
British Osteopathic Association, 8-10 Boston Place, London NW2, ph. (01) 262 1128, Runs clinic.

PRIMAL THERAPY
Reciport, 8 Princes Avenue, London N10 3LR, Individual and group therapy.

PYRAMID ENERGY
Pyramid Energy Products, Rectory Court, Chalvington, Hailsham, East Sussex BN27 3TD, ph. 032 183 579, Various pyramid sizes available for experiments.

RADIONICS
The Radionic Association, 16a North Bar, Banbury, Oxon OX16 OTF, ph. 0295 3183, Maintains register of practitioners. Publishes journal, runs lectures and conferences.
International College of Radionics, Highfield, Dane Hill, Haywards Heath, Sussex RH17 7EX, ph. 0825790 214, Correspondence courses in radionics, radiesthesia and dowsing
Delawarr Laboratories, Raleigh Park Road, Oxford. ph. 0865 48572, Information service, publishes newsletter. Sells diagnostic and treatment instruments.

REICHIAN THERAPY
Boyesen Centre for Biodynamic Psychology, Acacia House, Centre Avenue, The Vale, London W3 7JX, ph. (01) 743 2437 or (01) 749 4957, Runs courses and workshops.

REFLEXOLOGY
The International Institute of Reflexology, 32 Coppetts Rd, Muswell Hill, ph. (01) 444 6354 London N10 IJY. Runs seminars. Books available.
The Bayly School of Reflexology, Nicola M. Hall, Monks Orchard, Whitbourne, Worcester, ph. 08862 207, Runs courses in London and regionally.
Elizabeth Gillanders, 92 Sheering Road, Old Harlow, Essex, ph. Harlow 29060, Runs seminars and weekend courses.
The Portland Centre, 16 Preston Street, Brighton, Sussex, ph. 0273 27464, Facilities for treatment.
Wessex Healthy Living Foundation, 72 Belle Vue Road, Southbourne, Bournemouth BH6 3DX, Runs natural therapy clinic including reflexology.

SHIATSU MASSAGE
Community Health Foundation, 188 Old Street, London ECIV 9BP, ph. (01) 251 4076, Runs courses.

SPIRITUAL HEALING
The National Federation of Spiritual Healers, Old Manor Farm Studio, Sunbury on Thames, Middlesex, ph. Sunbury 83164, Maintains directory of healer members. Trains healers, publishes newsletter.
The Spiritualist Association of Great Britain, 33 Belgrave Square, London SW1, ph. 235 3351, Runs healing clinic.
The Harry Edwards Spiritual Healing Sanctuary Trust, Burrows Lea, Shere, Guildford, Surrey, ph. 048641 2054, Absent and contact healing. Publishes journal.

T'AI CHI CHUAN
British T'ai Chi Chuan Association, 7 Upper Wimpole Street, London W1, ph. (01) 935 8444, Runs beginners and advanced courses.
International T'ai Chi Chuan Association, 40 Hillcroft Crescent, Wembley Park, Middlesex, ph. (01) 905 2351, Runs group and individual sessions.
The London School of T'ai Chi Chuan, P.O. Box 363, London NW2 6AF, ph. (01) 586 7657, Runs courses.

VEGETARIANISM
The Vegetarian Society, 53 Marloes Road, London W8 6LA, ph. (01) 937 7739 or (01) 937 1714, Information about vegetarianism. Publishes journal.

YOGA
British Wheel of Yoga, Glyn Galleries, Glyn Ceiriog, Llangollen. Clwyd, ph. 0691 50912, Information on groups and courses.
Salisbury Centre, 2 Salisbury Road, Edinburgh EH16 5AB, ph. 031 667 5438, Runs groups.
Albion Yoga Movement, Flat 1a, 7 Rosecroft Avenue, London NW3, ph. (01) 435 3774, Runs courses, lectures, seminars.

Other organisations involved in natural healing and humanistic psychology

Healing Research Trust, c/o Heseltine Moss and co., 3/4 Trump Street, London EC2V 8DH. Promotes alternative medicine and research into healing methods.
Health for the New Age
1a Addison Crescent, London W14 8JP, ph. (01) 603 7751, Encourages growth of holistic health care. Publishes newsletter.
Wrekin Trust, Dove House, Little Birth, Hereford HR2 8BB, ph. 09814 224, Runs residential seminars, workshops and conferences on all aspects of health and healing. Publishes newsletter.
Friends of the Healing Research Trust, 1 Castle Street, Totnes, Devon, Promotes the growth of natural health centres.
Association for Humanistic Psychology, 62 Southwark Bridge Road, London SE1 OAU, ph. (01) 928 8254, Runs conferences, seminars and workshops. Open to all interested in human potential movement.
Antioch Centre for British Studies, 115 Shepherdess Walk, London N1, ph. (01) 250 4011, Runs courses related to humanistic psychology.

Contacts:

ALEXANDER TECHNIQUE
Frances Robinson, 45a Hampstead High Street, London NW3, ph. (01) 794 8403.

THE BACH REMEDIES
John Ramsell and Nickie Murray, The Dr Edward Bach Centre, Mount Vernon, Sotwell, Wallingford, Oxon. OX10 OPZ, ph. 0491 39489.

BATES METHOD
Evelyn B. Sage, 76 Twyford Avenue, Fortis Green, East Finchley, London N2 9NN.

BIOENERGETICS
Gerda Boyesen, Boyesen Centre for Biodynamic Psychology, Acacia House, Centre Avenue, The Vale, Acton Park, London W3 7JX.

COLOUR THERAPY
Theo Gimbel, Hygeia Studios, Brook House, Avening, Tetbury, Glos GL8 8NS, ph. Nailsworth 2150.

GESTALT THERAPY
Ursula Fausset, 7 Parliament Hill, Hampstead, London NW3, ph. (01) 794 6071.

HOMOEOPATHY
Peter Chappell, 59 Norfolk House Road, Steatham, London SW16, ph. 677 3260.

MACROBIOTICS
William Tara, Community Health Foundation, 188 Old Street, London EC1, ph. (01) 251 4076.

PRIMAL THERAPY
Dr Glyn Seaborn Jones, 8 Princes Avenue, London N10, ph. (01) 883 5418

PYRAMID ENERGY
Alan Geffin, Rectory Court, Chalvington, Hailsham, East Sussex, BN27 3TD, ph. 032 183 579

SPIRITUAL HEALING
Diana Craig, President, National Federation of Spiritual Healers, Old Manor Farm Studio, Church Street, Sunbury-on-Thames, Middlesex TW16 6RG, ph. 093 27 83164.

T'AI CHI CHUAN
Nancy Treharne, The London School of T'ai Chi Chuan, P.O. Box 363, London NW2 6AF, ph. (01) 586 7657.

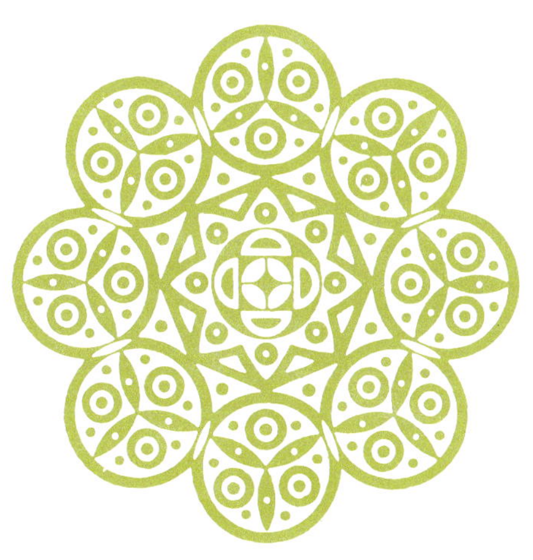

BIBLIOGRAPHY

Selected Sources for Further Reading

GENERAL

Berkeley Holistic Health Centre, *The Holistic Health Handbook*, Berkeley, California 1978, And/Or Press

Carlson, R. J. *The Frontiers of Science and Medicine*, Chicago 1975, Regnery

Eagle, R. *Alternative Medicine*, London 1978, Futura

Fadiman, J. and Frager, R. *Personality and Personal Growth*, New York 1976, Harper & Row

Grossinger, R. *Planet Medicine*, New York 1980, Doubleday

Hall, D. *The Natural Health Book*, Melbourne 1974, Nelson

Hill, A. *A Visual Encyclopaedia of Unconventional Medicine*, New York 1979, Crown

Hulke, M. *The Encyclopaedia of Alternative Medicine and Self-Help*, London 1978, Rider

Krippner, S. and Villoldo, A. *The Realms of Healing*, Millbrae, California, 1976, Celestial Arts

Law, D. *A Guide to Alternative Medicine*, London 1974, Turnstone

Regush, N. M. *Frontiers of Healing*, New York 1977, Avon

Stanway, A. *Alternative Medicine*, Adelaide 1979, Rigby

ACUPUNCTURE

Academy of Traditional Chinese Medicine, *An Outline of Chinese Acupuncture*, Peking 1975, Foreign Language Press

Croizier, R. C. *Traditional Medicine in Modern China*, Cambridge, Massuchusetts 1968, Harvard University Press

Duke, M. *Acupuncture*, New York 1977, Harcourt Brace Jovanovich

Mann, F. *Acupuncture, the Ancient Chinese Art of Healing*, London 1962, Heinemann
The Meridans of Acupuncture, London 1964, Heinemann
Treatment of Disease by Acupunture, London 1967, Heinemann

Season, S. M. Wong, *The Basic Knowledge of Acupuncture and Moxibustion*, Hong Kong 1975, Commercial Press

Stiefvater, E. W. *What is Acupuncture?* Sussex 1962, Health Science Press

ALEXANDER TECHNIQUE

Alexander, F. M. *Alexander Technique*, London 1974, Thames and Hudson

Barker, S. *The Alexander Technique*, New York 1978, Bantam

Barlow, W. *The Alexander Technique*, New York 1973, Random House

Byles, M. B. *Stand Straight Without Strain*, Essex 1978, Fowler

Maisel, E. *The Resurrection of the Body*, New York 1969, University Books

AROMATHERAPY

Lautie, R. and Passebecq, A. *Aromatherapy*, Northamptonshire 1979, Thorsons

Maury, M. *The Secret of Life and Youth*, London 1964, Macdonald

Tisserand, R. B. *The Art of Aromatherapy*, London 1977, C. W. Daniel

ASTROLOGY

Culpeper, N. *Astrological Judgment of Disease*, Tempe, USA nd, American Foundation of Astrologers

Garrison, O. *Medical Astrology*, New York 1971, Warner

Gauquelin, M. *The Cosmic Clocks*, London 1967, Peter Owen
Cosmic Influences on Human Intelligence, London 1974, Futura

Jansky R. *Modern Medical Astrology*, Van Nuys, California 1974, Astro-Analytics Publications

Rudyar, D. *An Astrological Mandala*, New York 1973, Random House

AURAS

Bagnall, O. *The Origin and Properties of the Human Aura*, New York 1969, University Books

Leadbeater, C. W. and Besant, A. *Man, Visible and Invisible*, Adyar Madras 1974, Theosophical Society
Thought Forms, London 1971, Theosophical Society

Kilner, J. W. *The Aura*, New York 1973, Weiser

BATES METHOD

Corbett, M. *Help Yourself to Better Sight* Los Angeles 1949, Wilshire

Huxley, A. *The Art of Seeing*, Washington 1975, Montana Books

BIOENERGY

Johnson, L. *Bioenergetics*, Houston 1974, Espiritu

Lowen, A. *Bioenergetics*, New York 1975, Viking
The Way to Vibrant Health, New York 1977, Harper & Row

BIOFEEDBACK

Blundell, G. and Cade, C. M. *Self Awareness and E.S.R.*, London nd., Audio Publications
Cade, C. M. and Coxhead, N. *The Awakened Mind*, London 1979, Wildwood House
Green, E. and A., *Beyond Biofeedback*, New York 1977, Delacorte
Karlins, M. and Andrews, L. M. *Biofeedback*, London 1973, Garnstone Press

BIORHYTHMS

Gittelson, B. *Biorhythm*, New York 1977, Warner

CHIROPRACTIC

Cannon, W. B. *The Wisdom of the Body*, New York 1939, Norton
Dintenfass, J. *Chiropractic: A Modern Way to Health*, New York 1977, Pyramid
Hassard, G. H. and Redd, C. L. *Elongation Treatment of Low Back Pain*. Springfield USA 1959, C. Thomas
Jause, Houser, Wells, *Chiropractic Principles and Technique*, Lombard, Illinois 1947, National College of Chiropractic
Sordoni, A. J. *Chiropractic in Industry*, Des Moines, Iowa 1962, American Chiropractic Association

COLOUR THERAPY

Anderson, M. *Colour Healing*, New York 1975, Weiser
Birren, F. *Colour Psychology and Therapy*, New York 1961, University Books
Clark, L. *Colour Therapy*, Old Greenwich USA 1975, Devon-Adair
Leadbeater, C. W. and Besant, A. *Man Visible and Invisible*, Adyar, Madras 1974, Theosophical Society

DIET AND HEALTH

Altman, N. *Eating for Life*, Illinois 1973, Theosophical Publishing House
Cilento, Lady, *Nutrition of the Child*, Sydney 1980, Blackmores Communications
Lesser, M. *Nutrition and Vitamin Therapy*, New York 1980, Grove Press
Phillips, D. *Guide Book to Nutritional Factors in Edible Foods*, Sydney 1977 Pythagorean Press
Stone, I. *The Healing Factor: Vitamin C Against Disease*, New York 1972, Grosset and Dunlap
Williams, R. *Nutrition Against Disease*, New York 1971, Bantam

ENCOUNTER THERAPY

Howard, J. *Please Touch*, New York 1970, McGraw-Hill
Rogers, C. *Carl Rogers on Encounter Groups*, New York 1970, Harper & Row
Schutz, W. *Here Comes Everybody*, New York 1971, Harper & Row

FASTING

Bragg, P. *The Miracle of Fasting*, Santa Ana, California nd., Health Science
Cott, A. *Fasting: The Ultimate Diet*, New York 1975, Bantam
Phillips, D. 'Fasting Can Save Your Life' in Drury, N. *Frontiers of Consciousness*, Melbourne 1975, Greenhouse Press
Shelton, H. *Fasting Can Save Your Life*, Chicago 1964, Natural Hygiene Press

FLOWER REMEDIES OF DR BACH

Bach, E. and Wheeler, F. J. *The Bach Flower Remedies*, New Canaan, Connecticut 1977, Keats
Chancellor, P. *Handbook of the Bach Flower Remedies*, London 1971, C. W. Daniel

GESTALT THERAPY

Naranjo, C. *The Techiques of Gestalt Therapy*, Berkeley 1973, SAT Press
Perls, F., *The Gestalt Approach*, Ben Lomond, California 1973, Science and Behaviour Books
Gestalt Therapy Verbatim, Lafayette, California 1969, Real People Press
In and Out of the Garbage Pail, Lafayette, California 1969, Real People Press

HERBALISM

Bethel, M. *The Healing Power of Herb*, Los Angeles 1974, Wilshire
Culpeper, N. *Culpeper's Herbal Remedies*, Los Angeles 1973, Wilshire
Grieve, M. *A Modern Herbal*, New York 1971, Dover
Hall, D. *Herb Tea Book*, Sydney 1980, Pythagorean Press
The Book of Herbs, Sydney 1972, Angus & Robertson
Hylton, W. *The Rodale Herb Book*, Emmaus USA 1974, Rodale
Kloss, J. *Back to Eden*, Santa Barbara 1972, Woodbridge
Law, D. *The Concise Herbal Encyclopaedia*, New York 1973, St Martins Press
Levy, J. *Common Herbs for Natural Health*, New York 1974, Schocken
Loewenfeld, C. and Back, P. *The Complete Book of Herbs and Spices*, London 1974, David and Charles; Sydney 1974, A. H. Reed
Lust, J. *The Herb Book*, New York 1974, Bantam
Rose J. *Herbs and Things*, New York 1974, Grosset and Dunlap

HOMEOPATHY

Coulter, H. L. *Homeopathic Medicine*, St Louis 1972, Formur
Gibson, D. M. *First Aid Homeopathy in Accidents and Ailments*, London 1975, British Homeopathic Association
Hahnemann, S. *The Chronic Diseases*, New Delhi 1898, Jain Publishers
The Organon of Medicine, Boulder, Colorado 1977, Hermes Press
Ross, A. C. Gordon, *Homeopathy*, Northamptonshire 1976, Thorsons
Sharma, C. H. *A Manual of Homeopathy and Natural Medicine*, New York 1976, Dutton
Vithoulkas, G. *Homeopathy: Medicine of the New Man*, St Louis 1975, Formur

The Science of Homeopathy, New York 1980, Grove

HYPNOTHERAPY

Meares, A. *A System of Medical Hypnosis*, Philadelphia 1960, W. B. Saunders

Rhodes, R. H. *Therapy Through Hypnosis*, Los Angeles 1975, Wilshire

Spiegel, H. and D., *Trance and Treatment*, New York 1978, Basic Books

Van Pelt, S. J. *Hypnotism and the Power Within*, London nd., Skeffington

IRIDOLOGY

Hall, D. *Iridology*, Melbourne 1980, Nelson

Jensen, B. *The Science and Practice of Iridology*, Solana Beach, California 1974, Jensen's Nutritional and Health Products

Kriege, T. *Fundamental Basis of Irisdiagnosis*, Essex 1969, Fowler

Lindlahr, H. *Irisdiagnosis and other Diagnostic Methods*, Mokelume Hill, California, Health Research Press

KIRLIAN DIAGNOSIS

Davis, M. and Lane, E. *Rainbows of Life*, New York 1978, Harper & Row

Krippner, S. and Rubin, D. *The Kirlian Aura*, New York 1974, Anchor/Doubleday

Moss, T. *The Body Electric*, Los Angeles 1979, J. P. Tarcher

MACROBIOTICS

Abehsera, M. *Cooking For Life*, New York 1972, Avon

Kushi, M. *The Book of Macrobiotics*, Tokyo and New York 1976, Japan Publications

Ohsawa, L. *The Art of Just Cooking*, California 1974, Autumn Press

MEDITATION

Abdullah, S. 'Meditation: Achieving Internal Balance' in E. Goldwag *Inner Balance*, New Jersey 1979, Prentice-Hall

Dass, B. R. 'Relative Realities' in R. Walsh and F. Vaughan *Beyond Ego*, Los Angeles 1980, J. P. Tarcher

Goleman, D. 'A Map for Inner Space' in R. Walsh op. cit.

Griffith, F. 'Meditation Research' in J. White, *Frontiers of Consciousness*, New York 1975, Avon

Johnston, W. *Silent Music: The Science of Meditation*, London 1974, Collins

Kiefer, D. 'Meditation and Biofeedback' in J. White, *The Highest State of Consciousness*, New York 1972, Anchor/Doubleday

Naranjo, C. *The One Quest*, London 1972, Wildwood House

Russell, P. *The TM Technique*, London 1977, Routledge and Kegan Paul

Walsh, R. N. 'Meditation Research' in R. Walsh op. cit.

NATURAL BIRTH CONTROL

Billings, E. and Westmore, A. *The Billings Method*, Melbourne 1980, Ann O'Donovan and New York 1981, Random House

Ewy, D. *Preparation for Childbirth*, New York 1976, New American Library

Hazell, L. *Commonsense Childbirth*, New York 1976, Berkley

Kitzinger, S. *The Experience of Childbirth*, New York 1972, Viking

Thompson, J. *Healthy Pregnancy the Yoga Way*, New York 1977, Doubleday

NATUROPATHY

Benjamin, H. *Everybody's Guide to Nature Cure*, Northamptonshire 1961, Thorsons

Berkeley Holistic Health Centre *The Holistic Health Handbook*, Berkeley California 1978, And/Or Press

Hall, D. *The Natural Health Book*, Melbourne 1974, Nelson

NEGATIVE IONS

Krueger, A. P. 'Are Negative Ions Good For You?' *New Scientist* (UK), June 14, 1973

Soyka, F. and Edmonds, A. *The Ion Effect*, New York 1977, Bantam

OSTEOPATHY

Hoag, J. M. et al. *Osteopathic Medicine*, New York 1969, McGraw Hill

Stoddard, A. *Manual of Osteopathic Technique*, London 1962, Hutchinson
Manual of Osteopathic Practice, London 1969, Hutchinson

PAST LIFE THERAPY

Hagon, M. *Journey Within*, Sydney 1981, Iona Sanctuary

Netherton, M. and Shiffrin, N. *Past Lives Therapy*, Melbourne 1978, Compendium

Ramster, P. *The Truth About Reincarnation*, Adelaide 1980, Rigby

Stevenson, I. *The Evidence for Survival from Claimed Memories of Former Incarnations*, Tadworth, Surrey 1961, privately published *Twenty Cases Suggestive of Reincarnation*, New York 1966, American Society for Psychical Research; reissued by University of Virginia Press

Wambach, H. *Reliving Past Lives*, New York 1978, Harper & Row

POLARITY THERAPY

Gordon, R. *Your Healing Hands: The Polarity Experience*, Santa Cruz 1978, Unity Press

Stone, R. *Energy: The Vital Principle in the Healing Art*, Chicago 1948, privately published
Health Building, Orange, California, 1978, Pannetier

PRIMAL THERAPY

Janov, A. *The Primal Scream*, London 1973, Abacus
The Primal Revolution, London 1975, Abacus

Janov, A. and Holden, E. *Primal Man: The New Consciousness*, New York 1975, T. Y. Crowell

Janov, A. *Prisoners of Pain*, New York 1980, Anchor/Doubleday

PSIONIC MEDICINE

Reyner, L. and V. *Psionic Medicine*, London 1974, Routledge and Kegan Paul

PSYCHIC SURGERY

Downs, C. 'My Meeting With Benji', Sydney 1976, *Simply*

Living, Vol. I, No. 2
Fuller, J. G. *Arigo – Surgeon of the Rusty Knife*, London 1977, Panther
Krippner, S. and Villoldo, A. *The Realms of Healing*, Millbrae, California 1976, Celestial Arts
Playfair, G. L. *The Indefinite Boundary*, London 1977, Panther
The Unknown Power, London 1975, Panther

PSYCHOMETRY
Hagon, M. *Journey Within*, Sydney 1981, Iona Sanctuary

PSYCHOSOMATIC HEALING
Carlson, R. J. *Frontiers of Science and Medicine*, Chicago 1975, Regnery

PYRAMID ENERGY
Rixon, G. *Discover Pyramid Power*, Sydney 1981, Pythagorean Press

RADIESTHESIA
Benham, W. and Williamson, J. *Handbook of the Aura Biometer*, London 1968, Society of Metaphysicians
Reyner, L. and V. *Psionic Medicine*, London 1974, :Routledge and Kegan Paul
Wethered, V. D. *An Introduction to Medical Radiesthesia and Radionics*, London 1974, C. W. Daniel

RADIONICS
Russell, E. *Report on Radionics*, London 1973, Spearman
'Radionics – Science of the Future', in J. White and S. Krippner *Future Science*, New York 1977, Anchor/Doubleday
Tansley, D. V. *Radionics and the Subtle Anatomy of Man*, Bradford, Devon 1972, Health Science Press

REFLEXOLOGY
Bergson, A. and Tuchak, V. *Zone Therapy*, New York 1975, Pinnacle
Ingham, E. D. *Stories The Feet Have Told Me*, Rochester NY.1951, Ingham
Kaye, A. and Matchan, D. C. *Reflexology for Good Health*, Los Angeles 1978, Wilshire

REICHIAN THERAPY
Boadella, D. *Wilhelm Reich – the Evolution of his Work*, London 1973, Vision Press
Mann, W. E. *Orgone, Reich and Eros*, New York 1973, Simon and Schuster

ROLFING
Pierce, R. 'Rolfing' in Berkeley Holistic Health Centre *The Holistic Health Handbook*, Berkeley 1978, And/Or Press

SEXUAL THERAPY
Kaplan, H. S. *The Illustrated Manual of Sex Therapy*, London 1981, Granada
Masters, W. H. and Johnson, V. E. *Human Sexual Response*, Boston 1966, Little Brown
Human Sexual Inadequacy, Boston 1970, Little Brown
Homosexuality in Perspective, Boston 1979, Little Brown
Pietropinto, A. and Simenauer, J. *Beyond the Male Myth*, New York 1977, Times Books; Sydney 1979, Harper & Row

Szasz, T. *Sex By Prescription*, New York 1980, Anchor/Doubleday

SHAMANIC HEALING
Drury, N. *The Shaman and the Magician*, London 1982, Routledge and Kegan Paul
Eliade, M. *Shamanism*, New Jersey 1964, Princeton University Press
Furst, P. T. *Flesh of the Gods*, London 1972, Allen and Unwin
Harner, M. *Hallucinogens and Shamanism*, New York 1973, Oxford University Press
The Way of the Shaman, San Francisco 1980, Harper] Row
Rios, M. de, *Visionary Vine*, San Francisco 1972, Chandler

SHIATSU AND ACUPRESSURE
Houston, F. M., *The Healing Benefits of Acupuressure*, Northamptonshire 1958, Thorsons
Masunaga, S., and Ohashi W. *Zen Shiatsu*, Tokyo 1977, Japan Publications
Ohashi, W. *Do-It-Yourself Shiatsu*, London 1977, Mandala/Unwin
Warren, F. Z. *Freedom From Pain Through Acupressure*, New York 1976, Frederick Fell
Yamamoto, S. *Barefoot Shiatsu*, Tokyo 1979, Japan Publications

SPIRITUAL HEALING
Edwards, H. *The Healing Intelligence*, New York 1965, Hawthorn
The Power of Spiritual Healing, London 1963, Herbert Jenkins
Hammond, S. *We Are All Healers*, London 1973, Turnstone
Worrall, A. and O. *The Gift of Healing*, London 1969, Rider

TONING
Keyes, L. E. *Toning: The Creative Power of the Voice*, Santa Monica 1973, De Vorss

TAI CHI
Horwitz, T. and Kimmelman, S., *Tai Chi Ch'uan*, London 1979, Rider
Huang, A. C. *Embrace Tiger, Return to Mountain*, New York 1978, Bantam
Khor, G. *Tai Chi*, Sydney 1981,Boobooks
Liang, T. T. *Tai Chi Ch'uan for Health and Self-Defence*, Boston 1974, Redwing
Maisel, E. *Tai Chi for Health*, New York 1963, Dell

YOGA
Chaudhuri, H. 'Yoga Psychology' in C. Tart *Transpersonal Psychologies*, New York 1975, Harper & Row
Eliade, M. *Yoga, Immortality and Freedom*, New Jersey 1969, Princeton University Press
Krishna, G. *Kundalini*, London 1971, Robinson and Watkins
Mumford, J. *Psychosomatic Yoga*, Northamptonshire 1979, Aquarian Press

INDEX

PEOPLE

SUBJECTS